Escaping From Predators

An Integrative View of Escape Decisions

When a predator attacks, prey are faced with a series of "if," "when," and "how" escape decisions – these critical questions are the foci of this book.

Cooper and Blumstein bring together a balance of theory and empirical research to summarize over 50 years of scattered research and benchmark current thinking in the rapidly expanding literature on the behavioral ecology of escaping. The book consolidates current and new behavior models with taxonomically divided empirical chapters that demonstrate the application of escape theory to different groups. The chapters integrate behavior with physiology, genetics, and evolution to lead the reader through the complex decisions faced by prey during a predator attack, examining how these decisions interact with life history and individual variation. The chapter on best practice field methodology and the ideas for future research presented throughout ensure this volume is practical as well as informative.

Electronic supplementary material is available for download at www.cambridge.org/9781107060548.

William E. Cooper, Jr. is Professor Emeritus of Biology at Indiana University-Purdue University Fort Wayne, and a Research Associate in the Department of Ecology and Evolution at University of Arizona. A behavioral ecologist by background, he has over 35 years of teaching and research experience in behavior, ecology, and evolution. He has specialized in escape behavior for the past 20 years, with particular interest in reptilian behavior.

Daniel T. Blumstein is Professor and Chair of the Department of Ecology and Evolutionary Biology at UCLA, and a Professor in UCLA's Institute of Environment and Sustainability. He has studied animal behavior throughout the world, with research focusing on the evolution of social and antipredator behavior and the effects that mechanisms of behavior have on higher-level ecological processes and for wildlife conservation.

Escaping From Predators

An Integrative View of Escape Decisions

EDITED BY

WILLIAM E. COOPER, JR.

Department of Biology, Indiana University–Purdue University Fort Wayne, and Department of Ecology and Evolution, University of Arizona, Tucson, USA

DANIEL T. BLUMSTEIN

Department of Ecology and Evolutionary Biology and Institute of the Environment & Sustainability, University of California, Los Angeles, USA

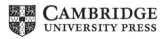

CAMBRIDGE
UNIVERSITY PRESS

University Printing House, Cambridge CB2 8BS, United Kingdom

One Liberty Plaza, 20th Floor, New York, NY 10006, USA

477 Williamstown Road, Port Melbourne, VIC 3207, Australia

314-321, 3rd Floor, Plot 3, Splendor Forum, Jasola District Centre, New Delhi - 110025, India

79 Anson Road, #06-04/06, Singapore 079906

Cambridge University Press is part of the University of Cambridge.

It furthers the University's mission by disseminating knowledge in the pursuit of
education, learning and research at the highest international levels of excellence.

www.cambridge.org
Information on this title: www.cambridge.org/9781107630635

© Cambridge University Press 2015

First published 2015
First paperback edition 2018

A catalogue record for this publication is available from the British Library

Library of Congress Cataloging in Publication data
Escaping from predators : an integrative view of escape decisions / edited by William E. Cooper, Jr.,
Department of Biology, Indiana University – Purdue University Fort Wayne, and
Department of Ecology and Evolution, University of Arizona, Tucson, USA, Daniel T. Blumstein,
Department of Ecology and Evolutionary Biology and Institute of the
Environment & Sustainability, University of California, Los Angeles, USA.
    pages   cm
Includes index.
ISBN 978-1-107-06054-8
1. Animal defenses.   2. Predation (Biology)   3. Escape (Psychology)
I. Cooper, William E., Jr.   II. Blumstein, Daniel T.
QL759.E833   2015
591.47–dc23

2014046687

ISBN 978-1-107-06054-8 Hardback
ISBN 978-1-107-63063-5 Paperback

Additional resources for this publication at www.cambridge.org/9781107060548

"Should I stay or should I go now?

If I go there will be trouble

An' if I stay it will be double"

The Clash, "Should I Stay Or Should I Go"

(*Lyrics reproduced with permission*)*

Contents

Contributors

Philip W. Bateman
Department of Environment and Agriculture, Faculty of Science
and Engineering, Curtin University, Perth, Australia

Guy Beauchamp
Faculty of Veterinary Medicine, University of Montreal, Canada

D. Caroline Blanchard
Pacific Biomedical Research Center, University of Hawaii at Manoa,
Honolulu, HI, USA

Robert J. Blanchard
Department of Psychology, University of Hawaii at Manoa, Honolulu,
HI, USA

Daniel T. Blumstein
Department of Ecology and Evolutionary Biology, University of California,
Los Angeles, CA, USA

Clint E. Collins
Department of Biology, University of California Riverside, Riverside,
CA, USA

William E. Cooper, Jr.
Department of Biology, Indiana University Purdue University Fort Wayne,
Fort Wayne, IN, USA and Department of Ecology and Evolution,
University of Arizona, Tucson, AZ, USA

Lawrence M. Dill
Department of Biological Sciences, Simon Fraser University, Burnaby,
British Columbia, Canada

Paolo Domenici
C.N.R. – Istituto per L'Ambiente Marino Costiero, Oristano, Loc.
Sa Mardini, 09170 Torregrande (OR), Italy

Esteban Fernández-Juricic
Department of Biological Sciences, Purdue University, West Lafayette, IN, USA

Patricia A. Fleming
School of Veterinary and Life Sciences, Murdoch University, Perth, Australia

Kathleen L. Foster
Department of Biology, University of California Riverside, Riverside, CA, USA

Timothy E. Higham
Department of Biology, University of California Riverside, Riverside, CA, USA

Theodore Garland, Jr.
Department of Biology, University of California Riverside, Riverside, CA, USA

Lesley T. Lancaster
School of Biological Sciences, University of Aberdeen, Abeerdeen, UK

Yoav Litvin
Laboratory of Neuroendocrinology, Rockefeller University, New York, NY, USA

Pilar López
Departamento de Ecología Evolutiva, Museo Nacional de Ciencias Naturales, CSIC. Madrid, Spain

José Martín
Departamento de Ecología Evolutiva, Museo Nacional de Ciencias Naturales, CSIC. Madrid, Spain

Anders Pape Møller
Laboratoire d'Ecologie, Systématique et Evolution, CNRS UMR 8079, Université Paris-Sud, France

Eigil Reimers
Department of Biosciences, University of Oslo, Oslo, Norway

Graeme D. Ruxton
School of Biology, University of Saint Andrews, Saint Andrews, Fife, UK

Diogo S. M. Samia
Departamento de Ecologia, Universidade Federal de Goiás, Goiânia, Brazil

Theodore Stankowich
Department of Biological Sciences, California State University Long Beach, Long Beach, CA, USA

Luke P. Tyrrell
Department of Biological Sciences, Purdue University, West Lafayette, IN, USA

Ronald C. Ydenberg
Department of Biological Sciences, Simon Fraser University, Burnaby, British Columbia, Canada

Foreword

Our 1986 paper "The economics of fleeing from predators" had a difficult birth. It was originally written for an edited volume on behavior, stillborn when the publisher reneged on the contract. Subsequently it was negatively reviewed for the *American Naturalist.* The reviewer's comments on the manuscript consisted of seven question marks, two marginal notes ("I disagree" and "too simplistic"), and the remark "The predictions are more extensions of the model's definitions than deductions" – which we still do not understand. Fortunately, others gave our model a more sympathetic hearing. Jay Rosenblatt and Colin Beer, who ran the annual publication *Advances in the Study of Behavior*, invited us to submit a manuscript after hearing LMD speak at the 1984 Animal Behavior Society meeting in Cheney, Washington. We accepted, and are still grateful to them.

In contrast to the frustration of pushing it out into the world, the gestation of the model was fun and exciting. The model's working title was "The economics of the third F," referring to the position of "fleeing" among the 4 Fs of behavior (feeding, fighting, fleeing, and reproduction). It was conceived at a time when behavioral ecology was just coming into its own at our university and at many others. As we noted in the introduction to the paper, "economic" (that is, costs and benefits in a fitness framework) ideas were being applied to feeding, fighting, reproductive and social behavior: the application to antipredator behavior seemed to us a natural step.

It was a happy and busy time. The Behavioral Ecology Research Group (BERG) at SFU was coalescing, and we were engaged with plans to host in Vancouver the 1988 meeting of the brand new International Society for Behavioral Ecology. We would like to thank the many colleagues who gave us useful input on our model, and we submitted a manuscript to "*Advances*" in April 1985, which was duly published the following year.

Thereafter, things went quiet – for a decade. The paper was not cited at all for a few years, then sporadically, and did not receive more than ten annual citations until 1997. Thereafter it has been cited more often in each subsequent year, as in the mid-90s the number of papers on escape began to climb. This increase was just one part of the swelling interest in antipredator behavior.

In spite of having been cited many hundreds of times, the basic model in "The economics of fleeing from predators" has not received much rigorous scrutiny. It does so in this volume, and we are a little embarrassed to agree that, strictly speaking, it is wanting. Perhaps the referee whose comments we castigated above had a point after all! But if the criticisms were justified, they also missed the bigger picture, something that

Professors Rosenblatt and Beer saw more clearly. Our model expressed the predator–prey interaction in a simple way that captured the essence of an idea that was in the air. In spite of its shortcomings, it provided a conceptual framework and suggested an empirical approach in a way that inspired many investigators to undertake their own studies.

The benefit of escape from predators has always seemed obvious – in fact, blindingly so. Few thought of fleeing as a "decision," or saw that there were costs, most notably lost opportunity, i.e., a fleeing animal cannot perform other fitness-enhancing activities. Many prey escape to a refuge, and it seemed natural to us to use the same approach to ask how long animals should remain before re-emerging. This interesting question requires a game theoretic approach, of which we anticipate much more in future work.

These two prey decisions – flight initiation distance and hiding time – have been the subject of most work and represent the majority of the research summarized in the present volume. But the field has expanded to consider other sorts of escape decisions, such as how far and in what direction to flee, prey strategies while being pursued by predators, and alternative tactics when fleeing is not feasible. The range of species in which these issues has been addressed is impressive, as Part II amply demonstrates. Particularly interesting is the recent work on genetics of escape, and the role of individual personality differences (the shy–bold continuum). Research described in Part III, on the physiology of escape, holds the promise of a more quantitative predictive theory than has existed to date. This will benefit the application of this work to animal welfare and conservation, as discussed in Chapter 16.

We are gratified that our work led to such an explosion of empirical and theoretical studies and contributed to the growth and maturation of an important subdiscipline of behavioral ecology. As the editors say in their introductory chapter, "The story is still unfolding, and many aspects of our topic have not yet been addressed theoretically and many generalizations and exceptions remain to be discovered through empirical studies." This book should go a long way to furthering the development of this exciting field.

We had always intended that "escape" be interpreted more broadly, as a general metaphor for decisions about antipredator behavior, with costs and benefits. The importance of antipredator behavior was first grasped in foraging, and is now beginning to be appreciated in the evolution of a broad range of phenomena including migration, metamorphosis, hibernation, clutch size, and others – classical topics that have rarely or never in their historical development considered that the risk of predation might be vital. Basic ecological topics such as population dynamics and community structure are being reshaped by the realization that facultative adjustments to danger have profound impacts that can be enormous in extent (kilometers and years) relative to the small (minutes and meters) behavioral changes that individuals make.

In closing we'd like to draw attention to an important point that continues to be misunderstood. How should "predation risk" be assessed? Many ecologists evidently think that risk can be assessed by the level of mortality. Accordingly, situations with low mortality are considered "safe." But, is this so? In previous commentaries we have made analogies with pedestrians (as prey) and cars (as predators), and noted that one could observe a busy downtown street for a long time and never observe a "predation event" (i.e., pedestrian struck by car). The situation is obviously dangerous for pedestrians, but they are struck infrequently because they are cautious. The analogy is imperfect (unlike real predators, drivers are generally careful of pedestrians) but it makes the point that mortality *per se* is a poor measure of risk. The "true" level of risk is the mortality that would occur if pedestrians were completely heedless. It must be assessed by techniques such as "flight initiation distance" or "giving-up density" (or, to pursue our analogy, how far a pedestrian would go to use a crosswalk rather than to jaywalk). This insight has turned the meaning of risk upside down. Rather than mortality setting the level of antipredator behavior, we see now that antipredator behavior sets the mortality rate. And because danger management also influences reproduction, an animal population, through the behavioral decisions of its members, in effect sets its own life table! It would be too much to claim that this startling conclusion could be deduced solely from our model's simple premises. As in all science, the cross-fertilization of ideas and data, such as those presented in this volume, is essential. However, we feel it is not too much to claim that this simple model, with all its shortcomings, opened a window that gave a different perspective on an everyday phenomenon. Read this volume and enjoy the view.

Ronald C. Ydenberg
Lawrence M. Dill

Acknowledgments

It has been extremely fun and educational to work with our contributors; we've learned a lot and we thank them for their contributions to what we believe is an exciting volume that summarizes past research and sets the stage for future discoveries! We're extremely grateful to Ron Ydenberg and Larry Dill for writing their historical preface that so nicely frames the book. Book chapters were thoughtfully reviewed by a mix of contributors and external reviewers (Peter Bednekoff, Don Kramer, Michael Jennions, Simon Lailvaux, Julien Martin, Sandrine Meylan, Mats Olsson, Terry Ord, and Matt Petelle). We are grateful for their incisive comments that helped us all improve individual contributions.

We were saddened by the passing of Robert J. Blanchard during the writing of this book. Bob was a pioneer in the field of defensive behavior and his loss is notable.

Of course, this book would not have seen the light of day without incredible support from Cambridge University Press. We're particularly grateful for guidance from Martin Griffiths, Megan Waddington, Ilaria Tassistro, and Renee Duncan-Mestel.

Bill appreciates the support of his wife who thought he had retired. Dan thanks Janice and David for tolerating the all too often "please wait just a minute longer while I respond to Bill!"

William E. Cooper, Jr.
Daniel T. Blumstein

Philip W. Bateman thanks Curtin University for financial assistance.

D. Caroline Blanchard thanks the National Science Foundation for supporting some of the work reported (NSF IBN97-28543).

Robert J. Blanchard was supported in preparation of Chapter 13 by the National Institutes of Health (R01MH81845).

Daniel T. Blumstein thanks the Australian Research Council, the US National Science Foundation (current support through NSF DEB-1119660), Macquarie University, and the University of California Los Angeles for support over the years. Long-term collaborations and conversations with my colleagues and co-authors Esteban Fernández-Juricic, Theodore Stankowich, Anders Pape Møller, William E. Cooper, Jr., and Diogo S. M. Samia have been invaluable.

Clint E. Collins thanks UCR and The Desert Legacy Fund for supporting his work.

William E. Cooper, Jr. is grateful for support for portions of the work represented here by Indiana University, Indiana University Purdue University Fort Wayne, the Cleveland Zoo, the John Ellerman Foundation, and my generous colleagues.

Esteban Fernández-Juricic thanks the National Science Foundation for support of his work by grant IOS-1146986 and thanks Daniel T. Blumstein and William E. Cooper for useful comments on drafts of Chapter 12.

Patricia A. Fleming thanks Murdoch University for financial assistance.

Kathleen L. Foster is grateful for support from NSERC (postgraduate scholarship 405019-2011).

Timothy E. Higham thanks the National Science Foundation for supporting this work (NSF IOS-1147043).

Theodore Garland, Jr. thanks the National Science Foundation for past support that was essential for development of ideas presented in this volume.

Pilar López thanks "El Ventorrillo" MNCN field station for use of their facilities and financial support provided by the project MICIIN-CGL2011-24150/BOS.

José Martín thanks "El Ventorrillo" MNCN field station for use of their facilities and financial support provided by the project MICIIN-CGL2011-24150/BOS.

Anders Pape Møller would like to thank Daniel T. Blumstein, L. Z. Garamszegi, J. T. Nielsen and numerous other collaborators for inspiration over the years. Esteban Fernández-Juricic kindly helped find some papers; comments by Diogo S. M. Samia helped improve the manuscript.

Diogo S. M. Samia is very grateful for support from CAPES and to Thiago Rangel and Ronaldo Bastos Francini for constant inspiration over the years and for fruitful discussions.

Theodore Stankowich thanks California State University Long Beach for support and Diogo S. M. Samia, Daniel T. Blumstein, and William E. Cooper, Jr. for helpful comments on previous versions of Chapter 3.

Part I

Overview and behaviors preceding and following initiation of escape

1 Escape behavior: importance, scope, and variables

William E. Cooper, Jr. and Daniel T. Blumstein

1.1 Escape, fitness, and predator–prey encounters

Prey that do not escape when attacked by lethal predators die. Even prey that suffer non-lethal injuries inflicted by predators may incur substantial costs, such as reduced ability to reproduce, reduced social status, reduced ability to forage, and reduced ability to escape in later encounters with predators. Unsuccessful escape reduces fitness. A prey that is killed by a predator loses all fitness that might have been obtained in the future. More technically, residual reproductive value (expected remaining reproductive output over a lifetime) becomes zero when a prey is killed. Therefore predator–prey interactions have been a major force driving evolutionary changes to reduce the likelihood of predation. Numerous, often spectacular, antipredatory adaptations have evolved, including morphological defenses such as shells and other armature, weaponry, camouflage, and the ability to shed tails or other expendable body parts.

In addition to such adaptations, prey that rely on escape to avoid predation must be able to make appropriate escape decisions when confronted by predators. The degree of predation risk posed by a predator that is approaching or is immobile nearby determines expected loss of fitness if the prey does not flee, i.e., the cost of not fleeing. This cost of not fleeing varies with distance between predator and prey when escape begins, and in some cases with the length of time that the predator approaches or is immobile nearby. Besides avoiding being eaten, prey must do many things to maintain themselves and increase their fitness, such as foraging and defending foraging grounds, courting, mating, and aggressively interacting with sexual rivals. When fleeing interrupts an activity that increases fitness, it imposes a cost of fleeing. Therefore each time a prey encounters a predator, the prey has a current level of fitness. The greater its fitness, the more the prey has to lose if killed.

In everyday usage, escape seems to be a simple term, but misleadingly so. If we think of a prey and predator that meet, the prey may flee and/or enter refuge to escape. However, prey may employ other defenses that allow them to escape in a broad sense, including avoiding areas where predators occur, avoiding detection by predators, and a variety of chemical, mechanical, and aggressive defenses that come into play when a prey has been overtaken by a predator. These are all fascinating topics, but are not included in this book.

Predator–prey encounters are sometimes described in terms of sequential stages from a predator's perspective, beginning with detection by the predator, identification, approach, subjugation, and consumption (Endler 1986). Other descriptions of encounters take into account both the predator's and the prey's awareness and actions (Lima & Dill 1990). From the prey's perspective, the encounter begins when the prey detects the predator and ends when the predator moves away or when the prey has escaped or been killed. The defenses used by prey vary during the stages from predator's viewpoint. Camouflage and immobility, for example, are important for reducing the likelihood of being detected or identified, whereas autotomy and weapons are used during the subjugation stage, and defenses such as spines and biting of tails to roll into a ball too large to be swallowed are employed to prevent consumption.

Material in this book is limited to prey behaviors that occur during brief predator–prey encounters. Thus occupation of predator-free habitats to avoid predators is excluded. When it has detected a predator, a prey monitors the predator during the approach stage. Alternatively, monitoring may occur as the prey approaches the predator or when both are immobile. The prey may at some time begin to flee. If it flees, it may or may not be pursued by the predator. The prey may enter a refuge where it is safe from the predator. If it enters, the prey must decide how long to stay in the refuge before emerging. If the predator overtakes the prey, the prey may deploy one or more of several defenses in response to imminent or actual physical contact with the predator. The latter defenses are not discussed in this book. In this book the focus is on escape behavior and processes leading to escape decisions. The processes leading to escape decision begin when the prey detects and starts to monitor the predator and last throughout the monitoring phase. When the decision to flee and initiation of escape behavior have occurred, further evaluative processes must occur related to the prey's strategies to evade the predator during pursuit, refuge entry, and time spent hiding in refuge.

All times and defenses outside the above intervals are omitted, but have been discussed elsewhere. Three excellent recent books review knowledge of them. *Antipredator Defenses in Birds and Mammals* (Caro 2005) describes the broad range of these defenses for two taxa. In *Animal Camouflage: Mechanisms and Function*, Stevens and Merilaita (2011) describe evidence for several means of avoiding detection by predators. Importantly for our discussion, the probability of being detected is reduced by camouflage, which should influence the decision by prey to flee. Because risk of being detected is lower for camouflaged prey, they should permit closer approach before fleeing than more conspicuous prey. In *Avoiding Attack: the Evolutionary Ecology of Crypsis, Warning Signals and Mimicry*, Ruxton et al. (2004) discuss ways in which prey avoid being detected, avoid being attacked if detected, and some defenses that may be used when contact with the predator is unavoidable. Some of the defenses treated by Ruxton et al. (2004) affect the probability of being detected or of being attacked and are important for our topic because they affect predation risk, which in turn affects decisions to flee and hide.

1.2   Focus and goals of this book

This book fills the gap left by the three recent books between defenses used to avoid being attacked and defenses used when contact with the predator is unavoidable. Interest in escape behavior has grown steadily since publication of the first model that predicts how closely a prey will allow a predator to approach before fleeing based on costs to fitness of not fleeing and of fleeing (Ydenberg & Dill 1986).

Both theory and data have been accumulating a quickening pace. Several new models of escape, refuge use, and related behaviors that appeared during the 1990s and 2000s are discussed in some detail in a chapter on escape theory (Chapter 2). Numbers of publications recovered in a citation analysis search for a few of the major escape terms (approach distance, flight initiation distance, flush distance, hiding time, and latency to emerge) showed that numbers of publications and citations increased more than twenty-fold in a search spanning the years 1994 to 2013 (Figure 1.1).

The bulk of research by the editors has been about evolutionary and ecological aspects of escape decisions, and the development and testing of models predicting effects of various factors on escape variables. The core of the book that reflects our research interests is in Part II, which presents economic and other models of escape and refuge use, and empirical data that tests their predictions. However, a full understanding of escape behavior requires a broader approach. In addition to the focus on economic escape decisions, the book presents an integrative view of escape behavior, refuge use, and prey behavior during pursuit. This material follows the chapters on theory and factors affecting escape decision in a series of chapters about behaviors that occur before escape that may affect it, determinants of locomotor performance that is crucial to escape, physiological under-pinnings of escape, maternal and genetic influences, personality traits, and use of information about escape behavior to inform wildlife management and conservation practices.

Our goals are to present the accumulated knowledge gained from these and earlier studies in an accessible form, interpret the findings using current theory, and to synthesize work to date. We sincerely hope that this book will stimulate new research. The interplay between theoretical and empirical studies of escape is a major success story in behavioral ecology because theory now permits many testable predictions that have been extensively verified. The story is still unfolding, and many aspects of our topic have not yet been addressed theoretically and many generalizations and exceptions remain to be discovered through empirical studies. Studying escape and refuge use in the field is fun and has provided us many memorable experiences. Laboratory experiments on these behaviors can also be exciting and satisfying to conduct. Developing new theoretical models of escape behavior often leads to very rewarding moments of insight. Join us in this research endeavor.

1.3   Escape theory and data

The interplay and trade-offs among factors that affect predation risk, cost of fleeing, and the prey's current fitness are the core features of theoretical models of escape and related

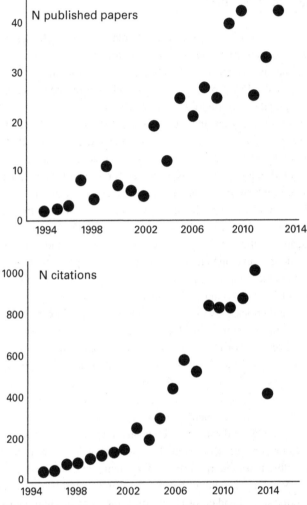

Figure 1.1   Citation analysis shows increasing numbers of articles and citations on escape behavior since the early 1990s. An ISI Web of Science search conducted on July 21, 2014 searching the terms following terms: "flight initiation distance" or "flush distance" or "hiding time" or approach distance" or "latency to emerge". Citations for 2014 appear to be fewer because the analysis was done mid-year.

behaviors. These models predict decisions by prey about whether to flee, how close to allow a predator to approach before fleeing, or how long to keep still before fleeing when an immobile predator is nearby, how far to flee, and how long to hide in a refuge. In Chapter 2, Cooper presents a number of graphical models, optimality models, and game theoretical models of escape behavior, hiding time in refuge, and related behaviors. Some of the models are highly successful at predicting important, yet limited, features of escape behavior, especially decisions about when to start fleeing. Other models are novel.

Predictions of cost–benefit models of escape and refuge use have been tested extensively and permit interpretation of the effects of numerous factors that affect predation
risk, cost of fleeing or emerging, and the prey's fitness at the outset of the encounter on
escape and emergence decisions. In addition, variables not predicted by current economic theory affect the trajectories adopted when fleeing begins and changes in trajectory and speed used to foil pursuit.

In Chapters 3 to 9 we summarize our empirically obtained knowledge about economically based escape. Major taxa differ in many ways that may affect escape capacities
and decisions. In Chapters 3 to 7 we present our empirical knowledge of escape in major
taxa: Theodore Stankowich and Eigil Reimers (mammals), Anders Pape Møller (birds),
William E. Cooper, Jr. (reptiles), Philip W. Bateman and Patricia A. Fleming (fish and
amphibians, and, in a separate chapter, invertebrates). These chapters emphasize decisions about how close to let the predator approach before fleeing, how long to remain
close to an immobile predator before fleeing, how far to flee before stopping if not
pursued, and whether to enter refuge. In addition to these variables, factors influencing
the initial direction of fleeing are discussed for some prey. In Chapter 8 Paolo Domenici
and Graeme D. Ruxton present information about initial directions of escape flight
and about strategic changes in prey escape behavior during active pursuit by predators.
In Chapter 9 Jose Martín and Pilar López detail decisions about time spent hiding in
refuge. Slight overlap occurs among certain taxonomically oriented chapters and
Chapters 8 and 9, and the cases of overlap are cross-referenced.

1.4   The rest: related behaviors, locomotor performance, physiology, genetic and maternal influences, personality difference, best practices for field studies, and conclusions

Whereas most of the material in the preceding chapters deals with ultimate causes, i.e.,
those having been molded by evolutionary processes, Chapters 10 to 15 discuss a
mixture of factors affecting escape. In Chapter 10, Guy Beauchamp discusses behaviors
including vigilance, alarm calling, predator inspection and monitoring, and pursuit-
deterrent signaling. All of these behaviors can affect the ability of prey to make
economic assessments of risk or the likelihood that a predator will attack. Therefore
they can affect escape decisions. These behaviors have been naturally selected, and
effects of all of them except perhaps vigilance on escape decisions have ultimate
interpretations. Natural selection favors vigilant prey, but prey that are not vigilant
may be forced to flee when the predator is closer than the optimal distance for initiation
of escape.

Proximate causes of escape behavior are discussed in Chapters 11 to 15. In
Chapter 11, Kathleen L. Foster, Clint E. Collins, Timothy E. Higham, and Theodore
Garland, Jr. present determinants of locomotor performance. Variation in the physiological capacities of prey to flee may explain variability in escape decisions among
individual prey, populations, and species. Running, swimming, or flying speeds, acceleration, climbing and jumping ability, and endurance all are variable and should be taken

into account by prey in assessing risk of being captured. Locomotor capacities place physiological limits of escape speed and other aspects of escape locomotion, and in this sense may be considered to be proximate causes of such aspects of escape behavior. In addition, these limits presumably affect escape decisions as ultimate causes because the risk assessment process must evolve to take locomotor abilities into account. Chapter 12, by Luke P. Tyrrell and Esteban Fernández-Juricic, covers aspects of sensory ecology important for escape decisions.

In Chapter 13 Yoav Litvin, D. Caroline Blanchard, and Robert J. Blanchard discuss the physiological bases of escape response. Physiological factors in escape behavior include neuroendocrine mechanisms of escape, including sensory bases of fleeing, and energetic costs of fleeing. Less is known regarding maternal and genetic effects on escape behavior, but some laboratory studies have begun to examine the development of escape behavior and to separate effects of the maternal environment from genetic transmission of escape traits. These topics are discussed by Lesley T. Lancaster in Chapter 14. Animal personalities have received increasing attention in recent years. A frequent finding has been that some individuals are consistently shyer or bolder than others, i.e., flee sooner or later during approaches or emerge later or sooner from hiding, respectively. In some species shyness and boldness are correlated with a variety of other traits to form adaptive suites of behaviors. In Chapter 15, Pilar López and Jose Martín discuss the literature on these personality traits and avenues for future research.

In Chapter 16, Daniel T. Blumstein, Diogo S. M. Samia, Theodore Stankowich, and William E. Cooper, Jr. discuss best practice for conducting field studies of escape behavior, a topic that we hope will be useful given differences in methods reported in the literature among investigators and recent findings that require new methods. In the final chapter the editors summarize and synthesize what we have learned about the diverse escape topics.

1.5   A standardized terminology for escape and time spent hiding in refuge

1.5.1   Current ambiguity in escape terminology

Studies of escape behavior and refuge use have often been done by investigators interested in a particular prey taxon. In some cases traditions using different terms for identical variables have developed for different taxa. The distance between a prey and an approaching predator when the prey starts to flee has been called reaction distance in many studies of fish; flush distance or flight distance, in studies of birds and mammals; and approach distance or flight initiation distance in studies of various taxa. Different terms for the same variable may be used in different subfields of escape studies, particularly between wildlife biologists and behavioral ecologists. In some cases, a single term may have multiple meanings. For example, flight distance is used to mean both predator–prey distance when escape begins and how far the prey flees before stopping.

Use of these diverse, conflicting, or ambiguous terms for different t taxa and in different conceptual fields of biology has at least two detrimental effects. One is confusion. Readers may be misled if they do not carefully examine the definitions of variables in methods sections. Sometimes the variables are not defined clearly, requiring the reader to assess the meaning from the study's context. The other primary problem with current terminology is that it makes literature searches difficult. This has affected researchers who were unaware of some synonyms.

In this section we hope to ameliorate such terminological problems by recommending a set of terms for standardized usage. We follow this terminology throughout the book and recommend that the terms defined be used in future publications on escape behavior and refuge use. Additional terms specific to their topics will be presented in Chapter 10 for escape trajectories and pursuit. In Chapter 17 we discuss set-back distance, one of several terms used in conservation biology and wildlife management.

1.5.2   Terminology for distance variables and proportions

Standing distance is the distance between an immobile prey and a predator that is immobile nearby. This term originated in studies in which researchers simulating predators stand still at some distance from a prey.

Starting distance (SD) is the distance between prey and predator when the predator begins to approach. Synonym – start distance.

Detection distance is the predator–prey distance when the prey detects the predator. Detection may be cryptic if it occurs before alert (see alert distance). For experiments in which prey are aware of the predator when approach begins, detection distance may be considered to be greater than or equal to starting distance. However, such experiments are of no value for determining detection distance.

Pre-detection distance is starting distance minus detection distance. This the distance approached by the predator before it is detected by the prey.

Alert distance (AD) is the distance between a prey and an approaching predator when the prey responds overtly to the predator by change of posture or orientation to monitor the predator. Synonym – alerting distance.

Minimum bypass distance (MBD) is the predator–prey distance at the point on the predator's path closest to the prey. This is zero for direct approaches that lead to contact with the prey. It increases as the approach angle (see below) increases to a maximum of 90° and increases as starting distance increases. Minimum bypass distance is greater than zero for all indirect, i.e., tangential, approaches.

Proportion (or percent) that flee (or fled). This refers to the proportion of individuals. Synonym – responsiveness. Proportion that flee is preferred because responsiveness, despite having the advantage of brevity, is not specific to escape and has multiple possible interpretations.

Flight initiation distance (FID) is the distance between a prey and an approaching predator when the prey begins to flee. Synonyms – approach distance, escape distance, fleeing distance, flight distance, flush distance, minimum approach distance, and reaction distance. Flight initiation distance is preferred as the clearest term. Approach distance was used frequently in the literature on economic escape, but might be confused with the distance the predator travels during its approach. Flight distance was recommended by Taylor and Knight (2003), but it is ambiguous and has been used to mean both flight initiation distance and distance fled. Flush distance is too specific for general use, being restricted to prey taxa. Escape distance and fleeing distance might also be misinterpreted to mean distance fled. Reaction distance has been used in recent reviews of escape by fish, but is less informative than flight initiation distance and might apply to other phenomena.

Buffer distance is alert distance minus flight initiation distance (Fernández-Juricic et al. 2002). This term suggests that long alert distance provides greater distance (and time) for risk assessment prior to fleeing. This term is distinct from buffer zone, which is the space within which human activity is restricted to reduce disturbance to wildlife (Camp *et al.* 1997). Synonym – assessment distance would highlight the relationship with assessment time, but we prefer buffer distance because it is established.

Margin of safety (MOS) is the distance that would separate an approaching predator from its prey when the prey reaches refuge. A refuging prey must select a flight initiation distance that will permit it to reach refuge before the predator. The margin of safety is the predator's distance to refuge when the prey enters the refuge.

Distance fled (DF) is the distance between a fleeing prey's starting and ending points if the prey is not pursued by a predator. Synonyms – escape distance, flight distance. Distance moved is preferred by Taylor and Knight (2003), but is not specific to studies of escape. A literature search for distance moved revealed thousands of papers that included distance moved, but the vast majority were irrelevant for escape.

Nearest approach distance is the distance between an immobile predator and a prey that is approaching it when the prey stops approaching. This term applies to prey that typically flee away from predators. Some prey may approach predators to counterattack or distract them, such as crabs that bite, autotomize the biting leg, and then flee (Robinson 1970). Others may approach to mob predators (Owings 1977; Gehlbach and Leverett 1995). Approaching to deploy a defensive alternative to fleeing is excluded from our topic. Nearest approach distance as used here is inappropriate to describe such behaviors. For prey that approach approaching predators to escape, nearest approach distance may also be an appropriate, accurate term.

Proportion (or percent) of individuals that enter refuge. This refers to the proportion of the individuals observed.

Proportion (or percent) of individuals that emerge before a trial is terminated after a predetermined time in refuge. Self evident.

1.5.3   Terminology for temporal variables

Detection latency is the time between the beginning of the predator's approach and its detection by the prey.

Escape latency is the time between onset of a sudden startling stimulus and the prey's first detectable reaction. In fish this occurs on a scale of milliseconds.

Latency to flee has different meaning in different contexts. When a predator approaches an immobile prey, latency to flee is the elapsed time between starting time and the time when the prey begins to flee. When an immobile prey has detected an immobile predator nearby, latency to flee is the time between detection of the predator and initiation of escape behavior. In experiments in which a predator approaches and stops near a prey that has detected it, this is the time when the prey flees minus the time when the predator stops.

Assessment time is the time spent monitoring the approaching predator before fleeing. For prey that exhibit alerting responses, assessment time is defined operationally as the time between alerting and initiation of fleeing. However, a prey may have detected a predator and have been monitoring its approach prior to adopting an alert posture. In many experiments using prey that do not show alerting, the prey may detect the predator before approach begins. Even if prey do not become aware until after the approach begins, assessment time is problematic for prey species that do not show overt alerting behaviors.

Margin of safety (temporal margin of safety) is the expected time between arrival at a refuge by a fleeing prey and arrival by the predator. Maintaining a margin of safety requires prey to assess arrival times based on relative velocities of predator and prey.

Hiding time (HT) is the elapsed time between entry into a refuge and emergence from the refuge. In typical experiments, trials are terminated if a prey does not emerge within a fixed maximum time. Therefore estimates of mean hiding time often underestimate the true mean hiding time and longer mean hiding times may be found using longer cut-off times. Synonyms – emergence time, latency to emerge, submergence time. Hiding time is preferred because it is used relatively widely and does not present numerous false positives during literature search, which is a problem that plagues searches for the synonyms that have alternate meanings unrelated to escape behavior.

1.5.4   Terminology for directional variables

Ideally, escape paths would be measured by vectors giving speed and direction throughout the encounter and would be related to similar information for the predator. This is not generally done and such vectors are more difficult to measure than the two-dimensional directions usually presented. We often measure only initial directions with no indication of escape speed. To indicate directions in Euclidian space when no information about speed is available, unit vectors could be used. In most studies of escape by non-volant terrestrial prey and even by some prey that escape in three dimensions, only two-dimensional angles have been measured. However, take-off angle, the vertical angle above horizontal, is an important aspect of the initial escape response by birds, grasshoppers, and presumably other insects. For prey escaping in air or water, the dive (swooping) angle or ascent angle of the predator is very likely to affect the degree to which the prey flees upward or downward. Prey that jump also may vary their vertical take-off angles. Climbing and descent angles of terrestrial and arboreal prey on slopes, logs, and trees may affect both escape speed and the speed and ability of predators to follow, both of which may affect predation risk, and, therefore, escape decisions. Other prey might vary the angle of rapid burrowing in sand or loose dirt. The terms listed below are the two-dimensional angles used in escape studies.

Approach angle has three distinct meanings. One is the difference in degrees between two predators simultaneously approaching a single prey. The other use of this term occurs in studies of effects of directness of approach by a predator on escape decisions. In the latter case approach angle is the angle from the apex point where the predator begins to approach between a line of direct approach and the actual linear approach path. In the third case, approach angle refers to the angle between the line of attack by the predator and the body orientation of the prey. We prefer the following two terms in this case.

Attack angle is the angle between the predator's line of approach and the body orientation of the prey. It has range of 0 to 180°. The attack angle is 0° when the prey is directly facing the predator and 180° when the prey is oriented directly away from the predator.

Stimulation (or stimulus) angle is equivalent to attack angle, but is used in situations in which the stimulus does not approach the prey, such as when a sudden sound is presented experimentally.

Direct approach is movement by the predator on a straight line toward the prey; the approach angle is 0°.

Tangential approach is movement by the predator along a straight path that does not lead to contact with the prey, but bypasses it. For tangential approaches, a minimum bypass distance (see above) is associated with each combination of starting points and approach angles. Synonym – indirect approach. Tangential approach is preferred because it emphasizes that the tangent line from the prey intersects the predator's path at the its closest point to the prey. Indirect approach may be used for contrast with direct approach, but the tangential nature of approach should be made clear.

Escape trajectory (ET) is the path taken by a fleeing prey. In typical studies, the initial escape trajectory is linear at a fixed angle in relation to the direction of the predator's position. Escape trajectory is often defined as this initial angle of fleeing. However, the prey's path may change during pursuit, as in classical mathematical models and cases in which prey make evasive maneuvers such as gradual or rapid turns, or even if no pursuit occurs. An escape trajectory of 180° is directly away from the predator; an escape trajectory of 0° is directly toward the predator. In some studies escape trajectories are considered to span 0 to 360°. In that case a distinction between sides may be made in one of two ways. In one, the right side of a circle corresponds to 0 to 180° and the left side to 180 to 360°. In the other, when a prey turning to flee ends with the threat on the opposite side of the prey's body than before the turn, escape trajectory falls in the range 0 to 180°; when turning to flee ends with the threat of opposite side opposite side of the prey's body than before the turn, the trajectory lies in 180 to 360°. Thus there are three commonly used measures of escape trajectory, two measured on a normal 360° scale and one on an axial (180°) scale. It is important to distinguish between these two interpretations of the escape direction and between circular (360°) and axial (180°) scales, which require use of different circular statistics. For detailed descriptions of the three types of ET, see Chapter 8. Synonyms – flight angle, escape angle. We prefer escape trajectory because this term has long been used in mathematical models of pursuit and in studies of escape by fish. Escape angle and flight angle may vary during pursuit, differing among the prey's positions along the path, the angular changes through space defining a trajectory. Because most studies have measured only the initial direction taken by the prey, the escape angle and escape trajectory defined as a direction for brevity are identical.

Escape angle is the angle of the prey's initial escape with respect to the predator's approach path. It is typically measured on an axial scale of 0 to 180° as discussed for escape trajectory. As noted, these angles may change during escape, in which case the path, or trajectory is altered. Synonyms – escape trajectory, flight angle. Escape angle is preferred over flight angle because flight angle may also refer to aerial flight in contexts other than escape.

Turn angle is the angle between the prey's body axis before the attack and its path during the initial phase of fleeing. It usually spans 0 to 180°, but can be larger if, for example, the prey turns in circles.

Directionality is the proportion of prey that rotate or bend their bodies in a direction directed away from the predator or predatory stimulus during the initial phase.

1.6   Electronic supplementary material

For several chapters space did permit full coverage of certain topics or data that may be useful to researchers. These files are available online at www.cambridge.org/9781107 02060548 (additional resources appear under the "Resources" tab). In the printed chapters and on the website, the electronic supplementary files are identified by chapter and number. For example, ESM 5.2 is the second electronic file for Chapter 5.

References

Camp, R. J., Sinton, D. T. & Knight, R. L. (1997). Viewsheds: A complementary management approach to buffer zones. *Wildlife Society Bulletin*, **25**, 612–615.

Caro, T. M. (2005). *Antipredator Defenses in Birds and Mammals*. Chicago: University of Chicago Press.

Endler, J. A. (1986). Defense against predators. In *Predator–prey Relationships: Perspectives and Approaches from the Study of Lower Vertebrates*. Chicago: University of Chicago Press, pp. 109–134.

Fernández-Juricic, E., Jimenez, M. D. & Lucas, E. (2002). Factors affecting intra- and inter-specific variations in the difference between alert distances and flight distances for birds in forested habitats. *Canadian Journal of Zoology*, **80**, 1212–1220.

Gehlbach, F. R. & Leverett, J. S. (1995). Mobbing of eastern screech-owls: Predatory cues, risks to mobbers, and degree of threat. *Condor*, **97**, 831–834.

Lima, S. L. & Dill, L. M. (1990). Behavioral decisions made under the risk of predation: a review and prospectus. *Canadian Journal of Zoology*, **68**, 619–640.

Owings, D. H. (1977). Snake mobbing by California ground squirrels: Adaptive variation and ontogeny. *Behaviour*, **62**, 50–69.

Robinson, M. J., Abele, L. G. & Robinson, B (1970). Attack autotomy: A defense
against predators. *Science*, **169**, 300–301.

Ruxton, G. D., Sherratt, T. N. & Speed, M. (2004). *Avoiding Attack: The Evolutionary
Ecology of Crypsis, Warning Signals and Mimicry*. Oxford: Oxford University Press.

Stevens, M. & Merilaita, S. (2011). *Animal Camouflage: Mechanisms and Function*.
Cambridge: Cambridge University Press.

Taylor, A. R. & Knight, R. L. (2003). Behavioral responses of wildlife to human activity:
Terminology and methods. *Wildlife Society Bulletin*, **32**, 1263–1271.

Ydenberg, R. C. & Dill, L. M. (1986). The economics of fleeing from predators.
Advances in the Study of Behavior, **16**, 229–249.

Part II

Escape and refuge use: theory and findings for major taxonomic groups

IIa Escape theory

2 Theory: models of escape behavior and refuge use

William E. Cooper, Jr.

2.1 Introduction

Despite its crucial role in surviving attacks by predators, escape behavior has received far less theoretical attention from animal behaviorists than other topics, such as foraging and social behavior. Nevertheless, our understanding of escape decisions by prey in certain contexts has been advanced greatly by considering the fitness costs and benefits of escape. Because these costs and benefits of fleeing and hiding have not been measured in fitness units, the models do not permit precise quantitative predictions. They do allow predictions at the ordinal level about effects of greater and lesser levels of factors that affect predation risk and factors that make fleeing costly. Several economic models of escape behavior now routinely provide qualitatively accurate predictions about aspects of fleeing and refuge use. Here, I review these models, develop a model for a scenario not previously treated theoretically, and develop a rubric in which models are placed according to the relative movements of predator and prey. I also discuss alternative approaches to modeling escape decisions and models of behaviors during predator–prey encounters that occur before fleeing.

2.2 First economic models of escape and time spent hiding in refuge

2.2.1 Escape

Much theoretically based empirical research on escape has focused on flight initiation distance (FID), the distance between a prey and an approaching predator when the prey begins to flee (Lima & Dill 1990; Lima 1998; Stankowich & Blumstein 2005). Several other terms are synonyms of FID in some publications, most notably approach distance, flush distance, and flight distance (Chapter 1). Flight initiation distance is the least ambiguous of these terms and is now the most prevalent. The term "flight distance" should be avoided in future research because it is sometimes used to mean flight

Escaping From Predators: An Integrative View of Escape Decisions, ed. W. E. Cooper and D. T. Blumstein. Published by Cambridge University Press. © Cambridge University Press 2015.

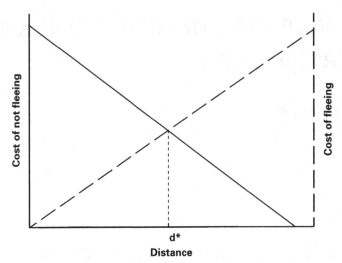

Figure 2.1   Ydenberg and Dill's (1986) graphical model of flight initiation distance (FID) when a predator approaches an immobile prey that monitors its approach. The horizontal axis is the distance between predator and prey. The vertical axes are the cost of not fleeing, which is primarily expected loss of fitness due to predation risk, and the cost of fleeing, which is incurred when fleeing leads to loss of opportunities to enhance fitness at the prey's current location. The predicted FID, d*, occurs at the distance where the cost of not fleeing and cost of fleeing curves intersect. Modified from Ydenberg and Dill (1986)

initiation distance, but in other cases denotes distance fled by the prey. Although escape initiation distance might be preferable to flight initiation distance because some readers might think that flight refers to flying, flight initiation distance is the best of established terms and will be used here.

Economic modeling of escape behavior began with a graphical model by Ydenberg and Dill (1986) that remains useful over 25 years later. Ydenberg and Dill (1986) assumed that prey often do not flee immediately upon detecting (and becoming aware of) an approaching predator, but monitor the predator's approach until fleeing becomes advantageous. As the distance between predator and prey decreases, the cost of not fleeing increases because the risk of predation increases. Many factors affect the degree of risk at a particular distance. These include the predator's speed and directness of approach, body size, the prey's detectability, and body armor (Stankowich & Blumstein 2005; Cooper 2010a). The cost of fleeing is primarily a consequence of losing opportunities to feed, engage in social activities such as courtship, mating, and territorial defense, and to perform other activities that increase fitness. Although usually small, energetic costs of fleeing and risk of injury as a consequence of fleeing are other costs of fleeing. As the predator–prey distance decreases, the opportunity cost of fleeing decreases. This is because less must be foregone by fleeing because the prey has had more time during the predator's approach to feed, drink, or engage in social activities.

Ydenberg and Dill (1986) proposed that prey begin to flee when cost of not fleeing and cost of fleeing are equal. In their graphical model, flight should occur at the intersection of the falling cost of fleeing and rising risk curves (Figure 2.1). As long as the cost of fleeing is greater than the cost of not fleeing, the prey remains where it is. When the cost associated with predation risk and cost of fleeing are equal, the prey begins to flee because in the next instant cost of not fleeing becomes greater than the cost of fleeing and thereafter the cost of not fleeing grows increasingly larger than the cost of fleeing.

If the costs were known in exact fitness units, it would be possible to predict flight initiation distance exactly. Ydenberg and Dill's (1986) model and subsequent economic models are useful because they permit us to make ordinal level predictions about which of two risk levels or which of two costs of fleeing is associated with greater FID. Cost of not fleeing is expressed as cost associated with predation risk or, in shorthand, predation risk.

Many factors affect predation risk (*sensu* the danger of being killed if no antipredatory behavior is used; Lank & Ydenberg 2003) at a given distance between predator and prey. If two identical predators approach at different speeds, the risk to the prey at any particular distance is greater during the faster approach. If the cost of fleeing is the same in both cases, the cost of not fleeing and cost of fleeing curves intersect farther from the prey when the cost of not fleeing curve is higher (i.e., FID is longer when cost of not fleeing is greater, Figure 2.2b).

If a prey has a feeding opportunity (or other opportunity to enhance fitness), its cost of fleeing is greater at all non-zero distances than that of a prey without a feeding opportunity (Figure 2.2a). Consequently, if the two prey have the same cost of not fleeing curve, the predator is closer to the prey at the intersection of the cost of not fleeing and cost of fleeing curves for the prey having the higher cost of fleeing curve (i.e., FID is shorter when cost of fleeing is greater).

The Ydenberg and Dill (1986) model has been modified by Blumstein (2003) to include three zones (Figure 2.3a). At the shortest predator–prey distances, prey flee as soon as they detect a predator. The shortest zone of predator–prey distance, zone I, extends from distance $d = 0$ to d_{min}, the shortest distance at which prey assess risk rather than fleeing immediately upon detecting the predator. In a range of longer distances, zone II, prey make economic decisions based on costs of fleeing and not fleeing as described by Ydenberg and Dill (1986). Zone II extends from d_{min} to d_{max}, the maximum distance at which cost–benefit considerations affect escape behavior. (Equivalently, d_{max} is the maximum distance at which prey assess risk either because they cannot detect the predator or the predator isn't relevant/poses no risk at longer distances.) Zone III includes all distances longer than d_{max}. Prey in zone III do not flee. Stankowich and Coss (2007) recognize the same three zones (see also Chapter 3).

Reasons for non-responsiveness by prey in zone III include failure to detect the predator, inattentiveness to activities at long distance, and the perception that predator–prey distance is too great for the predator to pose an immediate threat (Blumstein, 2003). Stankowich and Coss (2007) added that risk is not assessed in zone III. This is clearly so when the predator is not detected, but is trivial because there has been no predator–prey encounter from the prey's point of view. On the other hand, prey might appear to be inattentive because perceived risk is too low to justify incurring monitoring

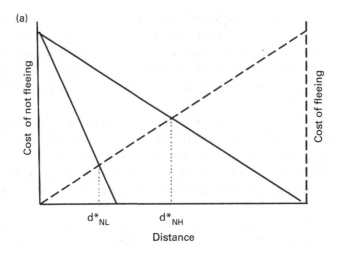

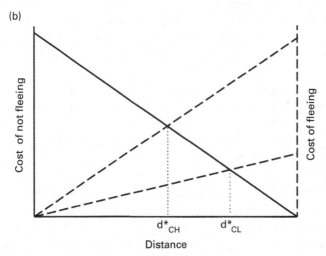

Figure 2.2   The predicted FID, d*, is (A) longer for the higher of two cost of not fleeing curves when there is a single cost of fleeing curve and (B) longer for the lower of two cost of fleeing curves when there is a single cost of not fleeing curve. Terms are d*$_H$ for high cost and d*$_L$ for low cost. Modified from Ydenberg and Dill (1986)

costs. An interesting possibility is that prey in zone III that assess risk as being very low nevertheless monitor the activities of predators there, but appear to be inattentive because they monitor predators at intervals rather than continuously, reducing monitoring costs. More empirical work is required to understand the proximate processes occurring in zone III.

Prey are always expected to flee immediately if a predator is detected closer than the economically predicted FID. Therefore the regression of predator–prey distance when the predator is detected on FID should have a slope of 1 on predator–prey distance in the range 0 to d*, the economically predicted FID. A slope that did not differ significantly

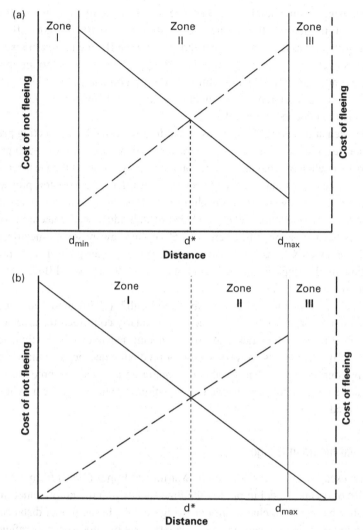

Figure 2.3   Responses of prey to predators differ in three ranges of distance. (A) In Blumstein's (2003) version, prey flee immediately without assessing risk and cost when they detect predators at close range in zone I. Assessment occurs in zone II, which begins at d_{min} and continues at all distances in zone II, which ends at d_{max}. Modified from Blumstein (2003). Prey may or may not detect predators in zone III, but do not monitor them attentively. (B) If prey flee immediately in $0 \leq d \leq d^*$, as predicted by the models of Ydenberg and Dill (1986) and Cooper and Frederick (2007a, 2010), $d_{min} < d^*$ does not exist. Therefore, zone I extends from $0 \leq d \leq d^*$, zone II from $d^* < d \leq d_{max}$ and zone III is where $d > d_{max}$.

from 1.0 was observed in the teiid lizard *Aspidoscelis exsanguis* for approaches starting between 0 and 1.5 m (Cooper 2008). The intercept, too, did not differ significantly from 0 (Cooper 2008). As zone I has been conceived, assessment occurs in the interval between d_{min} and d^*. However, if escape occurs immediately when at $d < d^*$, $d_{min} = d^*$. In that case zone I is 0 to d^*.

If flight begins immediately for $d \leq d^*$, the zones are modified (Figure 2.3b). Zone 1, the zone of immediate flight, includes distance 0 to d^*. In zone II, the zone of monitoring and assessment, $d^* < d \leq d_{max}$. In zone III, the non-response zone, the predator is even farther from the prey at $d > d_{max}$. Non-response to an approaching threat may indicate either (1) an inability to detect a predator beyond d_{max}, (2) detection with true lack of any consequent alteration of behavior, or (3) less intense monitoring than occurs in zone II.

Stankowich and Coss (2007) proposed that for prey capable of detecting predators at long distances, higher values of d_{max} characterize more reactive prey. Such prey would begin cost–benefit assessments at longer predator–prey distances than less reactive prey. Among prey having similar reactivity, scanning rate affects the predator–prey distance at which prey become aware of approaching predators. In Columbian black-tailed deer (*Odocoileus hemionus columbianus*), 38.5% of individuals had detected investigators before they began to approach, whereas 61.5% became aware some time after approach began (Stankowich & Coss 2007). Because awareness is inferred by an alert posture and orientation to the approacher, this finding is consistent with differences in either reactivity or scanning rate.

The qualitative predictions of Ydenberg and Dill's (1986) model and the optimal escape model described below have been spectacularly confirmed for diverse prey and factors affecting predation risk and cost of fleeing (Stankowich & Blumstein 2005; Cooper 2010). The models are very useful for predicting decisions about when to begin fleeing by immobile prey that are able to monitor an approaching predator's behavior and distance. Other models are needed for situations in which prey are moving and both prey and predator are still.

2.2.2   Time spent hiding in refuge

The basic escape model was adapted by Martín and López (1999) from Ydenberg and Dill's (1986) escape model to predict the time spent by a prey before emerging from a refuge after having been chased into one (Figure 2.4). In the model distance between predator and prey is replaced on the horizontal axis by time spent in refuge and the variable measured is latency to emerge, also called emergence time or hiding time. Hiding time is preferable to emergence time, which also refers to other phenomena, especially times of hatching or metamorphosis.

The vertical axes of this model are cost of emerging (risk) and cost of not emerging (Figure 2.4). Cost of emerging decreases as time spent in refuge increases because the predator is increasingly likely to have left the area as latency to emerge increases. Cost of not emerging increases as time spent in refuge increases because prey lose opportunities to conduct various activities and, in ectotherms, because body temperature falls during stays in cool refuges, requiring basking or other thermoregulatory behavior upon emergence and decreasing running speed and therefore escape ability (Martín & López 1999; Polo *et al.* 2005; Cooper & Wilson 2008). A prey is predicted to emerge when the risk of emerging equals the cost of not emerging.

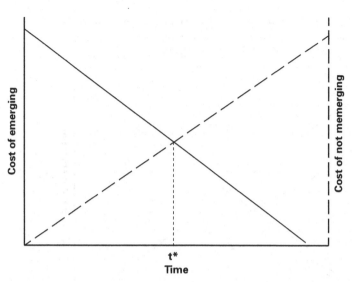

Figure 2.4   The latency to emerge from refuge after fleeing from an approaching predator (hiding time) is predicted to be t*, which occurs at the intersection of the cost of emerging and cost of not emerging curves. Modified from Martín and López (1999)

Many of the same predation risk factors and opportunity costs that affect flight initiation distance also affect hiding time. The hiding time model has been particularly successful in increasing our understanding of the effects of thermal costs of refuge use (Martín & López 1999; Polo *et al.* 2005; Cooper & Wilson 2008). Some empirical studies have shown that risk associated with entering a refuge associated with presence of a predator inside it affects decisions to enter the refuge (Amo *et al.* 2004).

The hiding time model can be generalized to include effects of the costs of emerging or not emerging due to presence of predators and opportunities outside the refuge, and costs of remaining in or leaving the refuge due to predation risk and opportunities in the refuge (Figure 2.5). In the expanded model, the cost of emerging includes predation risk present in the original model and an additional cost of losing benefits that might be obtained by staying in the refuge. The cost of remaining in the refuge includes both the loss of opportunity available outside the refuge and the risk inside the refuge, primarily due to presence of another predator.

The risk of emerging and loss of benefits in the refuge upon emerging decrease as hiding time increases. The opportunity cost and predation risk associated with remaining in the refuge increase as hiding time increases (Figure 2.5). The total cost of emerging is the sum of the cost of emerging due to outside risk and the loss of inside benefits. Similarly, total cost of remaining in the refuge is the cost of lost opportunities outside and predation risk inside the refuge. The predicted hiding time occurs when the total cost of remaining inside equals the total cost of emerging (i.e., at the intersection of the two total cost curves, Figure 2.5). All costs are in expected fitness units. It is apparent that the

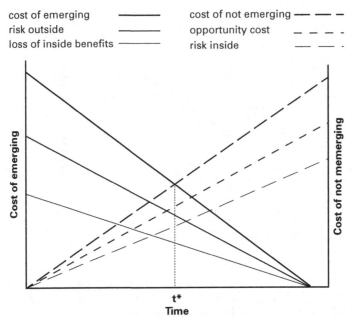

cost of emerging ———————   cost of not emerging — — —
risk outside ———————   opportunity cost — — — ·
loss of inside benefits ———————   risk inside — — — ·

Figure 2.5   If a predator is present outside the refuge and a different predator is inside the refuge, the cost of emerging and cost of not emerging curves each are given by the sum of two costs. The total cost of emerging is the sum of cost due to predation risk outside and loss of benefits that might have been obtained inside the refuge. The total cost of not emerging is the sum of the cost due to risk of predation inside and cost of losing opportunities outside the refuge. The predicted hiding time, t*, occurs at the intersection of the total cost of emerging and total cost of not emerging curves.

original hiding time model (Martín & López 1999) is a special case of the model in Figure 2.5 when there are no risks and no benefits to be gained inside the refuge.

2.2.3   Assumptions and restrictions

In both the escape and hiding time models, the cost functions are sometimes shown as linear and sometimes as curvilinear. The precise relationships between predator–prey distance and time spent in refuge and the costs of fleeing or emerging and of not fleeing or emerging are unknown, but the predictions hold for a wide range of functions. As predator–prey distance increases, cost of not fleeing is assumed to decrease and cost of fleeing to increase. However, because cost of fleeing is largely opportunity cost, the cost of fleeing curve may be horizontal or nearly so if opportunity is absent or meager.

Cooper and Vitt (2002) examined these assumptions for the Ydenberg and Dill (1986) model. Their findings are described here for escape, but similar considerations apply to emergence from refuge. Two or more cost of not fleeing curves are assumed to have identical values when predator–prey distance is zero. The cost of fleeing when predator–prey distance is zero is assumed to be zero. Exceptions may occur. If the risk factor is lethality of the predator, the expected loss of fitness is greater for more lethal predators or more vulnerable prey when the predator contacts the prey (Cooper & Frederick 2010). Cost of fleeing at distance zero may be greater than zero for prey that have some chance of surviving contact with a predator, and the cost may differ among predators that impose different opportunity costs, such as differing times spent in refuge.

Imagine that two predation risk curves intersect with each other and intersect at different points with a cost of fleeing curve and that investigators are unaware that the risk curves intersect. Predictions about relative FIDs for the two risk curves based on their magnitudes closer to d = 0 than their intersection would be erroneous because the lower risk curve in this interval intersects the cost of fleeing curve at a longer distance (unless there are multiple intersections between risk curves). For predictions to hold, the cost of fleeing and not fleeing must be monotonic or precisely known. If a non-monotonic cost of not fleeing curve intersects more than once with a risk curve or a non-monotonic risk curve intersects more than once with a cost of fleeing curve, multiple predicted flight initiation distances exist, each for some distance interval.

The graphical models of Ydenberg and Dill (1986) and Martín and López (1999) apply to a wide range of functions relating predator–prey distance or time in refuge to cost curves (Cooper & Vitt 2002). These models have had great heuristic value and have been very successful in empirical tests. Their main theoretical drawback is the require-ment that fleeing or emerging can occur only when the curve for cost of not fleeing intersects the curve for cost of fleeing, or the curves for cost of emerging and cost remaining in refuge intersect. This issue is addressed by optimality models.

2.3   Optimality models of escape and refuge use

Optimality models predict that animals select behavioral options that maximize their fitness. In the present context, this implies that prey decide to initiate escape behavior at the FID for which their fitness at the conclusion of the encounter is greatest or to emerge after the hiding time that maximizes fitness when the encounter has ended. Optimality models have been used extensively in studies of foraging behavior (Stephens & Krebs 1986), but only two optimality models of escape have been published, one for FID (Cooper & Frederick 2007a, 2010), the other for hiding time (Cooper & Frederick 2007b). As discussed below, the Ydenberg and Dill (1986) model is not an optimality model because the predicted FID may be associated with less than optimal fitness.

Optimality models of foraging fell out of favor in the mid-1980s for various reasons, especially the presumed inability of animals to make precisely optimal decisions (Stephens et al. 2007). However, they had enormous heuristic value and led to advances in our understanding of foraging behavior and social behavior. For the most part, optimal escape theory is used to make ordinal level predictions, not quantitative ones such as those made by optimal foraging theory. Nevertheless, at our current level of under-standing of escape behavior, optimality models, as well as simple cost–benefit models, remain very useful and have led to substantial improvement in our understanding of escape decisions.

In Cooper and Frederick's (2007a, 2010) optimality model for FID, the optimal FID is the product of predation risk (based on distance) and a term that includes the prey's initial fitness, benefits that it may gain during the encounter with the predator, and energetic cost of fleeing. All of these terms except initial fitness vary with predator–prey distance, permitting calculation of fitness associated with each flight initiation distance. The optimal flight initiation distance is the predator–prey distance with the highest expected fitness. If all benefits gained during the encounter are lost when the prey is killed, the sum of initial fitness, benefits, and energetic cost is multiplied by the probability of survival to determine expected fitness. However, if benefits are retained after death, as for successful reproduction, fitness is estimated by adding the benefits and energetic costs to the product of the sum of initial fitness and energetic cost with probability of survival.

The prey begins with initial fitness F_0. In both the optimality and Ydenberg and Dill (1986) models of FID, benefits are zero at distance d_d at the outset of the encounter. The benefit function $B(d)$ increases as the predator draws nearer (i.e., as d decreases). The maximum benefit that may be obtained during the encounter is B*, which is obtained at $d = 0$. This is because the prey has additional time during the approach to obtain benefits when it allows the predator to come closer. The benefit function in the model is $B(d) = B*[1 - (d/d_d)^n]$, where d_d is the distance at which the prey detects the predator and beyond which benefits cannot be obtained, n is the exponent setting the rate of change in B with respect to d. The benefit function and other terms in the fitness equation might have various mathematical expressions. The energetic expense of fleeing is $E(d) = fd^m$, where d distance, m is the exponent relating expense to d, and f is a proportionality constant that is the slope if $m = 1$. The probability of survival is $1 - e^{-cd}$, where c is the rate constant for exponential decay, if contact with the predator is always lethal. These variables and parameters are summarized in Table 2.1.

When all benefits obtained during the encounter are lost if the prey is killed, the prey's expected fitness if it starts to flee at distance d is $F(d) = [F_0 + B(d) - E(d)][1 - e^{-cd}]$, $0 \leq d \leq d_d$. If the prey obtains reproductive benefits or augments

Table 2.1 Parameters and variable for the optimal flight initiation distance model.

B	benefits in fitness units obtained by the prey during the encounter
$B(d)$	function relating benefits obtained to predator–prey distance d
B*	maximum possible benefits, which are attained at $d = 0$
c	rate constant for exponential decay in probability of survival as d decreases
d	predator–prey distance
d_d	distance at which the prey detects the predator and at which benefits may start to accumulate
$E(d)$	energetic expenditure required to flee when the predator–prey distance is d
f	proportionality constant affecting energetic expense
F_0	the prey's initial fitness (when the encounter begins)
m	exponent setting the change in energetic expense in conjunction with d
n	exponent setting the rate of change in benefits with distance

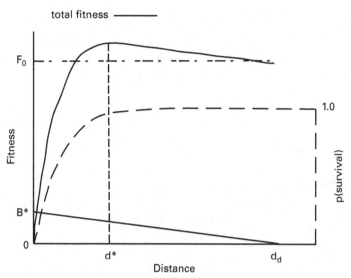

Figure 2.6   In optimal escape theory the prey's expected fitness increases as benefits that it obtains during the predator's approach increase. In the absence of predation the total fitness would be the prey's initial fitness, F_0, plus benefits gained at distance d. This total fitness is discounted by the increasing probability of being captured as the predator draws nearer. The distance at which expected fitness is maximized is the optimal flight initiation distance, d*, which decreases as the maximum benefit, B* (obtained by not fleeing), increases and increases as initial fitness increases. The remaining parameter is d_d, the predator–prey distance when the prey detects the predator and can start accumulating benefits. Modified from Cooper and Frederick (2007a)

fitness by kin selection that are retained if the prey is killed, the equation becomes $F(d) = [B(d)] + [F_0 - E(d)][1 - e^{-cd}]$, $0 \leq d \leq d_d$. In the latter equation initial fitness is lost, but the benefits remain.

The optimal FID occurs at the distance where the derivative $F'(d) = 0$ (and the second derivative < 0, Figure 2.6). Because no analytical solutions for $F'(d)$ exist, the effects of varying model parameters must be studied by simulation. The model predicts that the optimal FID increases as initial fitness and predation risk increase and decrease as benefits increase. The optimal FID decreases as the constant f and the exponent m in the escape cost term decrease due to increasing energetic cost. Only the model that allows retention of benefits predicts that prey should accept great risk or death if benefits are large enough and increase rapidly when the predator is very close.

The optimal FID model has been generalized to account for the degree of predator lethality (Cooper & Frederick 2010) by modifying the term for survival to $(1 - L(e^{-cd}))$, where L is the proportion of fatalities among prey contacted physically by the predator. The optimal FID increases as lethality (L) increases (Figure 2.7). The generalized model can predict FID for factors having complex influences on escape. Consider autotomy, the voluntary shedding of a body part to facilitate escape when overtaken by a predator. Autotomy of the tail by lizards is beneficial because it increases the probability of escape.

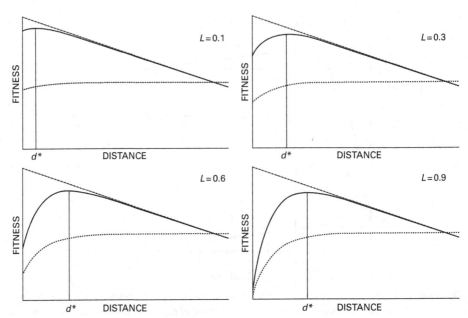

Figure 2.7   For fixed initial fitness, predation risk curve and benefit curve, the optimal FID (d^*) increases as the lethality (= L, the proportion of prey that the predator kills upon contact) increases. Modified from Cooper and Frederick (2010)

However, in subsequent encounters with predators, initial fitness is lowered for autotomized individuals because they have decreased reproductive output and growth. Also, lizards that have lost a portion of the tail are less able or unable to use autotomy unless and until the tail has regenerated. Thus predator lethality is greater for autotomized than intact individuals. Decreased ability to obtain benefits and slower running speed by autotomized lizards are predicted to increase FID. Formerly, it was widely believed that FID should increase after autotomy. However, the optimal escape model shows that FID may increase, decrease, or be unaffected by autotomy depending on the balance of effects of autotomy on fitness, lethality, running speed, and ability to obtain benefits.

The optimal hiding time and FID models are isomorphic. In the optimal refuge use model, time since entering refuge replaces distance as the horizontal axis and in all variables affecting survival and benefits. Optimal hiding time increases as predation risk upon emerging and initial fitness increase and decreases as benefits obtainable upon emerging increase (Cooper & Frederick 2007b).

2.4   Comparison of the graphical and optimality models

Simulations using a range of values for costs, benefits, and initial fitness show that prey can increase their fitness at the end of the encounter to a value greater than their fitness at the outset of the encounter by selecting the optimal FID or hiding time (Cooper & Frederick 2007a,b). This is not possible according to the graphical models discussed above.

The best that a prey can do in the graphical models of FID and hiding time is to flee or emerge when the costs of performing the activity equal the costs of not performing it. These graphical models and their mathematical equivalents (Cooper & Frederick 2007a) have been characterized as break-even models to contrast the fitness consequences of the predicted behavioral decisions with those of optimality models, which allow more profitable decisions.

The graphical models do not explicitly consider the prey's initial fitness, which is an important omission because FID and hiding time are predicted to increase as initial fitness increases according to the asset protection principle (Clark 1993). However, initial fitness could be considered a predation risk factor because more is at risk when initial fitness is greater. Using that approach, graphical models predict longer FID for greater initial fitness, as does optimal escape theory. Qualitative predictions about effects of initial fitness are identical for the break-even and optimality models. Moreover, qualitative predictions of the two types of models are identical for all factors affecting predation risk and cost of fleeing or cost of not emerging.

The two types of models are equally useful for predicting FID and hiding time in almost all circumstances. The only exception occurs when prey can perform activities during the approach or upon emerging from a refuge that allow them to increase their fitness after the encounter to a value greater than its initial level. In some extreme cases this occurs even if the prey dies because it does not flee or because it emerges too soon. For example, a prey might enhance its lifetime fitness by obtaining fertilizations during an approach even at the cost of not fleeing and being eaten. This accounts for prey, such as male black widow spiders (*Latrodectus* spp.) and male preying mantises (*Mantis* spp.), that, rather than fleeing, approach their predators to trade their lives for fertilizations.

Cooper and Frederic (2007a) suggested that such cases cannot be accommodated by the Ydenberg and Dill (1986) model because fitness cannot be increased if prey flee when the two cost curves intersect. Consider a graphical model similar to the Ydenberg and Dill model except that cost curves do not intersect. Such cases could be represented by a cost of fleeing curve on which cost of fleeing is greater than the cost of not fleeing at all distances or vice versa (Figure 2.8). Suppose that there is no cost of fleeing or that the cost of fleeing is always less than the cost of not fleeing (Figure 2.8a). Such cases may not exist in zone II. Any intersection would fall in zone III, but would not affect risk assessment. This situation, which may occur when a lethal, efficient predator approaches and no large benefits can be obtained during the encounter. Immediate fleeing is required upon detecting a predator in zone II despite the absence of intersection of the cost curves. This prediction is similar to that of the original zone model (Blumstein 2003) when prey detect predators in zone II closer than the intersection where cost of not fleeing exceeds cost of fleeing. Alternatively, it is similar to the prediction of modified zone model presented above when prey detect predators closer than the optimal FID. The possibility that zone II is longer for more efficient predators has not been studied. The lack of intersection in Figure 2.8b can be interpreted as predicting zero flight initiation distance because cost of fleeing is greater than cost of not fleeing at all distances, which might

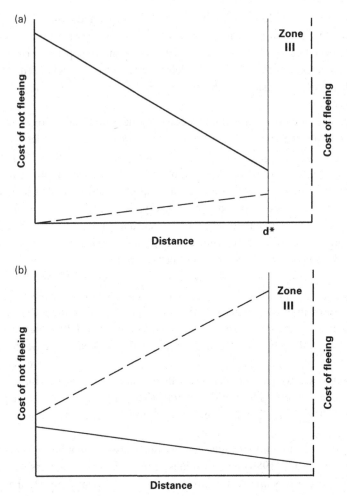

Figure 2.8   Ydenberg and Dill (1986) envisioned cost of not fleeing and cost of fleeing curves whose intersection determined d*, the predicted FID. However, if the curves do not intersect (at least in zone II, the assessment zone) the model applies to broader circumstances. (A) If the cost of not fleeing curve is above the cost of fleeing curve everywhere in the assessment zone, prey should flee as soon as a predator is detected at the boundary of zones II and III, $d_{max} = d*$. (B) If the cost of fleeing curve is always higher than the cost of not fleeing curve when $d \geq 0$, prey should allow the predator to overtake it. This corresponds to the case in optimal escape theory in which the prey gains enough fitness through reproduction during the predator's approach to justify loss of fitness expected by contact with the predator.

occur when prey can obtain large reproductive benefits and/or the predator has low lethality or its approach implies low risk.

With the addition of predictions about prey behavior in the cases of non-intersection of the cost curves depicted in Figure 2.8, the Ydenberg and Dill (1986) model and its later modifications discussed above become much more flexible. They apply to all of the situations in the optimality models and make the same qualitative predictions. Quantitative predictions of the graphical and optimality models differ, but that currently is inconsequential because we cannot determine the relevant fitness values. Given fitness values, the relative merits of the models would become an empirical matter. Until the relevant fitness components can be measured, the two types of models may be used interchangeably. The term break-even model, implying that prey flee when expected loss of fitness due to predation risk equals expected fitness gained during the encounter, applies to the graphical models only if the two curves intersect.

2.5   Flushing early: effects of starting distance and alert distance on flight initiation distance

2.5.1   Starting distance: an unexpected challenge to economic escape theory

Starting distance (SD), the predator–prey distance when the predator begins to approach, has an effect on FID that is highly variable and has been difficult to explain. Blumstein (2003) found that FID increased as SD increased in many birds. Since then, SD has been shown to affect FID in mammals (Stankowich & Coss 2007), a crab (Blumstein 2010), and some lizard species (Cooper 2005, 2008; Cooper *et al.* 2009; Cooper & Sherbrooke 2013a). Among lizards FID did not vary with SD in several species of ambush foragers that were approached slowly (Cooper 2005; Cooper & Sherbrooke 2013a). However, FID increased markedly as SD increased in active foragers (Cooper 2008; Cooper *et al.* 2009) and, in one ambushing species, increased slightly at fast, but not slow, approach speeds (Cooper 2005).

The effect of SD on FID was difficult to understand, and its basis was controversial. Previously studied factors that affect escape have obvious effects on cost of remaining, cost of fleeing, or both, but the possible effect of SD was obscure. In economic escape theory, a prey monitors a predator as it approaches and decides to flee based on predation risk and cost of fleeing, neither of which are obviously affected by SD.

Blumstein (2010) proposed a possible economic basis in the flush early hypothesis: prey start to flee shortly after having detected a predator to lower the cost of monitoring the predator during its approach. Prey need not flush immediately upon detecting predators, but sometimes do. A recent model suggests that cryptic prey should flee immediately or not at all (Broom & Ruxton 2005). In contrast, in the flushing early model, FID increases as monitoring costs increase. Flushing early matches the effect of SD on FID for a prey that has detected a predator, but is reducing monitoring cost the cause of this relationship?

Spontaneous movement (i.e., leaving its earlier position before a prey detects a predator) might account for an increase in FID with increase in SD, especially for very long SDs. Spontaneous movement also might occur after detection of the predator, leading to increase in apparent FID as SD increases. Such spontaneous movements might generate artifactual increases in the estimates of FID, causing apparent FID to be longer than the FID based on economic decisions. Differences in spontaneous movement rates might account for the differences in effect of SD between ambushing and actively foraging lizards (Cooper 2008). Such differences probably explain some of the difference in effects between foraging modes, but not all, because rates of spontaneous movement by actively foraging lizards are very unlikely to be high enough to account for large effects at short SDs.

The artifactual portion of the effect of spontaneous movement may be reduced or eliminated in prey species that indicate awareness of a predator by staring at and orienting toward it. The predator–prey distance at which this occurs is the alert distance, AD (Blumstein *et al.* 2005). Because FID is correlated positively with alert distance (Stankowich & Coss 2007), the relationship between SD and FID cannot be entirely due to spontaneous movement by prey that have not detected predators.

Alert distance has its own limitations. Prey may be aware of predators before adopting alert postures and may monitor them less intently then. This may occur when prey detect predators in zone III (Fig. 2.2). Some prey deter pursuit by signaling that they have detected the predator (e.g., Ruxton *et al.* 2004; Caro 2005; Cooper 2010b, 2011a,b; Chapter 10) and in some cases the signals are alert postures (Holley 1993). In such cases effects of signaling and alert distance *per se* may be conflated, and this may reduce the apparent effect of alert distance because FID is shorter for signaling than non-signaling prey (Cooper 2011b).

After becoming alert, a prey monitors the predator approaching prior to fleeing. This interval between alerting and fleeing is assessment time (Stankowich & Coss 2007; Chapter 1). The spatial interval corresponding to assessment time is AD to FID (Chapter 1). Monitoring in these intervals matches the scenario of economic models. Alert distance is preferable to SD because larger artifactual effects due to spontaneous movement and statistical constraints (Dumont *et al.* 2012) occur for SD.

Dumont *et al.* (2012) examined the relationship between SD and AD for SD $\geq$ AD to assess the utility of SD as a proxy for AD when AD is difficult to ascertain. By conducting traditional statistical analyses of data for the marmot *Marmota marmota* using AD as a covariate, they showed that AD and the previous activity of marmots interactively affected FID. Similar analysis using SD as the covariate revealed no such effect. When the assumption that SD $\geq$ AD $\geq$ FID ≥ 0 is incorporated into the null hypothesis, SD and AD were unrelated. Dumont *et al.* (2012) suggested that there is no biologically meaningful relationship between SD and AD. They concluded that SD may be a misleading substitute for AD, but there is no evidence that this conclusion applies widely. They claim that the effect of SD in the range from SD to AD is entirely artifactual. This agrees with the interpretation that spontaneous movements account for any effects of SD in that distance range. However, when SD is short enough for prey to be aware of the predator before the approach begins, the artifact is absent. At longer SDs, use of SD as a proxy for AD is currently the only option when AD cannot be ascertained. As discussed below, it is a viable alternative.

2.5.2   Model of effects of starting distance on flight initiation distance: monitoring costs and spontaneous movements

To examine effects of spontaneous movement and monitoring costs on the relationship between SD and FID, Chamaillé-Jammes and Blumstein (2012) developed a model that predicts two distances, the predator–prey distance where spontaneous movement occurs and FID based on monitoring cost. Recall that d_{min} in Blumstein's (2003) model separates zone I where flight is immediate from zone II where escape decisions are based on costs and benefits. Starting distance might or might not affect economic assessment leading to FID in zone II. To allow both possibilities, Chamaillé-Jammes and Blumstein (2012) assumed that the predator–prey distance where monitoring cost elicits escape is proportional to SD. In the equation $d^* = d_{min} + \beta SD$, d^* is the distance at which prey flee based on monitoring cost and β is the proportionality constant. When $\beta > 0$, only spontaneous movement can affect the relationship between SD and FID.

Spontaneous movement was assumed to have a random Poisson distribution with rate $\lambda(s^{-1})$, which can also be expressed in m^{-1}. Prey are allowed to move spontaneously when $d^* <$ SD. The probability of spontaneous movement increases exponentially as the distance approached by the predator increases. The predicted distance for spontaneous movement is $d_{spon} = \alpha e^{\lambda d}$, $0 < d^* \le d \le$ SD, where d_{spon} is the distance where spontaneous movement occurs and α is a proportionality constant. Thus the distance where spontaneous movement is predicted increases exponentially with distance with exponential rate constant λ.

Predicted FID is the longer of the distances predicted separately from monitoring cost and spontaneous movement. Chamaillé-Jammes and Blumstein (2012) applied the model to data from four avian species. They concluded that analysis using ordinary least squares (OLS) is appropriate only if prey move only in response to a predator's approach. In that case, the slope of the relationship between FID and SD can be tested against the null hypothesis that $\beta = 0$. This is an important case because in many studies prey are aware of predators only when an approach begins in zone II. During my extensive field work with lizards, I have the impression that spontaneous movements of many prey are suppressed while monitoring, presumably to reduce the likelihood of being detected and attacked due to their own motion. Suppression of movement during approach is supported by the observation that lizards approached tangentially often flee immediately after passing out of a predator's field of view (Cooper 1997). In such cases, which include most studies of lizards, OLS analyses are justified.

When the spontaneous (natural) leaving rate $\lambda > 0$ and FID is variable at each SD, quantile regression can be used because it permits heterogeneous variances due to differing effects of β and λ across SDs. In OLS procedures, the mean FID is estimated for each value of predator–prey distance. In quantile regression, the value of FID is instead estimated for various quantiles, such as the 10 or 20% of individuals with the lowest or highest values of FID at each SD. This requires a large data set.

For four species of birds with sufficient data using the lowest quantiles (e.g., 5 or 10% of FIDs for a particular predator–prey distance) provided the lowest and best estimates of β. This slope should be 1.0 at distances shorter than d_{min}, but such distances are excluded from analysis. As λ increases, the slope approaches 1.0. By restricting analysis to the lowest quantiles, many individuals that move spontaneously are excluded, giving a better estimate of the slope of d* on SD based on responses to predators. In two of the four bird species for which FID increased as SD increased using all data, FID was unrelated to SD in quantile regression. When spontaneous movement is frequent and sufficient data are available, quantile regression appears to have great promise (Chapter 17).

2.5.3   Starting distance, alert distance, and economic escape

2.5.3.1   Effects of monitoring predators on escape decisions

Cooper and Blumstein (2014) examined ways in which monitoring might affect FID and proposed novel effects of AD on FID in the context of economic escape theory. Monitoring occurs as part of the scenario in economic escape theory (Ydenberg & Dill 1986; Cooper & Frederick 2007a, 2010), but had not been thought to affect predation risk or cost of fleeing. However, the flush early hypothesis requires that increased monitoring cost associated with longer SD (or AD) causes longer FID (Blumstein, 2010; Chamaillé-Jammes & Blumstein 2012). This can occur only in a limited range of predator–prey distance. If a prey detects an approaching predator in the range $0 \leq d \leq d*$, economic escape models predict that it should flee immediately. No opportunity exists for dynamic adjustment of FID based on AD at these short distances; AD and related effects of monitoring the predator can affect FID only in zone II where $d* < d_{max}$.

The effect of monitoring on spontaneous movement can influence the degree to which spontaneous movement affects FID. If movement by the prey increases the likelihood that the predator will attack, spontaneous movements may be suppressed during monitoring. In that case, spontaneous movements occur and the natural rate of leaving, λ, is applicable only for long starting distances in zone III where $d > d_{max}$. Spontaneous movement in zone III does not affect estimates of FID in zone II where prey make economic escape decisions. Spontaneous movement occurs in the entire interval between the SD and FID in the model of Chamaillé-Jammes and Blumstein (2012). When this is so, spontaneous movement inflates estimates of FID and methods of removing its effect on FID would be valuable.

Monitoring might affect escape decisions in the cost–benefit escape models via costs of not fleeing and costs of fleeing. The cost of not fleeing is primarily a consequence of predation risk, and increases as the predator comes closer; cost of fleeing is primarily opportunity cost, and increases as FID increases because the prey has less time to complete beneficial activities. Effects of monitoring may be complex, affecting costs of fleeing, not fleeing or both, but have not been studied empirically. Cooper and Blumstein (2014) identified several ways related to SD that monitoring might influence FID. Any combination of the newly identified effects might contribute to flushing early.

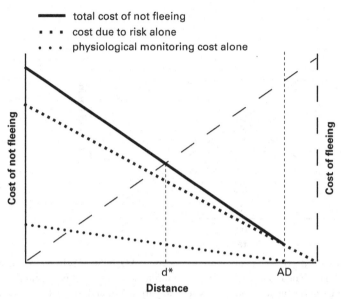

total cost of not fleeing
cost due to risk alone
physiological monitoring cost alone

Figure 2.9   Upon detecting an approaching predator at the alert distance, AD, the prey begins to monitor it. The physiological cost of monitoring increases as the duration and distance of approach increase. The sum of this physiological cost of monitoring and the cost due to predation risk is the total cost of not fleeing. The predicted FID, d*, occurs at the intersection of the total cost of not fleeing and cost of fleeing curves. The effect of physiological cost of monitoring is to increase d*. From Cooper and Blumstein (2014)

2.5.3.1.1 Cost of not fleeing

The physiological cost of monitoring is the energy expended to monitor the predator, presumably via neurological and sensory processes, that is over and above the energy that would be expended in the absence of monitoring. The physiological cost is greater when FID is shorter because the predator has been monitored for a longer time and over a longer distance. Although potentially measurable, it is presumably very small. The total cost of not fleeing is obtained by adding physiological cost to cost due to predation risk (Figure 2.9). Because physiological cost is very small, it can be omitted in empirical studies unless there is reason to believe that it differs among experimental treatments.

The other effect is a dynamic increase in assessed risk as the duration and length of the predator's approach increase, leading to assessment of greater risk than that attributable to predator–prey distance alone. This effect would lead to increase in FID as AD increases. Prey adjust assessed risk rapidly and dynamically to changes in the behavior of approaching predators (Cooper 2005). As the duration of approach increases, the probability that the predator has detected or will soon detect the prey and will attack increases. Effective risk assessments must account for increased duration/distance approached, which would lead to increase in FID as AD increases.

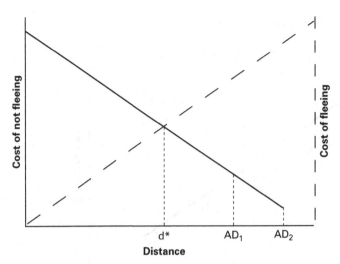

Figure 2.10   The predicted FID, d*, does not vary with alert distance, AD, if the ADs lie on the same cost of not fleeing curve. This would occur if ongoing monitoring does not affect perception of risk dynamically. By projecting the dotted lines vertically from AD_1 and AD_2 to the cost of fleeing line, it becomes apparent that AD does not affect cost of fleeing when there is a single cost of fleeing curve. This could occur if there is no cumulative cost of monitoring in addition to that incorporated in the cost of fleeing curve. From Cooper and Blumstein (2014)

Alert distance, which affects distance or duration approached, is very likely an important predation risk factor. Alert distance sets limits on the maximum FID and duration of approach during risk assessment. The length of approach and, therefore, assessed risk at any given predator–prey distance increase as AD increases. If duration of monitoring does not affect assessed risk, risk is on the same cost of not fleeing curve for all ADs (Figure 2.10).

A curve representing the case in which assessed risk increases with increase in duration of monitoring lies above the curve for no monitoring cost when $0 < d < AD$ (Figure 2.11a). Both curves have identical values at AD where assessment begins and at $d = 0$, where the cost of not fleeing is the expected loss of fitness upon contact with the predator. If the lower curve is linear, the higher risk curve is concave downward (Figure 2.11a). The predicted FIDs are $d*_N$ when duration of approach does not influence assessed risk and $d*_R$ when it does. The intersection of the cost of not fleeing and cost of fleeing curves occurs at a longer predator–prey distance when assessed risk increases as duration of approach increases than when duration of approach does not affect assessed risk, i.e., $d*_R > d*_N$. If assessed risk increases as duration of approach increases and AD differs, the curve for the longer AD, AD_2, is above the curve for the shorter AD_1 at all $d > 0$ (Figure 2.11b). In conclusion, when AD affects assessed risk, FID increases as AD increases.

2.5.3.1.2   *Cost of fleeing*

Alert distance might be related to opportunity cost of fleeing in several ways, especially if monitoring entails complete or partial reduction of fitness-enhancing activities.

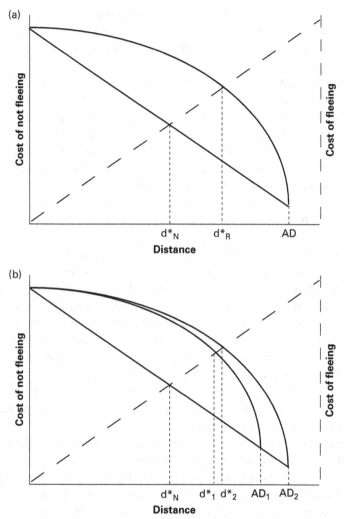

Figure 2.11 In both panels, let a line show the cost of not fleeing when the duration/distance that the predator approaches does not alter the prey's assessed risk. (A) The upper curve portrays an increase in assessed risk to its maximum at $d = 0$. For the upper curve, the assessed risk is greater than that in the cost of not fleeing line because the prey assess increasing predation risk as the duration/length of approach increases. The predicted FID, for a prey that that assesses increasing risk as the duration/distance approached increases, d^*_R, is longer than the predicted FID if alert distance, AD, does not affect assessed risk, d^*_N. (B) If assessed risk increases as AD increases, assessed risk is greater and the predicted FID is longer for the longer of two ADs. From Cooper and Blumstein (2014)

In certain conditions, monitoring does not affect ability to obtain other benefits. For example, basking lizards that have body temperatures too low for efficient locomotion may not feed or engage in social activities. In such cases, FID will not be affected by a monitoring cost associated with a cost of fleeing. This case can be represented by a single cost of fleeing curve with two ADs (Figure 2.10). Because opportunity cost increases as d increases, it is greater at the longer AD. However, the predicted FID is the same for both ADs because they lie on the same cost of fleeing curve (Figure 2.10). This relationship holds for prey that do not flush early because of the monitoring cost of fleeing.

While monitoring predators, prey may not be able to devote sufficient attention to efficiently detect their own cryptic prey (Dukas & Kamil 2000). Suppose that prey have an attentional cost of monitoring and the cost of fleeing curves for prey that do and do not have impaired ability begin at d = 0 and have identical values at AD (Figure 2.12a). The curve for a prey incurring no monitoring cost of fleeing is the highest of a family of such curves. For any two cost of fleeing curves, the curve will be lower for a prey incurring greater monitoring cost. Consequently, for a fixed alert distance, the predicted FID is longer for the curve with greater monitoring costs (Figure 2.12a). The cost of fleeing curve is lowered progressively as the degree of impairment of ability to obtain benefits while monitoring increases.

Monitoring cost begins at AD when the prey becomes aware of a threat. At this point, the opportunity cost OC_{AD} is equal for any two curves because no cost of monitoring has accumulated. The cumulative monitoring cost can be calculated by integrating the difference in cost of fleeing between a curve for no monitoring cost and a lower curve for prey having reduced ability to obtain benefits while monitoring between AD and FID. Opportunity cost for all curves at d = 0 is $OC_0 = 0$. Because benefits remaining to be obtained by a prey suffering monitoring cost decrease as predator–prey distance decreases, the total cost of fleeing at a given predator–prey distance is reduced as d decreases, whereas the accumulated cost of monitoring continues to increase. The difference between the two cost curves is progressively reduced toward the origin to account for decline in remaining benefits.

In the same scenario, let two cost of fleeing curves for prey that incur monitoring costs start at different ADs and intersect the cost of fleeing curve for a prey that has no attentional monitoring cost at their respective ADs (Figure 2.12b). The curve having the longer alert distance is always lower than the curve for the shorter alert distance if monitoring cost accumulates at the same rate during the predator's approach. Therefore the predicted FID is longer for the curve with longer AD (Figure 2.12b). Demonstrating the effects of monitoring and alert distance depicted in Figure 2.12 would provide strong support for the flush early hypothesis.

2.5.3.2   Spontaneous movement

Suppression of spontaneous movement during monitoring would eliminate its effect between AD and FID, but at SD > AD, spontaneous movement increases estimated FID. If prey move spontaneously even while monitoring, empirical estimates of FID will be inflated relative to the economically determined value. The extent of inflation is determined by the natural leaving rate, λ. Using an exponential function as in Chamaillé-Jammes and Blumstein (2012), the proportion of individuals that leave spontaneously between SD and d is $1 - e^{-\lambda(SD - d)}$, $\lambda \geq 0$. The estimated FID overestimates the economically based d^* by an increasing distance as λ increases and the difference between SD and d^* increases. Nevertheless, if AD is held constant in a single

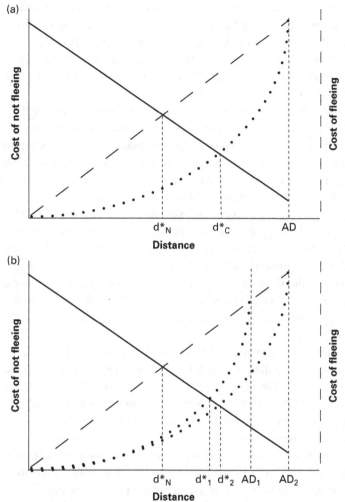

Figure 2.12   (A) Reduced rate of obtaining benefits while monitoring lowers the cost of fleeing and therefore increases FID. This plot shows an upper opportunity cost of fleeing line for a prey that incurs no monitoring cost and a lower curve. In the upper line the opportunity cost is OC_0 at $d = 0$ and OC_{AD} at AD. Monitoring cost is zero for both curves at the origin and at the alert distance (AD), but greater for the lower curve at all distances between them, which lowers opportunity cost of fleeing. In this case the cost of monitoring increases as the predator approaches, but its effect is diminished as benefits remaining to be obtained shrink as predator–prey distance decreases. The predicted FID is shorter for the upper line representing no monitoring cost (d^*_N) than for the curve in which monitoring impairs ability to obtain benefits (d^*_C). (B) For two alert distances lying along the line for which monitoring costs do not affect cost of fleeing, let monitoring cost increase at the same rate as duration of approach increases. The cost of fleeing discounted for monitoring cost and adjusted for decrease in remaining benefits as the predator approaches is shown as curves through the origin to two alert distances. The curve for the longer alert distance is always lower than that of the shorter alert distance in the interval $0 < d \le AD_1$, the shorter alert distance. Therefore d^* is greater for the longer alert distance. Confirmation of this effect of monitoring on cost of fleeing would strongly support the flush early hypothesis. From Cooper and Blumstein (2014)

population, spontaneous movement does not affect ordinal level predictions of FID for cost of not fleeing and cost of fleeing factors. At the longest observed FID, monitoring costs accumulated during approach are the same for prey that flee and do not flee. Therefore d* must be greater for the prey that flee. The same applies in succession at shorter observed FIDs. In comparative studies, though, differences in λ among species might lead to misinterpretation of findings.

For a prey that has not detected an approaching predator in zone II or III, spontaneous movements occur, but no monitoring costs are incurred before the prey is aware of the predator. For prey that detect the predator at AD, spontaneous movement might continue as monitoring cost is incurred before the predator reaches the economically predicted FID. A major advantage of using AD instead of SD is that spontaneous movements while the prey is not assessing risks and costs are excluded.

Several methods might be used to estimate an economically based FID from raw data that include effects of spontaneous movement. The only method employed to date is discussed in Chapter 16. Other possible methods are suggested here. For normally distributed FID, the highest frequency should occur at d*. The highest frequency should also identify d* if the distribution is skewed to the right as long as the rate of spontaneous movement is not so high that few prey remain when the predator reaches d*. For values of λ that do not drastically deplete prey before the predator reaches d*, the modal FID is presumably d*.

Another method of estimating d* excludes all data for long distances. When d < d*, spontaneous movement does not occur because prey flee immediately, yielding a slope of FID on SD of 1.0. The value of d* can be estimated as the maximum distance for which the slope of FID on SD is 1.0. Although using this method avoids adjustment for spontaneous movement, it would be preferable to estimate d* from data that include spontaneous movements.

Two other methods use data for distances > d*. If the natural rate of leaving is known, the expected proportion of individuals that move spontaneously in each distance interval can be calculated using the exponential relationship presented above. This requires field research to determine whether rates of spontaneous movement are constant across distances, and if so, to estimate λ. Given λ, the expected numbers of individuals that left spontaneously is calculated for distance intervals in which prey do not always flee immediately. Data for the numbers of individuals expected to move spontaneously could then be removed random from each distance interval. The mean FID for the remaining data is an estimate of d*.

A different method of estimating d* is to compare expected proportions of individuals that leave by spontaneous movements with the total proportions that leave in each interval. The longest interval in which the observed proportion that left exceeds the expected proportion to the greatest degree contains d*. In intervals shorter than d*, immediate movement occurs for all individuals, but this is irrelevant in $0 \leq d < d^*$.

2.5.3.3   Rapid advances in understanding effects of starting distance

In the short time since Blumstein (2003) reported the effect on SD on FID, SD and AD have been studied intensively. The causes, relationship to economic escape theory, and the effects of spontaneous movement have all been examined theoretically and empirically. Research on relationships among SD, AD, and FID has led to rapid progress in our understanding of these phenomena through the combined theoretical and empirical studies of several behavioral ecologists.

We now understand the basic underlying causes for effects of SD and AD on FID theoretically, but much remains to be discovered, especially about the possible effects of monitoring discussed here on cost of fleeing and on assessed predation risk, and their relationships to flushing early. Research is needed to gauge the importance of all of these potential costs, any or all of which may occur in some prey. Rates of spontaneous movement, their variation with predator–prey distance, and the magnitude of their effect on FID are important topics for future empirical research.

2.6   Other approaches to modeling escape decisions and refuge use

2.6.1   Effect of direction of approach by predator on flight decisions for escape to a fixed refuge

Prey often have options to select among multiple refuges, but in some circumstances only a single refuge is available. There might be only one burrow, tree, or crevice close enough for the prey to reach before being overtaken by a predator. In such cases the direction from which a predator approaches has a strong influence on the risk of being killed if the escape attempt begins at a fixed distance. If the prey is on a line connecting an approaching predator and the refuge, and is located between the predator and the refuge, it can flee directly away from the predator to the refuge (Figure 2.13a). If the prey is on the same line, but the refuge lies between it and the predator, the prey must flee toward the predator to reach the refuge.

Kramer and Bonenfant (1997) modeled the effect of the direction of approach in this situation. They assumed that for both directions, there is a critical predator–prey distance, AD_{crit}, at which a predator approaching at a fixed speed will reach the refuge at the same time as the fleeing prey. AD_{crit} stands for critical approach distance, where approach distance is a synonym of FID, and is not to be confused with alert distance. Kramer and Bonenfant (1997) also assumed that prey flee before the predator reaches AD_{crit} to allow the prey a margin of safety in arrival at the refuge before the predator. In the model, the margin of safety (MOS) is a fixed distance that, when added to AD_{crit}, gives the predicted FID.

If the prey is between the predator and the refuge, the predicted FID, d^*, is AD_{crit} + MOS – DP, where DP is the distance between the prey and its refuge (Figure 2.13a). If the predator is on the far side of the refuge, the prey must flee toward the predator, requiring a longer FID for equal AD_{crit} and MOS. The expected FID in this case is $d^* = AD_{crit}$ + MOS + DP (Figure 2.13a). Values of d^* vary with distance to refuge, the ratio of predator to prey velocity, and whether the prey is on the same or opposite side of the refuge (Figure 2.13a). Let AV be the velocity of the attacker and PV be the velocity of the prey. Then AD_{crit} = DP(AV/PV). The slope of the line in Figure 2.13b

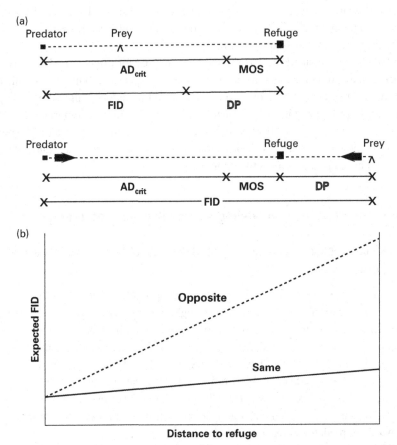

Figure 2.13   Flight initiation distance is shorter when a prey can flee directly away from a predator to a refuge than when it must flee toward a predator t reach refuge. (A)When the prey is between the predator and a refuge and its distance to refuge is DP, its expected FID, FID_{exp}, is the distance at which predator and prey are expected to reach the refuge simultaneously, AD_{crit}, plus the a margin of safety, MOS. When the refuge is between the predator and prey and DP and AD_{crit} are the same as in the previous case, FID_{exp} must be longer to reach the refuge with the same MOS. For a predator on the same side of the refuge as the prey, $FID_{exp} = AD_{crit} + MOS - DP$; for a predator on the opposite side of the refuge, $FID_{exp} = AD_{crit} + MOS + DP$. (B)The slopes of FID_{exp} on distance to refuge for predators approaching from the same (solid line) and opposite (dashed line) side of the refuge are shown for MOS = 8 and a predator 1.5 times faster than the prey. From Kramer and Bonenfant (1997)

when the predator and prey are on the same side of the refuge (Figure 2.13b) is $(AV/PV) - 1$, whereas the slope when both the prey and predator are on opposite sides of the refuge is $(AV/PV) + 1$. These values permit the prediction that these slopes differ by 2.0 slope units. In the only test of this prediction to date, the difference was 1.78 for woodchucks (*Marmota monax*), which did not differ significantly from 2.0 (Kramer & Bonenfant 1997).

This model complements the cost–benefit model of escape by being mechanistic. It applies only to the risk factors distance to refuge, relative velocities of the predator and prey, and the time/distance until the predator overtakes the prey. Nonetheless, the model makes the same general predictions as economic models (i.e., FID is longer when risk is greater in all three cases). No explicit MOS appears in current economic models, but one must exist for prey to escape contact with predators. Kramer and Bonenfant (1997) did not consider effects of cost of fleeing, but cost of fleeing can be considered to be nearly constant in the absence of social interaction and unusual opportunities by hungry prey to eat scarce food.

The model is remarkable for making predictions solely from readily measured variables, in contrast to economic models that make predictions based on fitness components that are extremely difficult to determine and in practice are not known above an ordinal scale. Further testing is required to determine whether an MOS is constant for a given predator/prey velocity ratio and for approaches from the same and opposite sides. Further testing is also required to determine whether the prediction of the difference of 2.0 slope units applies to other species. Other possibilities, not yet explicitly treated by this or other models, are that prey escape velocities differ when approaching or fleeing away from a predator, and that escape velocities are dynamically adjusted to changes in predator speed.

2.6.2 Game-theoretical model of escape decisions by cryptic prey

When a cryptic prey is approached by a predator, general economic models of FID treat crypsis as a predation risk factor that affects the cost of not fleeing. The more effective the crypsis, the shorter is the predicted FID. Broom and Ruxton (2005) developed a game-theoretical model that applies specifically to the effect of crypsis on FID. Here, the model's rationale will be discussed; its many equations and parameters can be consulted in the original article.

In the model the prey is aware of the predator before the predator detects the prey, but as the predator draws nearer, its probability of detecting the prey increases. The likelihood of being captured for the prey increases as the predator–prey distance where the predator detects the prey decreases. This scenario differs slightly from that of the Ydenberg and Dill (1986) and optimal escape (Cooper & Frederick 2007a, 2010) models. In those models the effect of decreasing predator–prey distance includes both the increase in probability of being detected and of being caught if attacked, and also allows the predator to have detected the prey before the prey has detected it. However, for a very cryptic prey that has been immobile, it is likely that the prey will detect the predator first.

If the prey flees before it has been detected, it may escape without being detected or its movement may draw the predator's attention, eliciting an attack. If the prey does not flee when it first detects the predator, but relies on crypsis to avoid being detected and attacked, the risk of being detected is lower than if it flees, but the risk of being captured if detected is greater when the predator is closer upon detecting the prey.

Table 2.2 Payoff matrix of Broom and Ruxton's (2005) model of escape by a cryptic prey. In the matrix c is the cost of surviving by outrunning the predator, which differs from the opportunity cost of fleeing in economic escape models. The probability that the predator captures if the predator initiates the attack from distance d when at point v on its trajectory is f[d(v)]. The advantage in distance gained by the prey by initiating escape before the predator attacks is Δ.

Situation	Prey's payoff	Predator's payoff
No chase	1	0
Attack-initiated chase	$(1 - c)(1 - f[d(v)])$	$f([d(v)]$
Fleeing-initiated chase	$(1 - c)(1 - f[d(v) + \Delta]$	$f[d(v) + \Delta]$

The game-theoretical model includes trajectories and speeds not explicitly stated in the other models and allows consideration of the effect of the prey's behavior on the predator's attack strategy. Broom and Ruxton (2005) considered cases in which a predator has passed the prey and can either still see the prey or not and can approach before attacking. Only the case in which the predator is approaching on a straight line and must attack as soon as it detects the prey is describe here.

The game matrix (Table 2.2) includes three possibilities and their payoffs. If no chase occurs, the prey's payoff is 1 and the predator's payoff is 0. If fleeing is elicited by attack, the payoffs depend on the predator–prey distance when attack begins, d, the cost of fleeing, c, and the probability of capture when the predator initiates the attack from distance d, f(d), when the predator is at point v on its trajectory. The prey's payoff is the product of $(1 - c)$ and $(1 - f[d(v)]$. The predator's payoff is f[d(v)]. If the prey begins to flee before it is attacked, it gains an advantage in distance covered, Δ, due to the delay in reactive attack by the predator. Therefore when escape is initiated before the predator attacks, the payoffs are $(1 - c)(1 - f[d(v) + \Delta]$ for the prey and f[d(v) + \Delta] for the predator. The situation in the crypsis model in which delayed escape occurs only when the predator attacks raises questions about how the prey might distinguish continued approach from attack. Prey rapidly adjust FID to changes in speed and directness of approach by predators (Cooper 1997, 1998, 2006), providing possible cues to permit the option of attack-initiated chases for d > 0.

The major conclusion of the model is that a cryptic prey should either flee immediately when it detects the approaching predator (that is still unaware of the prey) or postpone fleeing until the predator attacks. The prey should flee immediately when the predator has a low search rate (allowing escape with low probability of being detected), cost of escaping by outrunning the predator is low, probability of escaping if the prey initiates escape is greater than if it flees only in response to being detected and attacked, ability to detect the predator at a distance is low, the predator's ability to detect the prey is greater (ineffective crypsis), and capture rate when the predator attacks is high. In the opposite conditions, prey should postpone fleeing until attacked.

Are the predictions of Broom and Ruxton's (2005) model consistent with those of general economic escape models? In those models prey should flee immediately whenever the predator is detected closer than the economically predicted FID. If a predator is highly efficient at capturing the prey if it attacks and is unlikely to detect a prey fleeing due to low searching rate, fleeing immediately can be predicted. In the general models, lower cost of fleeing predicts longer FID, but the cost of fleeing is primarily opportunity cost, which is not considered in Broom and Ruxton's (2005) model. Nevertheless, if c in their model is considered to represent the sum of energetic cost of fleeing, cost of possible injury not inflicted by the predator while fleeing, and opportunity cost, the model is economic. In the general economic models, limited ability to detect the predator increases the likelihood that the predator will not be detected before it reaches the economically predicted FID, and high ability of the predator to detect the prey corresponds to a low degree of crypsis, which predicts longer FID due to greater risk of being detected and attacked.

In the model for cryptic prey, delaying escape attempts until attacked by the predator is favored by low capture efficiency by the predator, high probability of detecting and attacking the prey if it flees, high cost of fleeing if the prey outruns the predator, little or no advantage of initiating escape attempts rather than reacting to attack, strong ability of the prey to detect the predator at long distances, and limited ability of the predator to detect the prey at long distances. All of these factors are associated with shorter predicted FID in the general cost–benefit models through their effects on cost of not fleeing and cost of fleeing.

The predictions of Broom and Ruxton's (2005) escape model for immediate escape by cryptic prey are consistent with those of Ydenberg and Dill's (1986) and Cooper and Frederick's (2007a, 2010) cost–benefit models. The game-theoretical model includes a subset of the predation risk factors in those models. However, predictions of the model for cryptic prey when flight is triggered by attack differ from those of the more general models. The latter predict that prey monitor the predator until it closes to an economically predicted FID that is typically greater than zero. All of the models allow zero FID if crypsis is perfect. However, in the general models, the predicted FID may occur before or after the predator has detected the prey, depending on risk determined jointly by probability of being detected and attacked if detected, and by the predator's capture efficiency and lethality upon capture. Empirical studies of highly cryptic frogs and lizards (Cooper *et al.* 2008; Cooper & Sherbrooke 2010a,b) show that some individuals do not flee until overtaken; FID by horned lizards (*Phrynosoma cornutum*) increased as predation risk (approach speed and directness of approach) increased when the predator did not change speed or directness (Cooper & Sherbrooke 2010a). These findings support the general models in which FID increases with risk and challenge the crypsis model to identify a means of determining how prey assess when attack begins in a manner consistent with the data.

2.6.3   Game-theoretical approach to hiding time in refuge

When a prey flees into a refuge, it may gain safety, but lose information about the predator's location. A waiting game ensues in which the predator decides whether to stay in the area or seek other prey and the prey decides when to emerge. Emerging too soon may be disastrous for the prey, and waiting too long may be costly to the predator. Due to large differences in fitness consequences for predator and prey, prey are expected to win the waiting game by staying in refuge until after the predator has left the area (Hugie 2003).

Hugie's (2003) model establishes the existence of an evolutionarily stable strategy of waiting times for predator and prey, the prey's waiting time being hiding time. The predator's distribution of waiting times before leaving should resemble a negative exponential distribution, whereas prey should have more variable hiding times and a positively skewed distribution. The model predicts that predators will only rarely out-wait prey. The model does not permit predictions about the economic bases of latency to emerge from refuge, but does provides valuable insight into the process leading to successful refuge use.

2.6.4   Stochastic dynamic modeling of fitness consequences of hiding time in refuge

Stochastic dynamic modeling is a technique used to calculate the fitness of animals over some interval of time in which they have made various behavioral decisions (Mangel & Clark 1993), but this useful method of modeling has been applied to decisions about escape and refuge use only once. Rhoades and Blumstein (2007) conducted an empirical study of hiding time and modeled its consequences over the activity season in yellow-bellied marmots (*Marmota flaviventris*) that must gain sufficient body mass before entering hibernation in order to survive over winter.

The empirical study showed that marmots hide for longer times when approached slowly than rapidly, presumably because their most dangerous predators that stay longer in the vicinity when marmots enter refuge are stalking predators that search specifically for marmots. Hiding time decreased when food was placed outside the burrow. However, the effects of approach speed and added food interacted, being shortest when extra food was present after less risky approaches.

In the model, the ability of marmots to meet their energetic needs is improved, but predation risk is increased, by shorter hiding times. Daily weight gain by different age/sex groups and their asymptotic weights were used to calculate weight upon entering hibernation and daily energetic needs during the activity season. The probability of being killed was considered to be proportional to the amount of time spent outside refuge in each step (90 minute time interval). A proportionality constant, r representing the predation rate in the population was multiplied by the proportion of time in the open to give the probability of predation $P = r(t_0/t)$, where t_0 represent time in the open at each step. In the model runs, r was varied between 10 and 50% for the activity season.

Because marmots do not gain energy while in refuge, the amount acquired during each step (i.e., the gain) is $g(x) = [kn(t_0/t)^2]$, where k is a proportionality constant that was higher when extra food was present and n is units of need. Benefits for prey that emerge early from refuge are elevated by squaring the proportion of time outside refuge to account for high gain by early emergers and loss of the extra food to other group members by late emergers. The net energetic gain $G(x) = g(x) - c$, where c is the energetic cost (expenditure) in the step. Nine discrete levels of body condition of marmots ranged from 0 (dead) to 8 (able to hibernate without starving to death). Fitness of a marmot at the final step was represented by a sigmoidal function, $T (fit) = s^2/(4 + s^2)$, where s is the condition.

The model calculated the optimal hiding decisions for an individual over a given number of time steps. To examine effects of suboptimal hiding times on fitness, (1) predation was randomized to permit predation even on prey making optimal decisions and (2) populations of 100 marmots were simulated that used hiding times that were optimal, 50% of optimal, and 200% of optimal.

The consequence of shortened hiding time was drastic: all individuals were killed by predators. Individuals that hid too long lost condition over time, resulting in high mortality (*c.* 64 to 92%). Survival by prey making optimal decisions was 100% despite inclusion of randomized predation in the model. Thus the stochastic dynamic model highlights the crucial nature of making optimal decisions about hiding, decisions that balance the effects of predation risk against long-term energetic needs. The model revealed differences among age/sex groups in relative hiding times among combinations of approach speed and provision of extra food (or not). The rankings of hiding time for these combinations varied with body conditions both within and among age/sex groups (Rhoades & Blumstein 2007). The model was highly successful in identifying fitness consequences of suboptimal hiding times and revealed subtle variation among age/sex groups and states of body condition that correspond to testable predictions. Stochastic dynamic modeling shows great promise and could readily be applied to trade-offs between hiding time and reproductive and aggressive behaviors and to assessing fitness consequences of suboptimal escape decisions, especially about FID.

2.7   Behaviors prior to fleeing and flight initiation distance: vigilance, alarm calling, and pursuit-deterrent signaling

Several behaviors that may affect escape decisions are omitted or treated in less detail in this chapter, which is devoted to models of escape behavior and refuge use in which prey base decisions on economic considerations and to closely allied models. Vigilance, alarm calling, and pursuit-deterrent signaling are among these behaviors that occur prior to escape. They are considered here theoretically and discussed more comprehensively in Chapter 10. Vigilance affects escape decisions because less vigilant prey may permit predators to approach closer than more vigilant prey would before fleeing. In such cases, more vigilant individuals begin to escape at the longest predator–prey distance where cost of not fleeing outweighs the cost of fleeing. Less vigilant prey may fail to detect the predator until it is closer than the economically predicted distance where escape should begin.

In terms of escape theory, vigilant prey may detect an approaching predator in zone II, in which case it flees when the predator reaches the economically predicted FID, or in zone I, where immediate escape is predicted. A less vigilant prey may not detect the predator until it penetrates zone I, later than would occur for a more vigilant prey. Therefore FID is shorter for the less vigilant of two prey in zone I. Furthermore, predation risk is greater upon detection of a predator for the less vigilant prey. Not allocating time to vigilance can be catastrophic for a prey if it fails to detect the predator until captured. Even if a less vigilant prey flees when it detects a predator that is already close or that flees upon detecting a fleeing conspecific, the increase in risk compared to that for a more vigilant prey can be substantial (Lima 1994).

Many prey signal that they have detected a predator and are able to escape if attacked, or at least more able to escape than non-signaling prey. Nur and Hasson (1984) considered pursuit deterrence to be a case of the handicap principle (Zahavi 1975), which states that some traits that appear to be deleterious have evolved because they demonstrate that the bearer can overcome the handicap, which therefore indicates its superior fitness. Signaling to a predator might be considered a handicap that increases the likelihood of the signaler being detected and attacked. Nur and Hasson (1984) showed that if a signaler has a higher probability of escaping if attacked than nearby conspecifics, a predator should preferentially attack non-signalers. In Nur and Hasson's (1984) model and in other models unless stated otherwise, prey are aware that a predator is present and direct the signal to that predator.

Game theory is applicable to pursuit deterrence because the fitness consequences for the prey are affected by the predator's decision to attack or not and the predator's success depends on the relative escape ability of prey that signal and do not signal. Vega-Redondo and Hasson (1993) employed a game-theoretical approach to model a predator choosing which prey to attack from a herd. The herd includes individuals that have variable signal strength and non-signalers. The prey vary in ability to escape if attacked, which is honestly indicated by signal strength. The predator's choice also is affected by the frequencies of prey with high and low escape ability that is correlated signal strength. Given these conditions, an equilibrium favorable to both predator and prey exists, in part because a cheater whose signal indicates greater escape ability than it possesses is likely to be captured if attacked, which occurs at some probability greater than zero. At equilibrium, strong signalers are less likely to be attacked and predators gain attacking weaker signalers. The probability of successful cheating increases as herd size increases and the frequency of high-quality prey decreases, which affects the equilibrium probabilities of signaling and attacking.

Alarm calling by prey that detect predators may evolve by kin selection even if calling increases the chances of being detected and attacked. Signaling may also have a pursuit-deterrent function if the signaler is likely to escape because it is aware of the predator. In a game-theoretical model of alarm calling called the watchful babbler game (Bergstrom & Lachman 2001), the payoff matrix has separate entries when a predator is present and absent and, when a predator is present, separate entries for prey that do and do not signal (Table 2.3). When a predator is absent, uncertain prey may signal with payoff $1 - c$, where c is the prey's cost of signaling. If the prey does not signal, its payoff is one. In both cases the payoff for the predator is 0. If a predator is present and the prey signals, the prey's payoff is $(1 - c)(1 - t)$, where t is the probability of being captured if the predator attacks. The predator's payoff in this situation is $t - d$, where d is the cost to the predator of attacking. If the prey signals, but the predator does not attack, the prey's payoff is $1 - c$ and the predator's is zero. When the prey does not signal and the predator

Table 2.3 Payoff matrix of the watchful babbler game in which the prey can signal or not in the presence or absence of a predator and the predator can attack or not whether the prey signals or not. The prey's payoff is 1, its current fitness, if it does not signal and is not attacked. The predator's payoff is 0 if it does not attack and $t - d$ if it attacks, where t is the probability of capturing the prey that it attacks and d is the cost of attacking. The maximum payoff for the predator is the prey's fitness and can only be achieved if capture is certain and attack carries no cost.

	Predator present				Predator absent	
	Signal		No signal			
	Chase	No chase	Chase	No chase	Signal	No signal
Prey	$(1 - c)(1 - t)$	$1 - c$	$1 - t$	1	$1 - c$	1
Predator	$t - d$	0	$t - d$	0	0	0

Modified from Table 1 in Bergstrom and Lachmann (2001)

attacks, the payoff is $1 - t$ for the prey and $t - d$ for the predator. Finally, if the prey does not signal when a predator is present but fails to attack, the prey's payoff is 1 and the predator's payoff is 0. The predator's maximum possible payoff in this model is the same for prey and predator.

A key feature of this model is that the prey is uncertain whether a predator is present or not, and is more likely to signal when it assesses the probability of a predator being present to be higher. The model predicts that calls may not only inform conspecifics about the presence of a predator, but also honestly inform the predator that it has been detected and that the signaler is therefore more likely to escape if attacked. The signal does not indicate that signalers have greater physiological escape ability, only that they are aware. In Bergstrom and Lachmann's (2001) model, the cost of signaling is a consequence of alerting predators other than the one to which the prey is responding to the prey's presence. The watchful babbler game has a stable equilibrium at which predators are less likely to attack when prey signal. At equilibrium, prey benefit by being less likely to be attacked and killed, whereas predators benefit by not incurring cost of attacking when the probability of capture is too low.

An unpublished game-theoretical model by W. Cooper and W. Frederick examines effects of a predator on prey's decision to signal and of a solitary prey on the predator's decision to attack. The model makes four assumptions. First, signal strength does not vary. Second, the probability that a prey that has signaled will be killed if the predator attacks, K_s, is lower than that for a prey that does not signal, K_{ns}. Thus signaling is honest ($K_{ns} - K_s > 0$). If the term $K_{ns} - K_s$ is zero, signaling is not beneficial to predator or prey. Third, units in the payoff matrix are fitnesses for predator and prey normalized to 1. Fourth, the cost of signaling for the prey, C_s, is very small compared to the benefit of a kill for the predator, B (i.e., $C_s \ll B_k$). In effect, the benefit of the kill is unaffected by the signaling cost to the prey.

The game matrix (Table 2.4) excludes the case in which no predator is present that was in the payoff matrix of the watchful babbler game (Table 2.3). The model assumes that the predator has been detected with certainty. The optimal signaling strategy for the prey

Table 2.4 Payoff matrix of a game-theoretical model of pursuit deterrence for solitary prey that are certain that a predator is present. The predator attacks with probability p and does not attack with probability 1 – p. The prey signals with probability q and does not signal with probability 1 – q. For each combination of predator and prey actions, the payoff for the predator is shown first, separated by a comma from the payoff for the prey. B – the predator's benefit from killing the prey, C_a – the predator' cost of attacking, C_s – the prey's cost of signaling, K_s – the probability of killing a prey that has signaled if the predator attacks, K_{ns} – the probability of killing a prey that has not signaled if the predator attacks.

		Prey	
		Signal (q)	Not signal (1 – q)
Predator	Attack (p)	$(BK_s - C_a, 1 - K_s - C_s)$	$(BK_{ns} - C_a, 1 - K_{ns})$
	Not attack (1 – p)	$(0, 1 - C_s)$	$(0, 1)$

(Cooper & Frederick, unpublished)

depends on the probability that the predator will attack, and the optimal attack strategy by the predator depends on the probability that the prey signals. Thus the equilibrium strategies in the pursuit deterrence game are determined by mutual influences of predator and prey. The model is derived in ESM 2.1, which is available at www.cambridge.org/9781107060548.

Pursuit-deterrent signaling is relevant to escape decisions if signaling lowers the probability of being attacked and, therefore, predation risk. The models of pursuit deterrence show that honest signals that communicate the prey's likelihood of escaping when aware of the predator lead to a stable equilibrium of signaling and attack with reduced probability of attack on signalers. The reduced risk associated with signaling predicts that a prey should allow a predator to approach closer before fleeing when the prey signals than when it does not. This prediction was confirmed in the zebra-tailed lizard, *Callisaurus draconoides*, that lizards that signaled allowed predators to approach closer before they fled than did non-signaling individuals (Cooper 2011b).

2.8   Escape latency

The models considered thus far predict FID by an immobile prey being approached by a predator and hiding time in refuge when a predator was known to be nearby upon refuge entry. Two recent graphical models (Martín *et al.* 2009; Cooper *et al.* 2012) predict latency to flee by an immobile prey near an immobile predator. The former model is limited to predictions about effects of risk factors on escape latency. The latter model applies to predation risk factors and opportunity costs and is similar to the Ydenberg and Dill model of FID when a predator moves toward an immobile prey.

The escape latency model applies when a prey has moved toward an immobile predator before stopping or a predator has moved toward an immobile prey before stopping. If the prey has not detected the predator while approaching it or while the predator has approached the prey, the standing distance may be shorter than the

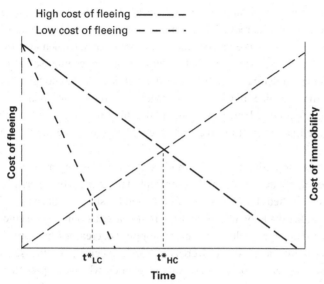

Figure 2.14   When an immobile predator is near an immobile prey, the probability that the predator will detect and attack the prey increases with time. Therefore the cost of fleeing incurred when movement causes the prey to be detected and attacked decreases as time increases. Cost of remaining immobile increases as time increases due to increasing loss of opportunities to enhance fitness that require movement. The predicted latency to flee, t*, occurs at the intersection of the two cost curves. Escape latency model. From Cooper *et al.* (2012). Predicted latency to flee, t*, is longer for the higher of two cost of fleeing curves. Although not shown, it also is longer for the lower of two cost of immobility curves intersecting a single cost of fleeing curve.

economically predicted FID when the prey has monitored the predator's approach. Therefore the escape latency model applies to a wide range of standing distances, the distance between the immobile predator and immobile prey. Because an immobile prey might approach the predator after a period of immobility, the prey's latency to approach might also be modeled and measured, but is not considered here beyond noting that a prey may assess the immobile predator as posing less risk as time spent immobile increases.

The encounter begins when the prey becomes aware that an immobile predator is nearby. Escape latency is the time between initial awareness and initiation of escape behavior. In the graphical model (Cooper *et al.* 2012; Figure 2.14) escape latency (time) is the horizontal axis and the cost of fleeing and cost of remaining immobile (not fleeing) are the left and right vertical axes, respectively. Cost of fleeing decreases as escape latency increases because the predator is increasingly likely to detect and attack the prey. Cost of immobility increases as time increases because opportunity cost increases. The predicted escape latency occurs at the intersection of the increasing cost of remaining immobile and the decreasing cost of fleeing curves.

Cost of fleeing decreases as risk increases. For two costs of fleeing (e.g. those for fast versus slow approach speeds by the predator), the latency to escape is predicted to be greater when predation risk is smaller (cost of fleeing is higher). Latency to flee is greater when standing distance is greater because risk is lower at longer standing distance due to longer time required by a predator to detect the prey and lower risk of being captured if attacked. Prey are predicted to move sooner when cost of remaining still is higher, preventing them from obtaining benefits of feeding, social behavior, or other activities that increase fitness. If expected benefits are large enough relative to risk, a prey animal may not flee, but instead approach the predator to obtain the benefit or move toward the source of benefit without approaching the predator. In such cases the variable measured is latency to move or latency to approach the predator, not escape latency.

Only a few tests of predictions of the models of escape latency have been conducted because the models are new; tests are thus far limited to lizards. However, all predictions tested have been verified. Escape latency is affected by standing distance and many of the predation risk factors known to affect FID. It increases as standing distance increases (six species), predator approach speed before stopping decreases (three species), direct-ness of approach by the predator decreases (three species), for the second of two consecutive approaches (two species), and is greater when the predator maintains eye contact with the prey than looks elsewhere (one species) (Martín et al. 2009; Cooper et al. 2012; Cooper & Sherbrooke 2013b). Escape latency decreases when opportunities to enhance fitness are present. It is shorter in the presence than absence of food (two species) or an unfamiliar female that may be courted by males (one species) (Martín et al. 2009; Cooper et al. 2012; Cooper & Sherbrooke 2013b). In all cases in which an effect has been observed in two or more species, two families and both active foraging and ambush foraging modes are represented, hinting that the predictions may apply to prey from diverse taxa having disparate ecological traits. More research is needed on additional taxa.

2.9   New model of nearest approach distance by a prey approaching an immobile predator

In a previously unmodeled scenario, a prey approaches an immobile predator that the prey has detected (Figure 2.15). As in Ydenberg and Dill's (1986) model of FID, the horizontal axis in the graphical model of nearest approach distance is distance between prey and predator. Left and right vertical axes are the cost of approaching and cost of not approaching, respectively. The cost of approaching due to predation risk increases as the distance from the predator decreases. The cost of not approaching, which is primarily an opportunity cost incurred when some benefit can only be obtained by approaching the predator, increases as distance from the predator increases. This model applies only to prey that have sensory systems and cognitive abilities that allow them to perceive an immobile preditor. The model is not applicable to prey that lack these abilities, such as some teiid lizards that often approach and walk on the feet of people who have remained immobile for some time.

The prey is predicted to stop approaching when the costs of approaching and not approaching are equal, which occurs at the intersection of the cost curves (Figure 2.15).

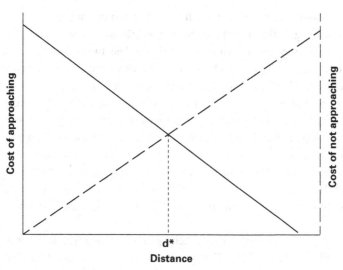

Figure 2.15   A prey approaching an immobile predator must balance the increasing cost of approaching (risk of predation) as it draws nearer against the cost of not approaching, which is primarily an opportunity cost. This model is isomorphic to Ydenberg and Dill's (1986) model of FID (Figure 1) with cost of approaching substituted for cost of not fleeing and cost of not approaching for cost of fleeing.

This may be accomplished by becoming immobile or moving in a different direction to avoid coming too close. The predictions for two cost of approaching or two cost of not approaching curves are similar to those of Ydenberg and Dill's (1986) FID model (Figure 2.2) and Cooper *et al.*'s (2012) latency to flee model (Figure 2.14). The higher of the two cost of approaching curves intersects with a single cost of not approaching curve at a greater distance, indicating that the predicted nearest approach distance is longer when predation risk is greater. The intersection of the higher of two cost of not approaching curves with a single cost of approaching curve is closer to the predator than that of the lower cost of not approaching curve. This comparison shows that the predicted nearest approach distance is shorter for higher cost of not approaching curves.

Mathematical expression of the Ydenberg and Dill (1986) model and related graphical models varies with the nature of cost curves. As a first approximation, linear cost curves can be used (Cooper & Frederick 2007a). The fitness cost of approaching the predator until distance $d = 0$ is the prey's initial fitness, F_0, multiplied by the predator's proportional lethality (L), which is LF_0. Let the cost of approaching be a negative linear function of predator–prey distance, $A(d) = LF_0 - ad$, where $a > 0$ is the slope of the fitness cost of approaching the predator on distance from the predator. The derivative is $A'(d) = -a$ and is the marginal cost of approaching, which increases from zero where the cost of approaching line intersects the distance axis to LF_0 when $d = 0$. The cost of not approaching, $N(d)$ is zero at $d = 0$ and increases linearly as predator–prey distance increases ($N(d) = nd$, where $n > 0$ is the slope of the cost of not approaching on predator–prey distance). The marginal cost of not approaching is $N'(d) = n$.

The prey should continue its approach while the cost of not approaching exceeds the cost of approaching. If the cost of approaching is greater than or equal to the cost of not approaching, the prey should stop approaching. The model predicts that approach continues until $A(d) = N(d)$, which occurs at the predicted nearest approach distance, d^*. For linear cost of approaching and not approaching curves, $d^* = LF_0/(n + a)$.

Greater cost of approaching at a particular distance corresponds to a higher cost of approaching curve and longer nearest approach distance, implying a lower absolute values of the slope a. Suppose that costs are linear and two cost of approaching lines have slopes $-a$ and $-a^\wedge$, and $a > a^\wedge$. The difference in predicted nearest approach distance for the lines that intersect a single cost of not approaching line is $d^{*\wedge} - d^* = LF_0(a - a^\wedge)/[(n + a)(n + a^\wedge)]$. The difference $a^\wedge - a$ is positive because $a^\wedge < a$, corresponding to greater nearest approach distance for the cost line having the lower slope, $a^\wedge$.

The greater of two costs of not approaching at a particular predator–prey distance is associated with the slope $n^\wedge > n$. For two cost of not approaching lines that intersect a single cost of approaching line, the difference in predicted nearest approach distances is $d^{*\wedge} - d^* = LF_0(n - n^\wedge)/[(n + a)(n^\wedge + a)$, where d^* is the predicted nearest approach distance for slope a. The nearest approach distance is shorter for a steeper cost of not approaching line ($n^\wedge > n$).

In the Ydenberg and Dill (1986) model of escape, the cost of not fleeing could be represented by any function that decreases monotonically or is non-increasing as predator–prey distance increases; similarly any monotonically increasing or non-decreasing function might be considered as a possible cost of fleeing curve (Cooper & Vitt 2002). Non-linear curves for cost of approaching must be described by monotonically decreasing or non-increasing functions of distance and those for cost of not approaching must be described by monotonically increasing or non-decreasing functions of distance.

Here, I describe one non-linear cost of approaching. As a prey approaches a predator, risk may increase slowly at long distances from the predator, but accelerate rapidly near the predator, resulting in a steeper rise in cost of approaching when nearing the predator. In such cases the cost of approaching may be a negative exponential function of distance, $A(d) = LF_0e^{-cd}$, where c is the rate constant for exponential decay. The cost of approaching is the expected fitness if contacted by the predator times the probability of being killed if the prey stops approaching at d. If cost of not approaching is linear and cost of approaching is negative exponential, the predicted nearest approach distance is $d^* = LF_0/n - d^*/e^{-cd} = d^*e^{cd^*}$. The solution of this equation is $d^* = \text{ProductLog}(cLF_0/n)/c$, where the function $\text{ProductLog}(z)$ in Mathematica is the principal solution for w in $z = we^w$. As when both cost functions are linear, d^* depends on lethality, initial fitness, and the rate constants for decrease in risk and increase in cost of not approaching as distance increases. Provided that risk approaches zero for a negative exponential cost where a linear cost reaches the distance axis, risk is lower for the negative exponential cost than the linear one at all distances except $d = 0$. Therefore the cost of approaching curve intersects the cost of not approaching line closer to the predator (i.e., nearest approach distance is shorter for the negative exponential than the linear cost of approaching).

An advantage of the model is that it allows many testable predictions to be made for diverse prey. The model permits a wide range of predictions to be made for many of the risk factors that affect decisions to flee or emerge from refuge in other scenarios. Each of the factors affects the degree of risk incurred by approaching the predator. Among these are longer nearest approach distance (1) for direct than indirect approach, (2) for prey that encounter predators infrequently than for prey habituated to the presence of potential predators that do not attack, (3) for the second of two approaches if attacked during the first approach, (4) for longer than shorter distance to refuge, (5) for longer than shorter starting distance, (6) for the more conspicuous prey or prey in less concealing cover, (7) for prey with less effective body armor or other effective defenses, and (8) for slower prey. Predictions are clear for other risk factors such as numbers of predators and prey, predator and prey sizes, direction of the predator's gaze, etc. Among factors affecting the cost of not approaching, shorter nearest approach distance is predicted for hungry prey in the presence than absence of food, for reproductively active prey in the presence than absence of mating opportunities, for thirsty prey in the presence than absence of water, and for hypoxic prey in a gradient of oxygen concentration that increases as distance from the predator decreases, and for prey that encounter more favorable thermal conditions nearer the predator.

The model's predictions may be more difficult to test than those of models for the scenarios discussed above. In the other escape scenarios, the prey is immobile, permitting a researcher or a model of a predator to approach the prey in various ways that affect risk or to approach to a desired position and then remain still. Collecting data on nearest approach distance in the field often may require a researcher to move to a location where prey are likely to approach and then remain immobile while waiting to be approached. Because there is no advantage of a researcher being able to move toward prey, predator models may be used more frequently. Tests of the model could be facilitated by studying highly mobile prey that spend a high proportion of the time moving, such as active foragers. If approaches by prey are infrequent, data could be accumulated by using motion-activated video recorders.

2.10   Relative movement of prey and predator: escape variables and models

Economic models of decisions about escape, refuge use, and approaching a predator share the perspective that prey adjust antipredatory behavior to both predation risk and costs of the antipredatory activities. Risk is traded for benefit in all of the models. Each model applies to a particular scenario defined by the movement of both predator and prey, and predicts a behavioral variable appropriate for the relative movements (Table 2.5). The first models described in this chapter were developed to predict FID when a predator approaches an immobile predator (Ydenberg & Dill 1986; Cooper & Frederick 2007a, 2010). More recently models were published that predict escape latency when both predator and prey are immobile (Martín *et al.* 2009;

Table 2.5 Models predicting escape decisions for various scenarios of relative movement and location of a prey and a single predator.

Movement/location		Variable	Model	Source
Prey	Predator			
still	moving	FID	graphical	Ydenberg and Dill 1986
			optimality	Cooper and Frederick 2007a, 2010
still	still	latency to flee	graphical	Martin *et al.* 2009,
				Cooper *et al.* 2012
		PAL	graphical	this publication
moving	still	NAD	graphical	this publication
moving	moving	not developed	none	none
in refuge	outside	hiding time	graphical	Martín and López 1999
			optimality	Cooper and Frederick 2007b

FID: flight initiation distance; MAD: nearest approach distance; PAL: prey approach latency.

Cooper *et al.* 2012). In the preceding section, I presented a model that predicts how closely a moving prey will approach an immobile predator before stopping or changing its direction of movement.

The only scenario not yet modeled is escape or approach by prey when both the predator and the prey are moving. This scenario is the most complex of the possibilities shown in Table 2.5. Relative speeds and directions of predator and prey are important when both are moving. If they are moving away from each other, risk decreases, requiring no additional behavioral alteration by the prey. If they are moving closer to each other, maximum risk is influenced by the minimum bypass distance between predator and prey if their trajectories are maintained. If the minimum bypass distance is long enough, prey may not alter their movements. When the minimum bypass distance is shorter, prey might be predicted to stop farther from the predator, as in the model of nearest approach distance, but the nearest approach distance should then be longer than if the predator were immobile. If the prey stops moving, the scenario shifts to that of FID models.

When both predator and prey are moving, prey have options other than stopping (which would shift the encounter to the original scenario of Ydenberg and Dill 1986), such as changing trajectories to avoid coming closer to predators, fleeing in various directions, and entering refuge. A prey might alter its speed rather than its trajectory to increase the minimum bypass distance, or alter both speed and trajectory. Degree of predation risk associated with the predator's speed relative to that of the prey, lethality, and other factors affecting risk may be predicted to affect the predator–prey distance at which prey change their speed, direction, or both, as well as the magnitude of the changes. The effects of foraging, social, and other opportunities should be to decrease the predator–prey distance when the prey's behavior is altered and decrease changes in speed and direction of movement. If the predator alters its movements to attack, the focus shifts from decisions by prey prior to being attacked to a later stage of predator–prey encounters, pursuit.

For linear trajectories, the slopes of the lines and the speeds determine whether, when, and where intersection occurs. Nearest approach distance can be calculated using parametric equations of the vector values to determine distances between predator and prey and then determine its minimum value, which occurs when the derivative of distance is zero. However, because predator and prey are free to change their trajectories, a linear model would have very limited applicability. On the other hand, it might be possible to use such a model to predict when a prey should alter its path and/or speed given a linear approach by the predator. We know little of such dynamics prior to pursuit. It would be worthwhile to use video recording to assess the responses of prey approaching a manipulatable model predator that in turn approaches the prey.

2.11   Conclusions

Theory is now available to guide empirical studies of many aspects of escape behavior. Cost–benefit models have been very successful in making predictions about effects of factors that influence cost of fleeing and cost of not fleeing on FID and latency to flee, and about costs of emerging and not emerging from refuge on hiding time. The new model I presented here provides similar predictions about the nearest approach distance for a prey approaching an immobile predator.

Some escape variables have been neglected in escape models, especially the distance fled, escape speed, escape trajectory when the predator does not pursue, and the probability of entering a refuge. Both distance fled and probability of entering refuge are expected to increase as predation risk increases and cost of fleeing decreases. However, the distance to the nearest refuge may affect both decisions. These relationships have not been modeled formally. Nevertheless, predictions for distance fled and refuge entry made using the logic of the economic models of FID have often been verified (Cooper 2009). However, there are exceptions (Cooper 2009). Although some exceptions could be consequences of unrecorded variation in distance to refuge, closer empirical examination of these variables is needed. Theory to guide research on relationships between these variables and costs and benefits would be very useful to inform such research.

Optimality models analogous to that for FID (Cooper & Frederick 2007a, 2010) and hiding time (Cooper & Frederick 2007b) could easily be developed for latency to flee and nearest approach distance. I have not done so here because almost all of their ordinal level predictions are the same as those of the graphical FID model by Ydenberg and Dill (1986). However, the optimality models allow the prey to make better escape decisions, and would be useful in theoretical studies of fitness.

Several other topics relevant to escape have received no theoretical attention. Models predicting the precise effects of alarm calling and other forms of pursuit-deterrent signaling on FID would be useful. Escape trajectories and speeds prior to pursuit have been largely ignored theoretically for terrestrial prey, but theory and empirical findings about trajectories are presented in Chapter 8, with emphasis on aquatic prey. The complex case in which both predator and prey are moving, but pursuit has not begun, will require explicit consideration of speeds and directions of movement by both predator and prey. Models and empirical studies of this scenario would greatly expand our knowledge of escape behavior. Another area in which our theoretical understanding is limited is the pursuit phase of predator–prey encounters, which is discussed in Chapter 8.

References

Amo, L., Lopez, P. & Martin, J.(2004). Multiple predators and conflicting refuge use in the wall lizard, *Podarcis muralis*. *Annales Zoologici Fennici*, **41**, 671–679.

Bergstrom, C. T. & Lachmann, M. (2001). Alarm calls as costly signals of antipredator vigilance: The watchful babbler game. *Animal Behaviour*, **61**, 535–543.

Blumstein, D. T. (2003). Flight-initiation distance in birds is dependent on intruder starting distance. *Journal of Wildlife Management*, **67**, 852–857.

Blumstein, D. T. (2010). Flush early and avoid the rush: A general rule of antipredator behaviour?*Behavioral Ecology and Sociobiology*, **21**, 440–442.

Blumstein, D. T., Fernández-Juricic, E., Zollner, P. A. & Garity, S. C. (2005). Inter-specific variation in avian responses to human disturbance. *Journal of Applied Ecology*, **42**, 943–953.

Broom, M. & Ruxton, G. D. (2005). You can run or you can hide: Optimal strategies for cryptic prey. *Behavioral Ecology*, **16**, 534–540.

Caro, T. M. (2005). *Antipredator Defenses in Birds and Mammals*. Chicago: University of Chicago Press.

Chamaillè-Jammes, S. & Blumstein, D. T. (2012). A case for quantile regression behavoral ecology: Getting more out of flight initiation distance data. *Behavioral Ecology and Sociobiology*, **66**, 985–992.

Cooper, W. E., Jr. (1997). Factors affecting risk and cost of escape by the broad-headed skink (*Eumeces laticeps*): Predator speed, directness of approach, and female presence. *Herpetologica*, **53**, 464–474.

Cooper, W. E., Jr. (1998). Direction of predator turning, a neglected cue to predation risk. *Behaviour*, **135**, 55–64.

Cooper, W. E., Jr. (2005). When and how does starting distance affect flight initiation distance. *Canadian Journal of Zoology*, **83**, 1045–1050.

Cooper, W. E., Jr. (2006). Dynamic risk assessment: prey rapidly adjust flight initiation distance to changes in predator approach speed. *Ethology*, **112**, 858–864.

Cooper, W. E., Jr. (2008). Strong artifactual effect of starting distance on flight initiation distance in the actively foraging lizard *Aspidoscelis exsanguis*. *Herpetologica*, **64**, 200–206.

Cooper, W. E., Jr. (2010a). Economic escape. In *Encyclopedia of Animal Behavior, Vol. 1*. London: Academic Press, pp. 588–595.

Cooper, W. E., Jr. (2010b). Pursuit deterrence varies with predation risks affecting escape behaviour in the lizard *Callisaurus draconoides*. *Animal Behaviour*, **80**, 249–256.

Cooper, W. E., Jr. (2011a). Influence of some potential predation risk factors and interaction between predation risk and cost of fleeing on escape by the lizard *Sceloporus virgatus*. *Ethology*, **117**, 620–629.

Cooper, W. E., Jr. (2011b). Pursuit deterrence, predations risk, and escape in the lizard *Callisaurus draconoides*. *Behavioral Ecology and Sociobiology*, **65**, 1833–1841.

Cooper, W. E., Jr. & Blumstein, D. T. (2014). Starting distance, alert distance and flushing early challenge economic escape theory: New proposed effects on costs of fleeing and not fleeing. *Behavioral Ecology*, **25**, 44–52.

Cooper, W. E., Jr. & Frederick, W. G. (2007a). Optimal flight initiation distance. *Journal of Theoretical Biology*, **244**, 59–67.

Cooper, W. E., Jr. & Frederick, W. G. (2007b). Optimal time to emerge from refuge. *Biological Journal of the Linnaean Society*, **91**, 375–382.

Cooper, W. E., Jr. & Frederick, W. G. (2010). Predator lethality, optimal escape behavior, and autotomy. *Behavioral Ecology*, **21**, 91–96.

Cooper, W. E., Jr. & Sherbrooke, W. C. (2010a). Initiation of escape behavior by the Texas horned lizard (*Phrynosoma cornutum*). *Herpetologica*, **66**, 64–71.

Cooper, W. E., Jr. & Sherbrooke, W. C. (2010b). Plesiomorphic escape decisions in cryptic horned lizards (*Phrynosoma*) having highly derived antipredatory defenses. *Ethology*, **116**, 920–928.

Cooper, W. E., Jr. & Sherbrooke, W. C. (2013a). Effects of recent movement, starting distance and other risk factors on escape behaviour by two phrynosomatid lizards. *Behaviour*, **150**, 447–469.

Cooper, W. E., Jr. & Sherbrooke, W. C. (2013b). Risk and cost of immobility in the presence of an immobile predator: Effects on latency to flee or approach food or a potential mate. *Behavioral Ecology and Sociobiology*, **67**, 583–592

Cooper, W. E., Jr. & Vitt, L. J. (2002). Optimal escape and emergence theories. *Comments on Theoretical Biology*, **7**, 283–294.

Cooper, W. E., Jr. & Wilson, D. S. (2008). Thermal cost of refuge use affects refuge entry and hiding time by striped plateau lizards *Sceloporus virgatus*. *Herpetologica*, **64**, 406–412.

Cooper, W. E., Jr., Caldwell, J. P. & Vitt, L. J. (2008). Effective crypsis and its maintenance by immobility in Craugastor frogs. *Copeia*, 2008, 527–532.

Cooper, W. E., Jr., Wilson, D. S. & Smith, G. R. (2009). Sex, reproductive status, and cost of tail autotomy via decreased running speed. *Ethology*, **115**, 7–13.

Cooper, W. E., Jr., López, P., Martín, J. & Pérez-Mellado, V. (2012). Latency to flee from an immobile predator: Effects of risk and cost of immobility for the prey. *Behavioral Ecology*, **23**, 790–797.

Dukas, R. & Kamil, A. (2000). The cost of limited attention in blue jays. *Behavioral Ecology*, **11**, 502–506.

Dumont, F., Pasquaretta, C., Réale, D., Bogliani, G. & Von Hardenberg, A. (2012). Flight initiation distance and starting distance: Biological effect or mathematical artefact. *Ethology*, **118**, 1051–1062.

Holley, A. J. F. (1993). Do brown hares signal foxes? *Ethology*, **94**, 21–30.

Hugie, D. M. (2003). The waiting game: A "battle of waits" between predator and prey. *Behavioral Ecology*, **14**, 807–817.

Kramer, D. L. & Bonenfant, M. (1997). Direction of predator approach and the decision to flee to a refuge. *Animal Behaviour*, **54**, 289–295.

Lank, D. B. & Ydenberg, R. C. (2003). Death and danger at migratory stopovers: problems with "predation risk". *Journal of Avian Biology*, **34**, 225–228.

Lima, S. L. (1994). On the personal benefits of vigilance. *Animal Behaviour*, **48**, 734–736.

Lima, S. L. (1998). Stress and decision making under the risk of predation: recent developments from behavioral, reproductive, and ecological perspectives. *Advances in the Study of Behavior*, **27**, 215–290.

Lima, S. L. & Dill, L. M. (1990). Behavioral decisions made under the risk of predation: a review and prospectus. *Canadian Journal of Zoology*, **68**, 619–640.

Mangel, M. & Clark, C. W. (1993). *Dynamic Modeling in Behavioral Ecology*. Princeton, NJ: Princeton University Press.

Martín, J. & López, P. (1999). When to come out from a refuge: Risk-sensitive and state-dependent decisions in an alpine lizard. *Behavioral Ecology*, **10**, 487–492.

Martín, J., Luque-Larena, J. J. & López, P. (2009). When to run from an ambush predator: Balancing crypsis benefits with costs of fleeing in lizards. *Animal Behaviour*, **78**, 1011–1018.

Nur, N. & Hasson, O. (1984). Phenotypic plasticity and the handicap principle. *Journal of Theoretical Biology*, **110**, 275–297.

Polo, V., López, P. & Martín, J. (2005). Balancing the thermal costs and benefits of refuge use to cope with persistent attacks from predators: A model and an experiment with an alpine lizard. *Evolutionary Ecology Research*, **7**, 23–35.

Rhoades, E. & Blumstein, D. T. (2007). Predicted fitness consequences of threat-sensitive hiding behavior. *Behavioral Ecology*, **18**, 937–943.

Ruxton, G. D., Sherratt, T. N. & Speed, M. (2004). *Avoiding Attack: The Evolutionary Ecology of Crypsis, Warning Signals and Mimicry*. Oxford: Oxford University Press.

Stankowich, T. & Blumstein, D. T. (2005). Fear in animals: A meta-analysis and review of risk assessment. *Proceedings of the Royal Society of London, Series B, Biological Sciences*, **272**, 2627–2634.

Stankowich, T. & Coss, R. G. (2007). Effects of risk assessment, predator behavior, and habitat on escape behavior in Columbian black-tailed deer. *Behavioral Ecology*, **18**, 358–367.

Stephens, D. W. & Krebs, J. R. (1986). *Foraging Theory*. Princeton, New Jersey: Princeton University Press.

Stephens, D. W., Brown, J. S. & Ydenberg, R. C. (2007). *Foraging*. Chicago: University of Chicago Press.

Vega-Redondo, F. & Hasson, O.(1993). A game-theoretic model of predator–prey signaling. *Journal of Theoretical Biology*, **162**, 309–319.

Ydenberg, R. C. & Dill, L. M. (1986). The economics of fleeing from predators. *Advances in the Study of Behavior*, **16**, 229–249.

Zahavi, A. (1975). Mate selection: A selection for a handicap. *Journal of Theoretical Biology*, **53**, 205–214.

IIb Escape decisions prior to pursuit

3 Mammals

Theodore Stankowich and Eigil Reimers

> Still prettier were the little oribi. These are grass antelopes frequenting much the same places as the duiker and stein buck and not much larger. Where the grass was long they would lie close with neck flat along the ground and dart off when nearly stepped on with a pig like rush like that of a reedbuck or duiker in similar thick cover. But where the grass was short and especially where it was burned they did not trust to lying down and hiding on the contrary in such places they were conspicuous little creatures and trusted to their speed and alert vigilance for their safety. They run very fast with great bounds and when they stand usually at a hundred and fifty or two hundred yards they face the hunter the forward thrown ears being the most noticeable thing about them. We found that each oribi bagged cost us an unpleasantly large number of cartridges.
>
> Theodore Roosevelt (1910)

3.1 Introduction

Very early in the formal study of mammalogy, scientists began describing "flight distances" estimated in the field, mainly in response to human approachers. Most were observational estimations of the distance at which big game animals fled from hunters, but some provided nuanced descriptions. In the quotation above, Roosevelt (1910), knowingly or not, tells the reader that escape behavior in oribis (*Ourebia ourebi*) is contextual: when they are afforded concealing vegetation, oribi adopt a strategy of crypsis with very short flight distances, and when they are encountered in more exposed environments, they take flight at much greater distances. In one of the first "comparative" studies of flight behavior, Swiss ethologist Heini Hediger (1964) compiled a list of examples of flight distances of various mammals, birds, reptiles, fish, and invertebrates; most of these entries were one-off observational statements of flight initiation distance (FID) in each species, but others compared FID in different contexts. For example, Kearton (1929) reported that giraffe (*Giraffa camelopardalis*) flee at 150 yards (135 m) from a man on foot but at only 25 yards (23 m) from a motor-car; Darling (1937) observed that red deer (*Cervus elaphus*) fled at 50 to 100 yards (46 to 91 m) when being fed but at 600 yards (549 m) when irritable. These and other early reports (Hone 1934; McMillan 1954; Denniston 1956; Altmann 1958; Estes & Goddard 1967) were obviously less rigorous than the hypothesis-driven, structured studies of today that incorporate strict approach protocols and statistical analyses, but they set the foundation for using escape responses as a proxy for animal stress and fear.

Escaping From Predators: An Integrative View of Escape Decisions, ed. W. E. Cooper and D. T. Blumstein. Published by Cambridge University Press. © Cambridge University Press 2015.

Seminal work by Fritz Walther (1969) on the escape behavior of Thomson's Gazelle (*Eudorcas thomsonii*) examined escape variation in response to variation in many different factors, including predator species, human activity, temperature, time of day, number of predators, and predator speed. This significant increase in rigor spawned a variety of similar studies in other ungulate species (as well as birds) throughout the 1970s and 1980s (reviewed in Stankowich 2008). By the 1980s, the first formal theories of escape behavior began to develop (Ydenberg & Dill 1986). Studies of escape responses in animals have become more and more commonplace, and we know animals pay attention to a wide variety of factors when deciding when to flee (Stankowich & Blumstein 2005). Despite a wealth of studies of the flight responses of birds (Chapter 4) and reptiles (Chapter 5), studies of flight responses in mammals have been historically limited to ungulates, marsupials, and a few sciurid rodents. Given the exhaustive review of the factors influencing flight responses in ungulates by Stankowich (2008), this chapter will not seek to list every study of escape behavior in mammals, but instead will outline the more significant factors influencing escape responses in mammals, what we can learn from them, what has limited inquiry on this topic in mammals, a case study of reindeer and caribou (*Rangifer tarandus*), and what our future goals should be in the study of mammal escape responses.

3.2   Predators of mammals and options for escape

Perhaps more than for any other group of vertebrates, risk of predation for mammals is largely based on body size: the larger a prey animal is, the fewer potential predators it will have. But the relationship is not strictly directional. Larger mammal prey are often more desirable targets for larger predators because of the greater energetic reward and smaller mammal prey are often better able to employ crypsis to avoid detection or make use of refugia (e.g., burrows, trees). This often leaves mammals of intermediate size (500 g to 10 kg) at greater risk due to the energetic rewards they confer and more limited ability to avoid detection due to small size; these intermediate-sized mammals tend to have lower metabolic rates, limiting their ability to rely on rapid escape, and are more likely to have morphological antipredator defenses (e.g., spines, quills, body armor) (Lovegrove 2001).

The primary predators of mammals are other mammals, birds of prey, snakes, and sharks (in marine environments) and the vast majority of what we know about mammal escape behavior comes from studies of predation by mammalian carnivores and birds of prey. Given their varied modes of locomotion and lifestyles, mammals show tremendous variation in how they flee from predators (Caro 2005): rapid running, jumping, dropping from trees to the ground, fleeing into a burrow or other cover, climbing trees, moving into water, and even flying away. Predator behavior, however, generally varies in two ways: hunting mode and pursuit duration. Many mammalian predators (e.g., felids), owls, and dangerous snakes hunt by stealth and may only successfully capture a prey animal by approaching very closely without being detected (these predators generally cannot sustain prolonged chases); if prey detect these predators within that range where capture is possible, escape likely immediately follows detection. If the predator is detected at a great enough distance where escape is highly likely, they will often simply monitor and possibly alert/harass the predator until it gives up. When models of large stealthy felid predators were exposed to Columbian black-tailed deer (*Odocoileus hemionus columbianus*) from 15 to 50 m away, they never fled immediately, but instead stayed alert, snorted, foot-stamped, and alarm walked in order to deter further approach by the potential predator and advertise awareness to the predator (Stankowich & Coss 2007b; Stankowich 2010). Note that mountain lions (*Puma concolor*) typically need to approach to within 5 to 10 m undetected in order to have a chance to capture a deer (Smallwood 1993). In fact, deer were most alarmed when the model was concealed following exposure (Stankowich, pers. observation); similar observations of heightened alarm responses when visual range is limited have been made in reindeer (*Rangifer tarandus*) groups interacting with humans (Reimers, pers. observations), and white-tailed deer fleeing in forests vs. pastures (*O. virginianus*) (Lagory 1987). Coursing predators (e.g., canids) and many diurnal birds of prey, on the other hand, can sustain prolonged chases and will initiate attack from longer distances; therefore prey should flee from such predators at greater distances in order to maintain a spatial margin of safety (Cárdenas *et al.* 2005). Yellow-bellied marmots (*Marmota flaviventris*) were much more likely to flee from a gray wolf (*Canis lupus*) model than they were a mountain lion model, which elicited mostly high levels of vigilance (Blumstein *et al.* 2009).

Mammals show tremendous variation in their escape strategies, but we can generally group them into four main categories: (1) flee at long range soon after detection and recognition; (2) observe the predator, assess the risk it poses, and decide when to flee in a way that optimizes fitness; (3) rely on crypsis until the last possible moment and then flee if necessary; and (4) hold one's ground and employ defensive strategies or morphologies (e.g., armor, fighting, toxins). These strategies, however, can vary both intraspecifically and interspecifically. Similar to Roosevelt's oribi observations, spiny mice (*Acomys cahirinus*) show dichotomous escape initiation strategies: they either flee early at a long distance, or, if an individual is agile enough, remain frozen and potentially cryptic until the last minute, fleeing only when the predator is very close (Ilany & Eilam 2008).

Wild ungulates are most vulnerable during their first few months of life and may suffer substantial calf losses to predators. This selection pressure has led to two different strategies, hiding and following, for neonatal defense or predator avoidance (Lent 1974). Followers, species in which the neonates accompany the mother within minutes or hours after birth, usually have highly developed social systems and inhabit open terrain with a low vegetative profile. Hiders, species in which the young do not accompany the mother for the first weeks of life, remain in seclusion, minimize their activity, and rely on cryptic coloration and a lack of scent glands to avoid predation. They often live in habitats of dense, high vegetation and respond with alarm bradycardia (decrease in heart rate) upon detecting alarm stimuli, e.g., red deer (*Cervus elaphus*) (Espmark & Langvatn 1979, 1985) and white-tailed deer (*Odocoileus virginianus*) (Jacobsen 1979). Deer fawns remain cryptic, hiding in vegetation, and only flee when a predator approaches to within a few meters, and mothers with vulnerable fawns nearby may remain motionless in the face of an approaching predator in an attempt to remain undetected. Detailed accounts of mothers defending their young come from early ethological studies of large ungulates fending off would-be or attacking predators (Lent 1974): mule deer, *O. hemionus* (Hamlin & Schweitzer 1979); white-tailed deer (Smith 1987); elk, *Cervus canadensis*, and moose, *Alces alces* (Altmann 1963); and pronghorn *Antilocapra americana* (Marion & Sexton 1979). When confronted with coyotes (*Canis latrans*), white-tails tend to flee, whereas sympatric mule deer are more likely to bunch together with other individuals and attack the predator (Lingle 2001; Lingle & Wilson 2001). Female mule deer with calves will run to and defend fawns that are being attacked by coyotes, using their powerful forelegs to kick and often injure the attackers. Even species with powerfully effective defenses against predators sometimes just turn and run: striped skunks (*Mephitis mephitis*) ran from approaching predators in nearly 44% of interactions (Larivière & Messier 1996).

Flocking behavior is widespread among mammals, is most conspicuous among larger herbivores, and is primarily influenced by resource availability and distribution (Matthiopoulos 2003), parasites (biting flies, warble flies, and parasitoids; Mooring *et al.* 2004), and predator pressure (Hamilton 1971). Flight is generally the response when herds interact with predators or humans. Muskoxen (*Ovibos moschatus*) and African savanna elephants (*Loxodonta africana*) are exceptions insomuch as their fluid fission–fusion social group system provides a cooperative defense of calves against predators (Lent 1991; Reynolds 1993; Archie *et al.* 2006).

3.3   Scanning for predators, risk assessment, and flight initiation distance

Prior to encounters with predators, mammals periodically scan their surroundings for potential threats that might be looming. This vigilance may be shared by members of a group, which would likely be more proficient at scanning than a solitary animal that must divide its time between scanning and other activities (e.g., foraging). There is a large literature suggesting that the distance at which a predator begins its approach toward an animal (starting distance: SD) and the distance at which the prey shows overt alertness to that predator (alert distance: AD) are usually strongly correlated with FID (Blumstein 2003; Stankowich & Blumstein 2005; Stankowich & Coss 2006). Theory suggests that the farther away a predator begins its approach and the farther away an animal becomes alert, the longer the distance at which the prey will flee: an animal does better by fleeing earlier to avoid further opportunity costs of staying and maintaining a larger margin of safety (Blumstein 2010; Cooper & Blumstein 2014).

The relationships between SD, AD, and FID, however, are not necessarily linear. Blumstein (2003) found that the relationship between SD and FID was logarithmic in some birds and linear in others, and Blumstein and Daniel (2005) found a strong effect of SD on FID in a comparative analysis of macropodid marsupials. Stankowich and Coss (2006) proposed that the relationship between SD and FID might be logarithmic or even quadratic due to suboptimal scanning rates by prey. If a predator begins its approach from well outside the zone of awareness of a prey (the maximum range at which a prey animal can detect or cares to attend to a predator) the predator may be able to approach

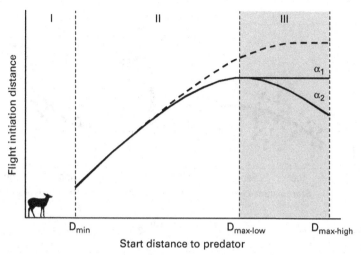

Figure 3.1 Predicted relationship between flight initiation distance (FID) and starting distance (SD), where D_{min} is the minimum distance at which prey might assess a predator before fleeing and D_{max} is the maximum distance at which prey can either detect predators or consider them threatening enough to attend to. To avoid opportunity costs, prey should flee at greater distance when they detect the predator at greater distances. When a predator starts from well outside the prey's zone of awareness (D_{min}–D_{max}), it might be able to approach more closely before detection due to suboptimal scanning (α_2). Some animals may also be more reactive than others and have a higher D_{max} (dashed curve). (Stankowich & Coss 2006)

closer to the prey before being detected (resulting in a lower FID) relative to an approach where the predator lingers at the edge of the zone of awareness prior to approach and may be detected earlier (Figure 3.1).

Due to suboptimal scanning (variation in α in Figure 3.1: prey cannot detect every predator that enters their zone of awareness the instant that the predator enters it), approaches with longer SD may have shorter FID than those with an SD at the limits of the zone of awareness. Finally, there is often tremendous individual variation in fearfulness or boldness within a population, with some more fearful animals likely having larger zones of awareness than others (Figure 3.1: dashed curve). Stankowich and Coss (2006) approached black-tailed deer from very long distances away, measuring SD, AD, and FID in order to test these hypotheses, and found that a quadratic model provided the best fit to the data (Figure 3.2a).

Animals that may have been more fearful of humans (those that were alert prior to approach) had greater FIDs, resulting in a logarithmic model providing the best fit and suggesting that they have a wider zone of awareness, as predicted. This suboptimal scanning hypothesis was further bolstered by the finding that the relationship between SD and AD was also non-linear, with the greatest SDs leading to somewhat shorter ADs than those trials where the approach began at the limits of the zone of awareness (Figure 3.2b). This suggests that the human was able to approach closer to the deer without being detected when he approached from greater distances. Finally, Stankowich

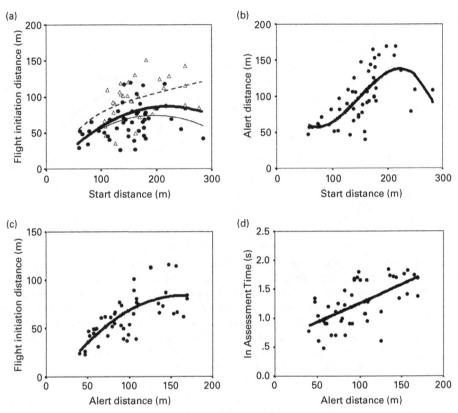

Figure 3.2   Scatterplots showing relationships between starting distance, alert distance, flight initiation distance, and assessment time of Columbian black-tailed deer in response to a human approacher. (a) Starting distance vs. flight initiation distance: black circles indicate deer that were not alert prior to approach (logarithmic model fit with thin black line), open triangles indicated deer that were alert prior to approach (logistic model fit with dashed line), thick black line indicates overall quadratic model fit (compare to Figure 3.1). (b) Alert distance vs. starting distance; thick curve is a cubic model fit suggesting that deer became alert later when approaches started from outside the zone of awareness. (c) Alert distance vs. flight initiation distance; thick curve is a logarithmic model showing that flight initiation distance increases with alert distance but levels off at D_{max}. (d) Alert distance vs. assessment time; deer that became alert earlier assessed the approacher for longer periods (there was no correlation between assessment time and flight initiation distance. (Stankowich & Coss 2006)

and Coss (2006) found a logarithmic relationship between AD and FID (Figure 3.2c): when deer became alert at very great distances, they typically did not flee immediately, instead waiting until the approacher came within 60 to 100 m before taking flight. This finding strengthens the argument that prey assess the threat posed by an approaching predator prior to flight in order to avoid potentially unnecessary and costly bouts of flight; when prey become alert at greater distances they have the luxury of assessing the threat for longer periods of time compared to when detection occurs at a very short distance (Figure 3.2d). Further analyses revealed effects of this pre-flight risk assessment on subsequent escape behavior (e.g., distance fled (DF), escape angle, running style) (Stankowich & Coss 2007a).

3.4   Factors influencing escape decisions in mammals

A huge number of biotic and abiotic factors are known to influence escape decisions in animals (Stankowich & Blumstein 2005) and most of these have been shown in some form in mammals. Stankowich (2008) provided a comprehensive review of escape behavior in ungulates and how it relates to conservation and management; therefore we will not perform a similar review here. Instead we will focus on some of the more important factors for mammals and then examine a case study of escape behavior in reindeer and caribou (*Rangifer* spp.) because a significant amount of research has been conducted in this system on flight decisions.

3.4.1   Effects of the environment and distance to refuge

Several non-predatory factors in the environment can affect escape decisions in mammals. Mammals appear to be very sensitive to small spatial variation in risk of capture in different environments. Stankowich (2008) found greater escape responses in ungulates in open environments compared to more densely vegetated areas; although some studies didn't find such an effect. Habitat cover also shortens FID in red kangaroos (*Macropus rufus*) and euros (*M. robustus erubescens*) (Wolf & Croft 2010) and brown bears (*Ursus arctos*) (Moen *et al.* 2012). In barren habitats one would expect that mammals that are unable to escape underground would seek higher country to improve visual control. Running upslope was the most common response in reindeer when disturbed (Baskin & Skogland 1997; Colman *et al.* 2001). For example, Reimers found that reindeer groups more often fled uphill (59%) compared to flat (20%) and downhill (21%) flight paths. (E. Reimers, unpublished data). The same data set shows that smell is an important sense for environmental control: the reindeer groups fled into headwind more often (51%) than crosswind (26%) or tailwind (23%). Wolves (*Canis lupus*) fled at shorter distances in stronger winds (Karlsson *et al.* 2007). Similar to other taxa (Stankowich & Blumstein 2005), many mammal species have been found to flee at greater distance when they are farther from refuge compared to when there is refuge nearby: woodchucks (*Marmota monax*; Bonenfant & Kramer 1996; Kramer & Bonenfant 1997), Eastern gray squirrels (*Sciurus carolinensis*; Dill & Houtman 1989), and degus (*Octodon degus*; Lagos *et al.* 2009); Stafl (2013) found no such effect in the American pika (*Ochotona princeps*).

Insect harassment has been shown to have profound effects on mammal behavior and morphology. For example recent evidence suggests that zebra stripes were favored by natural selection in environments with oppressive activity of biting flies for much of the year (Caro *et al.* 2014). Insect harassment may have even a greater effect on escape behavior in large mammals than both human infrastructure and predators. During the brief growing season in Arctic and high-mountain ecosystems, undisturbed grazing is crucial in order for reindeer to maximize growth and fattening. In particular warble flies

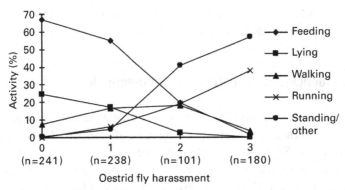

Figure 3.3   Activity budgets (means) of reindeer from scan sampling in relation to oestrid fly harassment
in Norefjell and Rondane wild reindeer areas inNorway in 1997. (0 = none, 1 = light,
2 = moderate, 3 = severe.) (Hagemoen & Reimers 2002)

(*Hypoderma tarandi*) and nose bot flies (*Cephenemyia trompe*; hereafter referred to as
oestrid flies) influence *Rangifer* behavior (Mörschel & Klein 1997; Anderson *et al.*
2001; Hagemoen & Reimers 2002) and may amplify or decrease response thresholds in
relation to human and predator activities. Throughout warm summers, reindeer are
exposed to vigorous oestrid fly harassment, which causes dramatic decreases in feeding
and lying, and increase in walking, running, and standing (Figure 3.3). Snow patches,
marshes, and windy mountain tops were used primarily to avoid oestrid fly harassment
and animals may flee long distances to avoid the insects. Even though *Rangifer* are
disturbed by human activities, they can increase their tolerance toward humans if insect
harassment is severe, as shown for domesticated reindeer (Skarin *et al.* 2004) and
caribou observed within the Prudhoe Bay oil field (Pollard *et al.* 1996). Oil-field gravel
pads and roads were used as insect relief habitats (Murphy & Curatolo 1987; Pollard
et al. 1996), as animals frequently occupy and take advantage of the shade of buildings
and pipelines.

3.4.2   Habituation to human disturbances and hunting

The vast majority of studies of the effects of human density and traffic on mammal
escape behavior have shown that mammals are able to habituate to humans in their
environment. Populations in areas with less exposure to humans (smaller populations,
less vehicle traffic) have greater FIDs than populations with more exposure to humans,
and this finding is robust across different mammalian taxa: ungulates (McMillan 1954;
Denniston 1956; Walther 1969; Rowe-Rowe 1974; Tyler 1991; Cassirer *et al.* 1992;
Recarte *et al.* 1998; Colman *et al.* 2001; Bekoff & Gese 2003), marmots (Louis & Le
Beere 2000; Griffin *et al.* 2007; Li *et al.* 2011), and squirrels (McCleery 2009; Chapman
et al. 2012). There may be, however, a sampling bias such that investigators have
preferentially focused their research on species that habituate easily to humans due to
ease of access. In fact, some studies have found no habituation effect (Alados & Escos

1988; Lehrer *et al.* 2011), and some mammals (especially predatory species) are known to not habituate well to humans. However, Wam *et al.* (2014) recorded a high level of individual plasticity in behavioral responses by protected, re-introduced wolves in Norway toward humans, suggesting that habituation to humans may occur over a longer period of time.

In a meta-analysis of ten studies, Stankowich (2008) found that populations of ungulates under hunting pressure had significantly greater flight responses than non-hunted populations, and more evidence from giraffes (Marealle *et al.* 2010) and reindeer (Baskin & Hjalten 2001) has supported this finding. The tendency to habituate in ungulates is so strong that the dis-habituating effects of seasonal hunting may not be strong enough to overcome the habituating effects of non-consumptive human exposure (e.g., recreationists) during the rest of the year (Reimers *et al.* 2009), and the interests of both hunters and wildlife watchers may be satisfied if a balance is struck between these practices.

3.4.3   Type of disturbance

The type of disturbance, be it anthropogenic or a non-human predator, has a significant impact on flight decisions in mammals. Stankowich (2008) found humans on foot to elicit stronger reactions from ungulates (meta-analysis of 11 studies) compared to other types of anthropogenic disturbance (e.g., automobiles, military noise, bicycles, snow-mobiles), but sometimes very large machines can be more evocative than pedestrians. Gray (1973) observed muskoxen to respond more strongly to aircraft than to humans, and harbor seals (*Phoca vitulina*) showed greater AD and FID to boats compared to pedestrians (Andersen *et al.* 2012). Past experience with such vehicles as a result of being chased by snow machines, helicopters, or fixed wing aircrafts (accidentally or for tagging or other purposes) can rapidly increase alertness and escape behavior. When humans have been a historical source of predation or disturbance, mammals clearly treat them as more dangerous than less threatening human transports (e.g., automobiles, bicycles), but the much greater size of some transports might override this effect and may engender greater fear than single humans on foot, similar to studies from other taxa indicating greater flight responses to larger rather than smaller predators (Stankowich & Blumstein 2005).

Different types of animal predators may also engender greater responses than others according to the relative predation risk they pose. Humans typically evoke a response greater than or equal to the response to domestic dogs (Hone 1934; Hamr 1988; Kloppers *et al.* 2005) and wolves (Bergerud 1974), but free-ranging dogs remain a significant source of disturbance and stress for wild mammals (Weston & Stankowich 2014). Reindeer had greater AD, FID, and DF in response to a human disguised as a polar bear (*Ursus maritimus*) than to a human in dark hiking gear (see case study). Finally, Thomson's gazelles (*Eudorcas thomsonii*) varied their FID dynamically in response to different species of mammalian predator. Wild dogs (*Lycaon pictus*) evoked the greatest FIDs, followed by cheetahs (*Acinonyx jubatus*), lions (*Panthera leo*), hyenas (*Crocuta crocuta*), and finally jackals (*Canis mesomelas*); this order closely agrees with the

Table 3.1 Flight initiation distances from different mammalian predators by Thomson's gazelles (expressed as percentage of cases).

Predator	5–50 m	51–100 m	101–300 m	301–500 m	501–1000 m	>1000 m	N
Jackal	85	15	–	–	–	–	66
Hyena	29	50	10	4	6	1	155
Lion	3	28	62	5	2	–	71
Cheetah	1	3	57	22	15	2	88
Wild dog	–	4	13	20	48	15	44

relative risk posed by each species to the gazelles (Table 3.1; Walther 1969). Jackals rarely ever attack adults and really are only dangerous to fawns. Hyenas kill more fawns than adults but packs of hyenas are far more dangerous to adults than solitary hyenas, resulting in significantly greater FIDs in response to hyena packs relative to solitary individuals. Gazelles flee from lions between 50 and 300 m, a comfortable distance given that lions will kill adults but prefer larger ungulates if they are available. Gazelles show mortal fear of wild dogs and cheetahs, which prefer to hunt gazelles, and to which they responded at the greatest distances (Walther 1969). Mammals clearly assess risk dynamically in response to the threat posed by different types of disturbances and predators, and the types of experiences individuals have with those predators also greatly influences flight decisions (Stankowich & Blumstein 2005; Stankowich 2008).

3.4.4   Effects of group size

Temporary or permanent aggregations commonly formed by mammals have a variety of potential benefits (enhanced vigilance, greater ability to find food or mates, group defense, etc.) and potential costs (easier to locate by predators, potential for disease transmission, interference effects during foraging, social agonism). Declining individual vigilance efforts with increasing group size has been widely reported for both mammals and birds (Elgar 1989; Lima 1995). Wild reindeer in Norway and also on Svalbard adhere to this effect (Reimers et al. 2011, .2012). The effects of group size on escape decisions in mammals, however, have been far less predictable. Stankowich and Blumstein (2005) found a positive effect of group size on FID in terrestrial organisms, but Stankowich (2008) found only a weak, non-robust positive effect ($r = 0.13$; $k = 21$ studies) in a meta-analysis on ungulates where heterogeneity among studies was enormous ($I^2 = 96\%$). Some studies showed large positive effects (Stankowich & Coss 2007a), while others showed strong negative effects (Matson et al. 2005). Wild reindeer in Norway conform to the latter strategy, FID and DF decreased with increasing group size (Reimers et al. 2012), but the insular wild reindeer of Svalbard have lost their group size effect (Colman et al. 2001; Reimers et al. 2011). Costly antipredator behavior such as these group size effects should not persist on islands once there is no net benefit (Blumstein & Daniel 2005). And indeed, the traditional grouping behavior that characterizes *Rangifer* elsewhere is absent in Svalbard, where animals live individually or in small groups. High vigilance rates will in most cases compromise feeding time, as suggested by (Laundre *et al.* 2001). The low scan frequency and total scan duration found in reindeer should not compromise feeding efficiency in any of the study herds. This intraspecific variation in the direction and effect size of group size on escape decisions suggests that group size effects likely interact with the history of the population, reproductive state of the group members, lethality and intensity of human exposure, or openness of the landscape to permit the benefits of collective vigilance (Stankowich 2008).

3.4.5   Effects of insularity and loss of predators

Many studies have shown that local extinction of predators for prolonged periods relaxes natural selection on predator recognition. Over hundreds or thousands of years, prey may lose the ability to recognize locally extinct predators as dangerous (Coss 1999; Berger *et al.* 2001; Blumstein & Daniel 2005; Blumstein 2006; Stankowich & Coss 2007b; Lahti *et al.* 2009). Tests of the effects of relaxed selection on escape behavior in mammals are more limited. For instance, Blumstein found that tammar wallabies (*Macropus eugenii*) living on predator-free islands allowed humans to approach much nearer than tammars living on mainland Australia (Blumstein 2002). In a broader comparative analysis of FIDs in macropodid marsupials, while insularity influenced foraging and vigilance behaviors, living on islands and loss of predators did not have significant effects on escape decisions (see group size discussion above; Blumstein & Daniel 2005), suggesting that effects of relaxed selection may vary between species or be more specifically correlated with time elapsed since isolation. Insular Svalbard reindeer and Greenland caribou show similar effects on foraging and escape decisions (see group size effects above and case study below). Generally, FID may be highly dependent on the individual experiences with predators and humans (Blumstein & Daniel 2005), and one significant traumatic event may be enough to restore recognition of, and responsiveness to, a previously absent predator (Berger *et al.* 2001).

3.4.6   Social and reproductive effects

Reproductive status influences the escape decisions of both sexes, but a paucity of studies limits our ability to make strong inferences. During times of peak mating (e.g., the rut in ungulates), males typically experience increased costs of fleeing (Ydenberg & Dill 1986) as it may mean abandoning an attractive high-quality territory or even a group of defendable females. This effect has been shown most convincingly in fish and lizards (Shallenberger 1970; Cooper 1997, 1999; Martín & López 1999), but less evidence exists for mammals. Moose and reindeer in rut are much more tolerant of an approaching human than they are just before the rut or when in velvet (Altmann 1958; Reimers *et al.* 2012), and territorial gazelles flee at shorter distances than solitary bachelors (Walther 1969). Rowe-Rowe (1974), however, found no effect of the rut on flight decisions in blesbok (*Damaliscus dorcas*). Similar effects of the costs of fleeing occur when individuals are forced to leave a profitable food patch: socially forging degus (*Octodon degus*) fled at shorter distances in food-rich patches, compared to patches with less food.

Female mammals tend to be warier than males (Stankowich 2008), suggesting that the costs of fleeing are greater for males and/or the benefits of fleeing in the form of protection of nearby offspring and future reproductive potential are greater for females. In fact, many ungulate studies have shown that females with calves flee at much greater distances and flee longer distances than those without calves (Stankowich 2008; Reimers *et al.* 2011). The presence of pups outside the burrow led to increased AD and FID in Alpine marmots (*Marmota marmota*) (Louis & Le Beere 2000). Females of some species may even dynamically assess the escape abilities of their young when deciding when to flee from predators: female red kangaroos (*Macropus rufus*) and female euros (*M. robustus*) fled at greater distances when they had young at foot compared to those carrying young in their pouch (Wolf & Croft 2010). In sum, both sexes have reproductive considerations during risk assessment, but the different roles that each sex plays in mating and parental investment influences their costs and benefits of fleeing in different ways.

3.4.7   Domestication effects

Price and King (1968) proposed that "domestication is an evolutionary process involving the genotypic adaptation of animals to the captive environment." There is limited experimental research on the evolution of different traits, including behavior, during domestication. However, there is sufficient evidence based on comparative studies of domestic stocks and their wild ancestors, to identify a number of typical domestication changes, including the following aspects (Jensen 2006): external and internal morphology, physiology, body development, and behavior, which in this context includes reduced fear, increased sociability, and reduced antipredator responses (Price 1997). Interestingly, this complex of changes may develop rapidly, in only a few generations, and in concert, even though only one of the traits is selected for. Belyaev *et al.* (1985) selected farm foxes only for reduced fearfulness toward humans, and found that the frequency of animals showing this complex of adaptations, including morphological and physiological changes, increased dramatically within 10 to 20 generations. Eurasian reindeer, which are the origin of caribou, may exemplify such complex and rapid adaptations (Reimers *et al.* 2012, 2014; Nieminen 2013). This subspecies was only recently domesticated by humans, with extensive control of specific herds first evolving during the sixteenth and seventeenth centuries (Mirov 1945). As is demonstrated in the case study, domestication of wild mammals can have significant effects on their escape behavior.

3.5   Case study: reindeer and caribou

3.5.1   Introduction

Reindeer and caribou belong to the same species (*Rangifer tarandus*), but different subspecies (Banfield 1961). Although the basic behavioral repertoire in the various subspecies appears fundamentally uniform (Thomson 1980), many differences in recorded behavior relate to degree of domestication and to variable factors in the physical and biological environment, herd size and structure, and past experience. While the caribou subspecies are wild, the Fennoscandian tundra reindeer include herds with both wild and domestic origin that vary in number and ecology. The relationship between life history strategies, behavior, and genetics in herds of reindeer that comprise contemporary wild and domestic stocks remains a focal research field. Hunting is the only important wild reindeer mortality factor, because traditional predators, although permanently present or present as stragglers, exert only minor predatory influence. All study herds in Norway are extensively hunted, but molecular genetic analyses (Røed *et al.* 2008, 2011) shows a clear genetic structure among the study herds that reflect varying degrees of domestic or wild ancestry. The insular Svalbard reindeer is the northernmost population of *Rangifer* inhabiting an environment without parasitizing insects and, except for a few observations of polar bear (*Ursus maritimus*) predation (Derocher *et al.* 2000), no predators (other than man). This situation has prevailed for at least 4000 years (Van der Knaap 1986; Tyler & Øritsland 1989). Unlike *Rangifer* subspecies elsewhere, Svalbard reindeer live individually or in small groups (Alendal & Byrkjedal 1976), are seasonally sedentary (Tyler & Øritsland 1989), and do not have the nomadic behavior known from other subspecies of *Rangifer*.

In the absence of four-legged predators, this case study deals with observations of *Rangifer* behavioral responses primarily to human disturbances in terms of direct provocations by individuals on foot, on ski, or on snowmobile. As a result of extensive field testing in a variety of populations with different degrees of genetic separation from wild reindeer and experiencing different levels of hunting and human recreation exposure, we begin to see how domestication, hunting, and habituation interact to influence escape decisions.

3.5.2   Habituation in relation to genetics, hunting and tourist activities

Assuming domestication selects for and supports tameness, researchers have investigated whether wild reindeer with some domestic ancestry and exposed to hunting remain tame or adopt wild behavior. In the past, restocking of previously wild reindeer habitats has occurred through release of reindeer from domestic herds under the assumption that "a reindeer is a reindeer" and that the introduced animals would eventually adopt behavior similar to wild animals (i.e., redevelop increased vigilance and fear responses). Contrary to expectations, extensive hunting (annual harvest around 30% of the winter herds) since 1956 in Forollhogna, 1967 in Ottadalen, and 1992 in Norefjell has only slightly altered the hard-wired behavioral traits indicative of their history of domestication (Figure 3.4a,b). The frequency of watching the person before flight (Figure 3.5) was 30 to 50% among the wild reindeer herds compared to 80 to 90% among the domestic herds (Reimers *et al.* 2012). Wild populations on Svalbard show equally weak escape responses, suggesting that factors other than domestication play a larger role in escape responses of *Rangifer*.

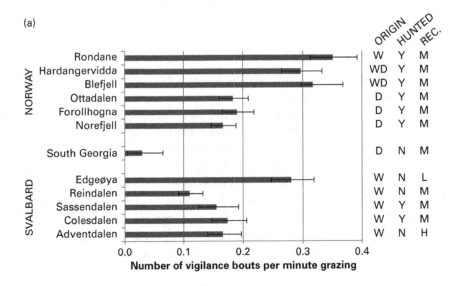

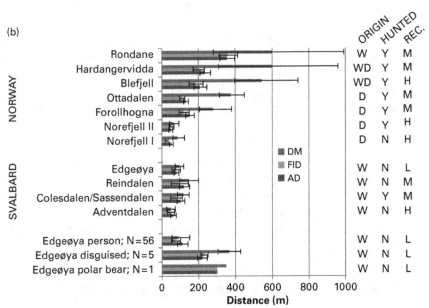

Figure 3.4 (a) Vigilance and (b) escape distances among wild reindeer herds in Norway and in South Georgia and Svalbard. Reindeer of mainly wild origin is denoted W, reindeer with mixed origin WD, and reindeer with domestic origin D. All herds in Norway are hunted on a sustainable basis (attempted kept at a carrying capacity level) while the two hunted herds in Svalbard (Colesdalen and Sassendalen) are subject to light hunting pressure. Hunting was initiated in 1992 in Norefjell and escape data were recorded the summer before hunt (Norefjell I) and again in 2002 to 2006 (Norefjell II). Recreational activities (REC.) are high (H) in Norefjell and Blefjell in Norway and Adventdalen in Svalbard, but moderate (M) in the other areas except in the remote Edgeøya (L) where reindeer rarely are exposed to humans. (X-axis in (b) is broken at 600 m for Rondane and Hardangervidda to allow for a closer inspection of the shorter distances in the other areas. Distance fled is 1722 m in Rondane and 1535 m in Hardangervidda; the SE are maintained in the figure). Recordings of vigilance in South Georgia were made before the eradication of the herd. In a few cases we were able to measure AD but not FID, and FID and not AD. The discrepancies are caused by these unbalanced samples. (Data from Reimers *et al.* 2009, 2010, 2011, 2012; Reimers & Eftestøl 2012, and unpublished.)

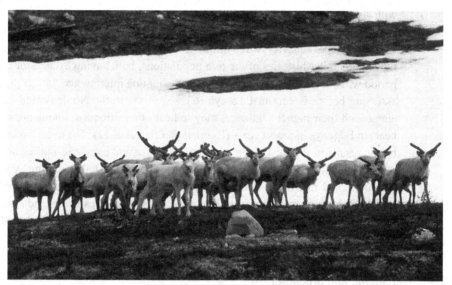

Figure 3.5   Alerted reindeer males in Ottadalen in May. Antlers in growth and in velvet.

As for the effects of extensive hunting, great differences in vigilance and escape responses persist between the populations despite similar levels of hunting (Figure 3.4). Rondane and Ottadalen are both hunted and experience moderate levels of human exposure, yet reindeer in Rondane show much greater escape responses than those in Ottadalen. Moreover, escape behavior in Norefjell did not change from before hunting was initiated (Norefjell I) after more than ten years of extensive hunting (Norefjell II). Finally, wild reindeer from Svalbard that are subject to light hunting or no hunting show similar vigilance and escape responses to many of the hunted populations of domestic origin in Norway.

As previously discussed, the frequency of encounters with humans may affect ungulate antipredator behavior (see reviews by Stankowich 2008; Tarlow & Blumstein 2007). Although disputed (e.g., Reimers & Colman 2006; Reimers *et al.* 2007), displacement is the effect most often predicted when recreational activities in wild reindeer are discussed (e.g., Vistnes & Nellemann 2008). While predator pressure is low for all herds, recreational activity has potentially influenced escape responses (Figure 3.4b): recreation and tourism are extensive in Norefjell but moderate in the other areas, and the lower vigilance rate and flight response distances in Norefjell compared to Ottadalen, in spite of comparable domestic origin and extensive hunting, may reflect habituation to the high level of recreational activities in the former. Wild reindeer in Blefjell are exposed to humans more frequently than in Hardangervidda, from which the Blefjell herd originates. The escape response distances (AD, FID, and DF) were shorter in Blefjell than in Hardangervidda, while the probability of assessing the observer before fleeing tended to be greater in Blefjell (Reimers *et al.* 2010). In Svalbard, Reimers and colleagues (2011) found that vigilance was higher in reindeer in Edgeøya than in the four Spitzbergen areas. Escape responses (AD, FID, and DF) were all shorter in Adventdalen, with its considerably higher amounts of human activities and infrastructure than the other study areas, a finding consistent with habituation toward humans. Greenland caribou escape behavior was similar to that of Svalbard reindeer (Aastrup 2000), reflecting similar histories of the two populations, both having existed for an extended period without large predators and with little hunting interference. Lower probability of assessing before fleeing in Edgeøya (63% vs. 94% in the Nordenskiöld Land areas), along with their higher vigilance, may indicate more frequent interactions with polar bears in Edgeøya in recent years (Reimers & Eftestøl 2012). The overall picture painted by the results in Figure 3.4 suggests that vigilance and escape responses are likely the result of an interaction between genetic origin, exposure to lethal hunting by humans and predators, and non-lethal human recreational activities. Areas lacking predation and having high exposure to humans show very weak escape responses and human recreation has been shown to cause moderate increases in escape responses due to short bursts of seasonal hunting (Stankowich 2008).

3.5.3   *Rangifer* and predators

Although the literature on *Rangifer* and their key predators is comprehensive, only two papers (Bøving & Post 1997; Aastrup 2000) address escape behavior and vigilance in caribou to predators. A short publication (Reimers & Eftestøl 2012) includes escape metrics. Female caribou in Alaska foraged in larger groups, displayed a higher rate of vigilance during feeding, and spent less time feeding than did female caribou in West Greenland without predators (Bøving & Post 1997). The results indicate that caribou, like several other species of ungulates, show behavioral adaptations to the risk of predation that are relaxed when this risk is reduced. Svalbard reindeer interact commonly with polar bears. Field work on Edgeøya, Svalbard, measured reindeer response distances from a stalking polar bear, approaches from a person disguised as a polar bear, and "normal" human encounters (Figure 3.4b). Alert and flight initiation distances and distance fled were 1.6, 2.5, and 2.3 times longer, respectively, when Svalbard reindeer were encountered by a person disguised as a polar bear compared to a person in dark hiking gear. Population increase of polar bears on Svalbard and decrease in sea-ice cover in the Arctic region during summer probably results in more frequent interactions with reindeer on the archipelago, indicating a predator–prey relationship between the two species on Edgeøya.

A key prediction of the multipredator hypothesis (Blumstein 2006) is that isolation from all predators may lead to a rapid loss of antipredator behavior, including loss of the group size effect and breakdown of predator recognition abilities. For example, both reindeer and caribou from predator-free regions (Svalbard and West Greenland) were about 3.5 times less vigilant to playback of wolf howling at control sites (Denali National Park and Tetlin Wildlife Refuge) (Berger 2007). Experience-dependent behavior may be lost after the first generation in the absence of predators, while more "hardwired" antipredator behavior may persist for thousands of years following isolation from predators (Byers 1997; Coss 1999). Domestic reindeer from Norway were introduced to South Georgia in 1911–12 and in 1925 (Leader Williams 1988). After 100 years in absence of predators, vigilance is strongly relaxed (Figure 3.4). On the other hand, experience-dependent behavior may be quickly restored the first time individuals encounter predators (Brown *et al.* 1997; Aastrup 2000; Berger *et al.* 2001). In accordance with this, vigilance rates displayed by Svalbard reindeer in Edgeøya, a location with a dense polar bear population, were 2.2 times higher than those of reindeer in Nordenskiöld Land that had fewer polar bears.

3.6   Conservation and management implications

Results from escape behavior studies have strong implications for conservation and management measures in land use planning. Stankowich (2008) makes several suggestions: (1) a broad understanding of how reproductive state and individual biology affects escape decisions is critical for predicting temporal variation in behavior; (2) the interaction between hunting and non-lethal recreation effects may allow consumptive management of populations and still permit convenient wildlife viewing opportunities for ecotourists; (3) knowledge of the extent to which other predators maintain antipredator responses may help predict how wild mammals will respond to human approach; (4) nearby alternative sites may allow wildlife to avoid high levels of human disturbance; and (5) wildlife may respond differently to humans depending on the openness of the environment and distance to potential refugia. Beyond these points, response distances may aid in establishment of buffer zones needed to maintain functional habitats for individual herds (Blumstein & Fernández-Juricic 2010).

3.7   Foci for the future study of mammal escape behavior

The theory and empirical study of escape behavior and risk assessment has been primarily driven by research on birds and reptiles, and, although there is an extensive literature on habituation to human disturbances in large mammals, we know comparatively little about the nuances of mammalian risk assessment. Given the depth of the current literature and the logistical difficulties of working on mammals, we suggest several areas of focus for future work on mammalian escape behavior.

Most studies of escape behavior in mammals examine a single factor or simply test for main effects of several factors. When animals pay attention to multiple factors simultaneously, different factors may interact to create non-additive effects on risk assessment and flight decisions. Some factors may only be important in certain contexts. The effect of distance to the burrow and food abundance only had significant effects on escape responses of degus when they were in social foraging groups, and not when solitary (Vásquez *et al.* 2002). Interaction effects may be exceedingly important to creating a deeper understanding of the risk assessment process – not just in mammals but in all animals. Potentially interesting interactions for investigation include sex × season, group size × season, and group size × habitat type or distance to refuge.

As previously mentioned, most studies of escape behavior in mammals have focused on ungulates, which tend to be easy to detect from long distance, habituate well to humans (and are thus easy to find), and are often targets of human hunting (making humans more relevant as potential predators). Ungulates are also frequently the focus of key conservation issues in land use conflicts. Broader taxonomic representation is needed, however, to test the same hypotheses regarding the factors influencing risk assessment. Medium-sized to large rodents, marsupials, armadillos, and rabbits could all prove to be tractable research subjects for studies of escape behavior given their visibility and lifestyle.

Similar to Møller's comparative studies of escape behavior in European and Asian birds (Chapter 4), evolutionary and comparative studies of risk assessment in mammals should be undertaken to understand which factors are most important across taxa and which are more important to individual species with unique ecologies. The taxa mentioned above would be excellent candidates for broad, potentially collaborative, taxon-wide studies of escape behavior using standardized approaches (Chapter 16). These data could also be compared to those from birds and reptiles and other taxa to understand how mammalian ecology influences the factors affecting risk assessment.

3.8   Conclusions

There is a rich history of studying escape behavior in wild mammals. Most of the original observations of flight initiation distance by Hediger (1964) and later workers were made on large, charismatic mammals, primarily to settle conservation conflicts. Nevertheless, while empirical work on flight decisions of birds and reptiles has flourished, similar studies in mammals have been limited primarily to ungulates (Reimers & Colman 2006; Stankowich 2008), for which humans are often a realized predator, and not just hypothetical proxy for a predator. Recent literature on escape behavior of mammals is slowly becoming more taxonomically diverse: brown bears (Moen *et al.* 2012) and squirrels and marmots (Griffin *et al.* 2007; McCleery 2009; Lehrer *et al.* 2011; Li *et al.* 2011; Chapman *et al.* 2012). Experience with predators, reproductive effects, and predator hunting behaviors have strong effects on mammalian escape responses. Future efforts should strive to test targeted interactions between factors to understand how species weigh the importance of each factor in different situations. Conducting comparative studies using standard approaches on a wide range of species will also promote an understanding of how morphological traits and ecological variables influence risk assessment.

References

Aastrup, P. (2000). Responses of West Greenland caribou to the approach of humans on foot. *Polar Research*, **19**, 83–90.

Alados, C. L. & Escos, J.(1988). Alarm calls and flight behaviour in Spanish ibex (*Capra pyrenaica*). *Biology of Behaviour*, **13**, 11–21.

Alendal, E. & Byrkjedal, I. (1976). Population size and reproduction of the reindeer (Rangifer tarandus platyrhynchus) on Nordenskiöld Land, Svalbard. *Norsk Polarinstitutt Årbok*, 1974, 139–152.

Altmann, M. (1958). The flight distance in free-ranging big game. *Journal of Wildlife Management*, **22**, 207–209.

Altmann, M. (1963). Naturalistic studies of maternal care in moose and elk. In Rheingold, H. L. (ed.) *Maternal Behavior in Mammals*. New York, NY: John Wiley & Sons, Inc.

Andersen, S. M., Teilmann, J., Dietz, R., Schmidt, N. M. & Miller, L. A. (2012). Behavioural responses of harbour seals to human-induced disturbances. *Aquatic Conservation: Marine and Freshwater Ecosystems*, **22**, 113–121.

Anderson, J. R., Nilssen, A. C. & Hemmingsen, W. (2001). Use of host-mimicking trap catches to determine which parasitic flies attack reindeer, *Rangifer tarandus*, under different climatic conditions. *Canadian Field-Naturalist*, **115**, 274–286.

Archie, E. A., Moss, C. J. & Alberts, S. C. (2006). The ties that bind: genetic relatedness predicts the fission and fusion of social groups in wild African elephants. *Proceedings of the Royal Society Biological Sciences Series B*, **273**, 513–522.

Banfield, A. W. F. (1961). A revision of the reindeer and caribou, genus *Rangifer*. *Bulletin of the National Museum of Canada, Biological Series*, **66**, 1–137.

Baskin, L. M. & Hjalten, J. (2001). Fright and flight behavior of reindeer. *Alces*, **37**, 435–445.

Baskin, L. M. & Skogland, T. (1997). Direction of escape in reindeer. *Rangifer*, **17**, 37–40.

Bekoff, M. & Gese, E. M. (2003). Coyote (*Canis latrans*). In Feldhammer, G. A., Thompson, B. C. & Chapman, J. A. (eds.) *Wild Mammals of North America: Biology, Management, and Conservation*. Baltimore: Johns Hopkins University Press.

Belyaev, D. K., Plyusnina, I. Z. & Trut, L. N. (1985). Domestication in the silver fox (*Vulpes fulvus* Desm): Changes in physiological boundaries of the sensitive period of primary socialization. *Applied Animal Behaviour Science*, **13**, 359–370.

Berger, J. (2007). Carnivore repatriation and holarctic prey: Narrowing the deficit in ecological effectiveness. *Conservation Biology*, **21**, 1105–1116.

Berger, J., Swenson, J. E. & Persson, I. L. (2001). Recolonizing carnivores and naive prey: conservation lessons from Pleistocene extinctions. *Science*, **291**, 1036–1039.

Bergerud, A. T. (1974). The role of the environment in the aggregation, movement and disturbance behaviour of caribou. In Geist, V. & Walther, F. (eds.) *The Behavior of Ungulates and its Relation to Management*. Morges, Switzerland: International Union for Conservation of Nature and Natural Resources (IUCN).

Blumstein, D. T. (2002). Moving to suburbia: ontogenetic and evolutionary consequences of life on predator-free islands. *Journal of Biogeography*, **29**, 685–692.

Blumstein, D. T. (2003). Flight-initiation distance in birds is dependent on intruder starting distance. *Journal of Wildlife Management*, **67**, 852–857.

Blumstein, D. T. (2006). The multipredator hypothesis and the evolutionary persistence of antipredator behavior. *Ethology*, **112**, 209–217.

Blumstein, D. T. (2010). Flush early and avoid the rush: a general rule of antipredator behavior? *Behavioral Ecology*, **21**, 440–442.

Blumstein, D. T. & Daniel, J. C. (2005). The loss of anti-predator behaviour following isolation on islands. *Proceedings of the Royal Society B*, **272**, 1663–1668.

Blumstein, D. T. & Fernández-Juricic, E. (2010). *A Primer on Conservation Behavior*, Sunderland, MA: Sinauer Associates, Inc.

Blumstein, D. T., Ferando, E. & Stankowich, T. (2009). A test of the multipredator hypothesis: yellow-bellied marmots respond fearfully to the sight of novel and extinct predators. *Animal Behaviour*, **78**, 873–878.

Bonenfant, M. & Kramer, D. L. (1996). The influence of distance to burrow on flight initiation distance in the woodchuck, *Marmota monax*. *Behavioral Ecology*, **7**, 299–303.

Bøving, P. S. & Post, E. (1997). Vigilance and foraging behaviour of female caribou in relation to predation risk. *Rangifer*, **17**, 55–63.

Brown, G. E., Chivers, D. P. & Smith, R. J. F. (1997). Differential learning rates of chemical versus visual cues of a northern pike by fathead minnows in a natural habitat. *Environmental Biology of Fishes*, **49**, 89–96.

Byers, J. A. (1997). *American Pronghorn: Social Adaptations and the Ghosts of Predators Past*. Chicago, IL: Chicago Univiversity Press.

Cárdenas, Y. L., Shen, B., Zung, L. & Blumstein, D. T. (2005). Evaluating temporal and spatial margins of safety in galahs. *Animal Behaviour*, **70**, 1395–1399.

Caro, T., Izzo, A., Reiner Jr, R.C., Walker, H. & Stankowich, T. (2014). The function of zebra stripes. *Nature Communications*, **5**, 1–10.

Caro, T. M. (2005). *Antipredator Defenses in Birds and Mammals*. Chicago, IL: University of Chicago Press.

Cassirer, E. F., Freddy, D. J. & Ables, E. D. (1992). Elk responses to disturbance by cross-country skiers in Yellowstone National Park. *Wildlife Society Bulletin*, **20**, 375–381.

Chapman, T., Rymer, T. & Pillay, N. (2012). Behavioural correlates of urbanisation in the Cape ground squirrel *Xerus inauris*. *Naturwissenschaften*, **99**, 893–902.

Colman, J. E., Jacobsen, B. W. & Reimers, E. (2001). Summer response distances of Svalbard reindeer *Rangifer tarandus platyrhynchus* to provocation by humans on foot. *Wildlife Biology*, **7**, 275–283.

Cooper, W. E. (1997). Factors affecting risk and cost of escape by the broad-headed skink (*Eumeces laticeps*): predator speed, directness of approach, and female presence. *Herpetologica*, **53**, 464–474.

Cooper, W. E. (1999). Tradeoffs between courtship, fighting, and antipredatory behavior by a lizard, *Eumeces laticeps*. *Behavioral Ecology and Sociobiology*, **47**, 54–59.

Cooper, W. E. & Blumstein, D. T. (2014). Novel effects of monitoring predators on costs of fleeing and not fleeing explain flushing early in economic escape theory. *Behavioral Ecology*, **25**, 44–52.

Coss, R. G. (1999). Effects of relaxed natural selection on the evolution of behavior. In Foster, S. A. & Endler, J. A. (eds.) *Geographic Variation in Behavior: Perspectives on Evolutionary Mechanisms*. Oxford: Oxford University Press.

Darling, F. F. (1937). *A Herd of Red Deer*. London: Oxford University Press.

Denniston, R. H. (1956). Ecology, behavior, and population dynamics of the Wyoming or Rocky Mountain moose, *Alces alces shirasi*. *Zoologica*, **41**, 105–118.

Derocher, A. E., Wiig, O. & Bangjord, G. (2000). Predation of Svalbard reindeer by polar bears. *Polar Biology,* **23**, 675–678.

Dill, L. M. & Houtman, R. (1989). The influence of distance to refuge on flight initiation distance in the gray squirrel (*Sciurus carolinensis*). *Canadian Journal of Zoology,* **67**, 233–235.

Elgar, M. A. (1989). Predator vigilance and group-size in mammals and birds: A critical review of the empirical-evidence. *Biological Reviews of the Cambridge Philosophical Society,* **64**, 13–33.

Espmark, Y. & Langvatn, R. (1979). Cardiac responses in alarmed red deer calves. *Behavioural Processes,* **4**, 179–186.

Espmark, Y. & Langvatn, R. (1985). Development and habituation of cardiac and behavioral responses in young red deer calves (*Cervus elaphus*) exposed to alarm stimuli. *Journal of Mammalogy,* **66**, 702–711.

Estes, R. D. & Goddard, J. (1967). Prey selection and hunting behavior of African wild dog. *Journal of Wildlife Management,* **31**, 52–70.

Gray, D. R. (1973). Winter research on the muskox (*Ovibos moschatus wardi*) on Bathurst Island, 1970–71. *Arctic Circular,* **21**, 158–163.

Griffin, S. C., Valois, T., Taper, M. L. & Scott Mills, L. (2007). Effects of tourists on behavior and demography of olympic marmots. *Conservation Biology,* **21**, 1070–1081.

Hagemoen, R. I. M. & Reimers, E. (2002). Reindeer summer activity pattern in relation to weather and insect harassment. *Journal of Animal Ecology,* **71**, 883–892.

Hamilton, W. D. (1971). Geometry for the selfish herd. *Journal of Theoretical Biology,* **31**, 295–311.

Hamlin, K. L. & Schweitzer, L. L. (1979). Cooperation by coyote pairs attacking mule deer fawns. *Journal of Mammalogy,* **60**, 849–850.

Hamr, J. (1988). Disturbance behavior of chamois in an alpine tourist area of Austria. *Mountain Research and Development,* **8**, 65–73.

Hediger, H. (1964). *Wild Animals in Captivity.* New York: Dover Publications, Inc.

Hone, E. (1934). The present status of the muskox in Arctic North America and Greenland. *Special Publications of the American Committee for International Wildlife Protection,* **5**, 1–87.

Ilany, A. & Eilam, D. (2008). Wait before running for your life: defensive tactics of spiny mice (*Acomys cahirinus*) in evading barn owl (*Tyto alba*) attack. *Behavioral Ecology and Sociobiology,* **62**, 923–933.

Jacobsen, N. K. (1979). Alarm bradycardia in white-tailed deer fawns (*Odocoileus virginianus*). *Journal of Mammalogy,* **60**, 343–349.

Jensen, P. (2006). Domestication: From behaviour to genes and back again. *Applied Animal Behaviour Science,* **97**, 3–15.

Karlsson, J., Eriksson, M. & Liberg, O. (2007). At what distance do wolves move away from an approaching human? *Canadian Journal of Zoology,* **85**, 1193–1197.

Kearton, C. (1929). *In the Land of the Lion.* London: National Travel Club.

Kloppers, E. L., St. Clair, C. C. & Hurd, T. E. (2005). Predator-resembling aversive conditioning for managing habituated wildlife. *Ecology and Society,* **10**, Online article 3, http://www.ecologyandsociety.org/vol10/iss1/art31/.

Kramer, D. L. & Bonenfant, M. (1997). Direction of predator approach and the decision to flee to a refuge. *Animal Behaviour,* **54**, 289–295.

Lagory, K. E. (1987). The influence of habitat and group characteristics on the alarm and flight response of white-tailed deer. *Animal Behaviour*, **35**, 20–25.

Lagos, P. A., Meier, A., Tolhuysen, L. O. *et al.* (2009). Flight initiation distance is differentially sensitive to the costs of staying and leaving food patches in a small-mammal prey. *Canadian Journal of Zoology*, **87**, 1016–1023.

Lahti, D. C., Johnson, N. A., Ajie, B. C. *et al.* (2009). Relaxed selection in the wild. *Trends in Ecology & Evolution*, **24**, 487–496.

Larivière, S. & Messier, F. (1996). Aposematic behaviour in the striped skunk, *Mephitis mephitis*. *Ethology*, **102**, 986–992.

Laundre, J. W., Hernandez, L. & Altendorf, K. B. (2001). Wolves, elk, and bison: reestablishing the "landscape of fear" in Yellowstone National Park, U.S.A. *Canadian Journal of Zoology*, **79**, 1401–1409.

Leader Williams, N. (1988). *Reindeer on South Georgia: the Ecology of an Introduced Population*. Cambridge: Cambridge University Press.

Lehrer, E. W., Schooley, R. L. & Whittington, J. K. (2011). Survival and antipredator behavior of woodchucks (*Marmota monax*) along an urban-agricultural gradient. *Canadian Journal of Zoology*, **90**, 12–21.

Lent, P. C. (1974). Mother-infant relationships in ungulates. In Geist, V. & Walther, F. (eds.) *Behavior of Ungulates and its Relation to Management of Nature and Natural Resources*. Gland, Switzerland: International Union for Conservation.

Lent, P. C. (1991). Maternal-infant behavior in muskoxen. *Mammalia*, **55**, 3–22.

Li, C., Monclús, R., Maul, T. L., Jiang, Z. & Blumstein, D. T. (2011). Quantifying human disturbance on antipredator behavior and flush initiation distance in yellow-bellied marmots. *Applied Animal Behaviour Science*, **129**, 146–152.

Lima, S. L. (1995). Back to the basics of anti-predatory vigilance: the group-size effect. *Animal Behaviour*, **49**, 11–20.

Lingle, S. (2001). Anti-predator strategies and grouping patterns in white-tailed deer and mule deer. *Ethology*, **107**, 295–314.

Lingle, S. & Wilson, W. F. (2001). Detection and avoidance of predators in white-tailed deer (*Odocoileus virginianus*) and mule deer (*O. hemionus*). *Ethology*, **107**, 125–147.

Louis, S. & Le Beere, M. (2000). Adjustment in flight distance from humans by *Marmota marmota*. *Canadian Journal of Zoology*, **78**, 556–563.

Lovegrove, B. G. (2001). The evolution of body armor in mammals: plantigrade constraints of large body size. *Evolution*, **55**, 1464–1473.

Marealle, W. N., Fossøy, F., Holmern, T., Stokke, B. G. & Røskaft, E. (2010). Does illegal hunting skew Serengeti wildlife sex ratios? *Wildlife Biology*, **16**, 419–429.

Marion, K. R. & Sexton, O. J. (1979). Protective behavior by male pronghorn, *Antilocapra americana* (Artiodactyla). *Southwestern Naturalist*, **24**, 709–710.

Martín, J. & López, P. (1999). Nuptial coloration and mate guarding affect escape decisions of male lizards *Psammodromus algirus*. *Ethology*, **105**, 439–447.

Matson, T. K., Goldizen, A. W. & Putland, D. A. (2005). Factors affecting the vigilance and flight behaviour of impalas. *South African Journal of Wildlife Research*, **35**, 1–11.

Matthiopoulos, J. (2003). The use of space by animals as a function of accessibility and preference. *Ecological Modelling*, **159**, 239–268.

McCleery, R. (2009). Changes in fox squirrel anti-predator behaviors across the urban-rural gradient. *Landscape Ecology*, **24**, 483–493.

McMillan, J. F. (1954). Some observations on moose in Yellowstone Park. *American Midland Naturalist*, **52**, 392–399.

Mirov, N. T. (1945). Notes on the domestication of reindeer. *American Anthropologist*, **47**, 393–408.

Moen, G. K., Støen, O.-G., Sahlén, V. & Swenson, J. E. (2012). Behaviour of solitary adult Scandinavian brown bears (*Ursus arctos*) when approached by humans on foot. *PLoS ONE*, **7**, e31699.

Mooring, M. S., Fitzpatrick, T. A., Nishihira, T. T. & Reisig, D. D. (2004). Vigilance, predation risk, and the allee effect in desert bighorn sheep. *Journal of Wildlife Management*, **68**, 519–532.

Mörschel, F. H. & Klein, D. R. (1997). Effects of weather and parasitic insects on behavior and group dynamics of caribou of the Delta Herd, Alaska. *Canadian Journal of Zoology*, **75**, 1659–1670.

Murphy, S. M. & Curatolo, J. A. (1987). Activity budgets and movement rates of caribou encountering pipelines, roads and traffic in Northern Alaska. *Canadian Journal of Zoology*, **65**, 2483–2490.

Nieminen, M. (2013). Response distances of wild forest reindeer (*Rangifer tarandus fennicus* Lönnb.) and semi-domestic reindeer (*R. t. tarandus* L.) to direct provocation by a human on foot/snowshoes. *Rangifer*, **13**, 1–15.

Pollard, R. H., Ballard, W. B., Noel, L. E. & Cronin, M. A. (1996). Summer distribution of Caribou, *Rangifer tarandus granti*, in the area of the Prudhoe Bay oil field, Alaska, 1990–1994. *Canadian Field-Naturalist*, **110**, 659–674.

Price, E. O. (1997). Behavioural genetics and the process of animal domestication. In Grandin, T. (ed.) *Genetics and the Behaviour of Domestic Animals*. Academic Press.

Price, E. O. & King, J. A. (1968). Domestication and adaptation. In Hafez, E. S. E. (ed.) *Adaptation of Domestic Animals*. Philadelphia, PA: Lea and Febiger.

Recarte, J. M., Vincent, J. P. & Hewison, A. J. M. (1998). Flight responses of park fallow deer to the human observer. *Behavioural Processes*, **44**, 65–72.

Reimers, E. & Colman, J. E. (2006). Reindeer and caribou (*Rangifer tarandus*) response towards human activities. *Rangifer*, **26**, 55–71.

Reimers, E. & Eftestøl, S. (2012). Response behaviours of Svalbard reindeer towards humans and humans disguised as polar bears on Edgeøya. *Arctic, Antarctic and Alpine Research*, **44**, 483–489.

Reimers, E., Dahle, B., Eftestol, S., Colman, J. E. & Gaare, E. (2007). Effects of a power line on migration and range use of wild reindeer. *Biological Conservation*, **134**, 484–494.

Reimers, E., Loe, L. E., Eftestol, S., Colman, J. E. & Dahle, B. (2009). Effects of hunting on response behaviors of wild reindeer. *Journal of Wildlife Management*, **73**, 844–851.

Reimers, E., Røed, K. H., Flaget, Ø. & Lurås, E. (2010). Habituation responses in wild reindeer exposed to recreational activities. *Rangifer*, **30**, 45–59.

Reimers, E., Lund, S. & Ergon, T. (2011). Vigilance and fright behaviour in the insular Svalbard reindeer. *Canadian Journal of Zoology*, **89**, 753–764.

Reimers, E., Røed, K. H. & Colman, J. E. (2012). Persistence of vigilance and flight response behaviour in wild reindeer with varying domestic ancestry. *Journal of Evolutionary Biology*, **25**, 1543–1554.

Reimers, E., Tsegaye, D., Colman, J. E. & Eftestøl, S. (2014). Activity patterns in reindeer with domestic vs. wild ancestry. *Applied Animal Behaviour Science*. **150**, 74–84.

Reynolds, P. E. (1993). Dynamics of muskox groups in northeastern Alaska. *Rangifer*, **13**, 83–89.

Røed, K. H., Flagstad, O., Nieminen, M., *et al.* (2008). Genetic analyses reveal independent domestication origins of Eurasian reindeer. *Proceedings of the Royal Society B-Biological Sciences*, **275**, 1849–1855.

Røed, K. H., Flagstad, Ø., Bjørnstad, G. & Hufthammer, A. K. (2011). Elucidating the ancestry of domestic reindeer from ancient DNA approaches. *Quarternary International*, **238**, 83–88.

Roosevelt, T. (1910). *African Game Trails: An Account of the African Wanderings of an American Hunter-Naturalist*. Scribner.

Rowe-Rowe, D. T. (1974). Flight behavior and flight distance of blesbok. *Zeitschrift für Tierpsychologie*, **34**, 208–211.

Shallenberger, E. W. (1970). *Tameness in Insular Animals: A Comparison of Approach Distances of Insular and Mainland Iguanid Lizards*. Ph. D. Dissertation, University of California, Los Angeles.

Skarin, A., Danell, Ö., Bergström, R. & Moen, J. (2004). Insect avoidance may override human disturbances in reindeer habitat selection. *Rangifer*, **24**, 95–103.

Smallwood, K. S. (1993). Mountain lion vocalizations and hunting behavior. *Southwestern Naturalist*, **38**, 65–67.

Smith, W. P. (1987). Maternal defense in Columbian white-tailed deer: When is it worth it? *The American Naturalist*, **130**, 310–316.

Stafl, N. L. (2013). *Quantifying the Effect of Hiking Disturbance on American Pika (Ochotona princeps) Foraging Behaviour*. MSc, University of British Columbia.

Stankowich, T. (2008). Ungulate flight responses to human disturbance: a review and meta-analysis. *Biological Conservation*, **141**, 2159–2173.

Stankowich, T. (2010). Risk-taking in self-defense. In Breed, M. D. & Moore, J. (eds.) *Encyclopedia of Animal Behavior*. Oxford: Academic Press.

Stankowich, T. & Blumstein, D. T. (2005). Fear in animals: a meta-analysis and review of risk assessment. *Proceedings of the Royal Society B*, **272**, 2627–2634.

Stankowich, T. & Coss, R. G. (2006). Effects of predator behavior and proximity on risk assessment by Columbian black-tailed deer. *Behavioral Ecology*, **17**, 246–254.

Stankowich, T. & Coss, R. G. (2007a). Effects of risk assessment, predator behavior, and habitat on escape behavior in Columbian black-tailed deer. *Behavioral Ecology*, **18**, 358–367.

Stankowich, T. & Coss, R. G. (2007b). The re-emergence of felid camouflage with the decay of predator recognition in deer under relaxed selection. *Proceedings of the Royal Society B*, **274**, 175–182.

Tarlow, E. M. & Blumstein, D. T. (2007). Evaluating methods to quantify anthropogenic stressors on wild animals. *Applied Animal Behaviour Science*, **102**, 429–451.

Thomson, B. R. (1980). Behaviour differences between reindeer and caribou (*Rangifer tarandus* L.). In Reimers, E., Gaare, E. & Skjenneberg, S. (eds.) *Second International Reindeer/Caribou Symposium, Røros, Norway.* Trondheim: Direktoratet for vilt og ferskvannsfisk.

Tyler, N. J. C. (1991). Short-term behavioral responses of Svalbard reindeer *Rangifer tarandus platyrhynchus* to direct provocation by a snowmobile. *Biological Conservation*, **56**, 179–194.

Tyler, N. J. C. & Øritsland, N. A. (1989). Why don't Svalbard reindeer migrate. *Holarctic Ecology*, **12**, 369–376.

Van Der Knaap, W. O. (1986). On the presence of reindeer (*Rangifer tarandus L.*) on Edgeøya, Spitzbergen in the period 3800–5000 BP. *Circumpolar Journal*, **2**, 3–10.

Vásquez, R. A., Ebensperger, L. A. & Bozinovic, F. (2002). The influence of habitat on travel speed, intermittent locomotion, and vigilance in a diurnal rodent. *Behavioral Ecology*, **13**, 182–187.

Vistnes, I. & Nellemann, C. (2008). The matter of spatial and temporal scales: a review of reindeer and caribou response to human activity. *Polar Biology*, **31**, 399–407.

Walther, F. R. (1969). Flight behaviour and avoidance of predators in Thomson's gazelle (*Gazella thomsoni* Guenther 1884). *Behaviour*, **34**, 184–219.

Wam, H. K., Eldegard, K. & Hjeljord, O. (2014). Minor habituation to repeated experimental approaches in Scandinavian wolves. *European Journal of Wildlife Research*, **60**, 839–842.

Weston, M. A. & Stankowich, T. (2014). Dogs as agents of disturbance. In Gompper, M. E. (ed.) *Free-Ranging Dogs and Wildlife Conservation.* Oxford: Oxford University Press.

Wolf, I. D. & Croft, D. B. (2010). Minimizing disturbance to wildlife by tourists approaching on foot or in a car: A study of kangaroos in the Australian rangelands. *Applied Animal Behaviour Science*, **126**, 75–84.

Ydenberg, R. C. & Dill, L. M. (1986). The economics of fleeing from predators. *Advances in the Study of Behavior*, **16**, 229–249.

4   Birds

Anders Pape Møller

4.1   Introduction

The study of flight initiation distance (FID) has a long history. Darwin (1868) described in detail how domestication resulted in loss of fear in birds and mammals, and that a number of different kinds of flight behavior seen in wild animals were lost when animals lived in human proximity. Hediger (1934) synthesized the literature on escape behavior including the distance at which animals became alert and that at which they fled an approaching predator, including humans, in a diverse array of organisms. The review by Hediger explicitly noted that different components of escape such as FID, flight direction, and alert distance (AD) reflected different aspects of flight behavior that could all, or in different combinations, change over the course of evolution. Hediger also pointed out how individuals, populations, and species differed in escape behavior, and that island populations showed less fear than mainland populations of the same or related species. Rand (1964) showed that FID was inversely related to body temperature in a lizard, implying that FID varied with risk of predation. Cooke (1980) noticed that urban birds had much shorter flight distances than rural populations of the same species, and that this difference depended on body size, the difference being larger in small species with high metabolism. This change in behavior was functional in the sense that it allowed birds to coexist with humans even at high human population densities that caused frequent disturbance. Burger (1981), Burger and Gochfeld (1981), and several others noticed that human disturbance affected FID at seabird colonies, and that such disturbance could result in habitat use alteration and reduced reproductive performance. These early studies placed research on escape behavior and FID firmly in the context of conservation biology, where it has remained ever since (Blumstein & Fernández-Juricic 2010).

In this chapter I use the definitions of FID and related terms as described in Chapter 1. Starting distance (SD) and AD are aspects of escape behavior that arise for methodological or biological reasons, and some of these components show significant covariation with FID (e.g., Blumstein 2003). Despite recent theoretical suggestions (Blumstein 2010; Cooper & Blumstein 2013) and empirical evidence (reviewed by Samia *et al.* 2013) that suggest biological mechanisms underlie covariation between AD (or SD) and FID, at least part of this covariation is artifactual (Dumont *et al.* 2012). In contrast to AD,

Escaping From Predators: An Integrative View of Escape Decisions, ed. W. E. Cooper and D. T. Blumstein. Published by Cambridge University Press. © Cambridge University Press 2015.

SD can be controlled experimentally in the field by keeping a fixed distance to animals before recording FID (e.g., Møller 2012) or by recording SD as part of the approach protocol (Blumstein *et al.* 2005). The remainder of this chapter focuses on FID and the factors that account for variation in FID within and among individuals, populations, and species.

Here I present an exhaustive review of research findings dealing with FID in birds. I judge the magnitude of effects of the covariates by relying on effect sizes estimated in terms of Pearson product-moment correlation coefficients because they have the intuitively simple property that the value squares reflects the amount of variance explained (Cohen 1988). I evaluate the strength of relationships between variables (preferably partial effects after adjustment for confounding variables) judging than an $r = 0.10$, accounting for 1% of the variance is small, $r = 0.30$, accounting for 9% of the variance is intermediate, and $r = 0.50$, accounting for 25% of the variance is a large effect (Cohen 1988). These three levels can be compared with mean effect sizes in biology in general. Møller and Jennions (2002) showed in a meta-analysis of all meta-analyses in biology that, on average, main effects accounted for 5 to 7% of the variance, thus constituting an intermediate effect. Test statistics were transformed into effect sizes using equations listed in Rosenthal (1994). I also report sample size to allow readers to estimate confidence intervals of the effect sizes. The effect sizes for interspecific comparisons were generally based on phylogenetically controlled analyses accounting for similarity among taxa due to common phylogenetic descent, while intraspecific studies simply represented relationships across individuals. A small number of studies could not be included because test statistics were not reported. I list all effect sizes and the associated sample sizes in the electronic supplementary material, while summary statistics including weighted means and 95% confidence intervals for different categories of effects are reported in Table 4.1. These estimates for categories of effects were derived from a non-phylogenetic, random effects meta-analysis comparing effect sizes for different categories of studies using the MetaWin 2.1 statistical software package (Rosenberg *et al.* 2000). The main text of this chapter only presents some representative examples of effect sizes, while a complete list of effect sizes can be found in the electronic supplementary material. Finally, readers should note that Pearson product-moment correlations as a measure of effect size may not always be the most efficient way to estimate relationships, and other methods for judging relationships between pairs of variables have been suggested (Koricheva *et al.* 2013).

To make a comprehensive review of studies of FID in birds, I searched the Web of Science using the key words FID, flight distance, and flight initiation distance. In the review, I start out by investigating (1) the frequency distributions of FIDs and their component parts. This part is based on a data set that I have collected, which comprises 9007 observations belonging to 181 species of European birds. Flight initiation distance was measured by having a fixed SD around 30 m to avoid covariation between FID and SD. Data collected from the same sites without the use of a fixed SD were very similar in terms of FID. Then I analyze (2) the phenotypic variation in FID and its environmental and genetic components, followed by (3) a summary of the different factors affecting FID, with a particular emphasis on life history because FID is squarely placed as the

Table 4.1 Summary statistics (mean effect size and 95% confidence intervals) for different categories of phenotypic traits for flight initiation distance (FID) based on a non-phylogenetic random effects meta-analyses weighted by sample size (Rosenberg *et al.* 2000). Effects differing significantly from zero are shown in bold font.

Category	Mean effect size	Lower 95% confidence interval	Upper 95% confidence interval	No. studies
Urbanization	**0.62**	0.50	0.74	20
Body mass	**0.39**	0.27	0.51	20
Predation	**0.37**	0.28	0.47	32
Range	**0.35**	0.19	0.52	11
Dispersal	0.31	−0.35	0.97	3
Sexual display	0.29	−0.05	0.63	5
Sociality	**0.26**	0.17	0.34	35
Parasitism	**0.22**	0.08	0.37	14
Life history	**0.20**	0.10	0.30	27
Disturbance	**0.19**	0.04	0.35	13
Habitat	**0.17**	0.05	0.28	20
Brain	0.09	−0.33	0.50	4
Personality	−0.16	−0.97	0.65	3

result of trade-offs between components of life history (Blumstein 2006; Møller & Garamszegi 2012). I then (4) analyze underlying assumptions linked to FID, such as its relationship with risk of predation and death, phenotypic adjustment related to predator avoidance, morphological adaptations, sensory organs related with (see also Chapter 12), and their cognitive aspects. Next, I (5) investigate the population consequences of disturbance on FID, and I finish (6) by providing some ideas for future prospects of research.

4.2   Frequency distributions of FID

Using the raw data of 132 to 181 species of European birds (depending on which statistical moment was analyzed; $N = 9007$ observations) I evaluated the frequency distributions of FID. I found that FID is characterized by a mean, and the moments that reflect variance, skewness, and kurtosis. The characteristics of the frequency distribution of FID are shown in Table 4.2 and Figure 4.1. There is considerable variation among species with a coefficient of variation of 108.

The frequency distributions of FID were significantly skewed toward the right and deviated significantly from the expected value of zero for normal distributions. In addition, there was significant leptokurtosis as reflected by the mean kurtosis value across species being positive. Wright (1968) showed, for the special case of a

Table 4.2 Characteristics of mean, variance, skewness, and kurtosis of FID for 132 to 181 (depending on variable) species of birds from Europe. $N = 9007$ observations. Skewness and kurtosis were tested against the null hypothesis of no significant difference from zero (i.e., the parameter-value expected assuming a normal distribution).

	Mean	SD	t	N	P
Mean	13.42	80.96		181	
Variance	100.09	1827.75		159	
Skewness	1.67	8.30	19.07	144	< 0.0001
Kurtosis	5.26	49.43	10.03	132	< 0.0001

(A. P. Møller unpublished data)

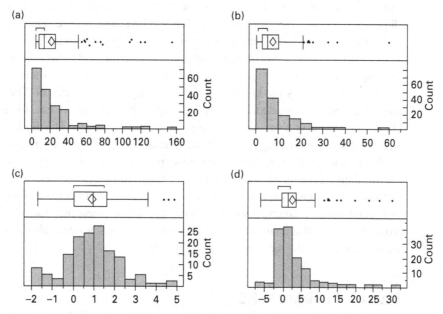

Figure 4.1 Frequency distributions of (A) mean (m), (B) standard deviation (m), (C) skewness, and (D) kurtosis of species-specific values of flight initiation distance in birds recorded by A. P. Møller. Sample size was 132 to 181 species depending on the moment. The box plots show means (diamonds), medians, quartiles, 95% confidence intervals, and extreme observations.

dichotomous individual difference, that the degree of leptokurtosis reflected the ratio of the variances of the two distributions. Hence species on average having leptokurtotic distributions imply that the overall population is composed of different subpopulations that differ inherently in degree of escape behavior. Thus the degree of leptokurtosis reflects heterogeneity in escape behavior among individuals, implying that a more heterogeneous population consists of more different kinds of individuals in terms of escape behavior.

4.3   FID and components of flight

Flying animals such as birds, bats and aquatic organisms are unique by moving in three dimensions, while all other organisms mainly move in two dimensions. This has important consequences for escape behavior (FID) because it is easier to escape in three than in two dimensions, since predators will have to pursue prey that can escape in one additional dimension. We should also expect that the horizontal and vertical components of FID should show design features that exploited these differences in escape propensity (Møller 2010b). Every single FID can be decomposed into its horizontal and vertical components, with the vertical component being zero in organisms moving in two dimensions (Blumstein *et al.* 2004; Fernández-Juricic *et al.* 2004). In a comparative study of 69 species of birds, Møller (2010b) showed that four times more variance in FID among species was due to the horizontal than the vertical dimension. The slope of the relationship between horizontal distance and FID (horizontal slope) increased with body mass, whereas the slope for the relationship between vertical distance and FID (vertical slope) decreased with body mass. In other words, large species rely more on the horizontal component of escape than small species, and this may be caused by the higher energy cost of flight in large species. The horizontal slope was negatively related to the vertical slope, albeit this negative relationship had a slope that was less than expected from a perfect trade-off. The horizontal slope decreased with increasing density of the habitat from grassland over shrub to trees, while that was not the case for the vertical slope. If the vertical slope provides a means for avoiding predation, we should expect adult survival rate to decrease with increasing vertical slope, which was indeed the case, while there was no relationship with the horizontal slope. In addition, species with a high rate of senescence had a high vertical slope, suggesting that an increase in vertical escape allowed for individuals of old age to accumulate due to the reduction in risk of predation.

4.4   Sources of variation in FID

4.4.1   Within- and among-individual variation

The variation within and among populations reflects differences among species (e.g., Blumstein *et al.* 2003). In a sample of 9289 FID estimates from Europe, 55% of the variance in FID occurred among species ($F = 59.83$, d.f. $= 186, 9103$, $P < 0.0001$). A model of mean FID weighted by sample size showed that 53% of the variance occurred among species ($F = 195.53$, d.f. $= 1, 176$, $P < 0.0001$). Thus more than half of the variance occurs among species with an almost similar fraction occurring within species.

4.4.2   Heritability, selection, and response to selection

Phenotypic variance in FID can be partitioned into environmental and genetic components, as well as gene × environment interactions (Falconer & Mackay 1996).

Table 4.3 Repeatability within and among years and habituation for FID in different species of birds.

Species	Repeatability within years	Repeatability among years	Habituation	Reference
Somateria mollissima	0.76–0.80	0.37–0.69	None	Seltmann *et al.* 2012
Athene cunicularia	0.84–0.92	_	None	Carrete & Tella 2010
Athene cunicularia	_	0.85–0.91	_	Carrete & Tella 2013
Numenius arquata	0.04	_	_	de Jong *et al.* 2013
Hirundo rustica	0.92	0.62	None	A. P. Møller unpublished data
Passer domesticus	0.79	_	None	Møller & Garamszegi 2012
Ficedula albicollis	_	_	None	Møller & Garamszegi 2012
Melospiza melodia	_	_	None	Scales *et al.* 2011
Dolichonyx oryzivorus	_	_	None	Keyel *et al.* 2012
Cardinalis cardinalis	_	_	None	Smith-Castro & Rodewald 2010

Repeatability sets an upper limit to heritability (Falconer & Mackay 1996). Differences in FID among sites can be due to learning, sorting of phenotypes (differential migration of specific phenotypes to particular areas), or local adaptation. Repeatabilities of FID (calculated using intra-class correlation coefficients; Falconer & Mackay 1996) were reported for five species, with all values except one being 0.76 to 0.92 (Table 4.3). Four out of five studies had significant repeatability. The exception was de Jong *et al.* (2013) who showed an absence of significant repeatability for breeding curlews (*Numenius arquata*, de Jong *et al.* 2013). Estimates of repeatability within individuals among years ranged from 0.37 to 0.62 in two species. I (unpublished data) estimated a repeatability of mean FID of 0.60 among individuals within 181species from Europe (SE = 0.04), and a repeatability for the standard deviation in FID among individuals within 159 species of 0.69 (SE = 0.12). This implies that particular species are consistent in their mean and variance in FID.

There is only weak evidence of habituation, with repeated estimates of FID not showing a decline with repeat tests in eight different species ranging from ducks and owls to passerines (Table 4.3). While some studies may suffer from short intervals between encounters resulting in individuals recognizing the experimenter as not being dangerous, other studies have carefully controlled for such effects. The literature on habituation effects is clearly in need of a general review (Blumstein, 2014).

Broad sense heritability is the proportion of phenotypic variance due to additive genetic effects (Falconer & Mackay 1996). Only a single study has estimated heritability for FID. Parent–offspring resemblance in the barn swallow provided a heritability of FID of 0.38 (0.07) for male parent–offspring and 0.46 (0.07) for female parent–offspring based on 191 individuals, and animal models provided similar estimates (Møller 2014a). Hence there is considerable additive genetic variance in FID.

Selection can be estimated as the change in standardized phenotype before and after selection (Falconer & Mackay 1996). Møller *et al.* (2013) provided estimates of FID in resident and migratory birds before and after a severely cold winter along a latitudinal gradient in Europe. They provided evidence of a reduction in FID before and after the cold winter, but only among resident species, and more so for rural than urban populations of the same species. This suggests that there has been directional selection on FID. Similarly, rapid change in FID between urban and rural populations of juncos (*Junco hyemalis*) suggests adaptation to an urban environment (Atwell *et al.* 2012).

If FID is heritable, and if there is directional selection, we expect the response to selection will be the product of additive genetic variation and selection. Hence, FID should change across selection episodes when the trait is heritable. I am unaware of any animal model or other studies providing evidence of such response to selection. In the scenario where we have prior estimates of FID and animals are subjected to an extremely cold winter, we should expect a reduction in FID after the cold winter, with the phenotype changing over time toward the value recorded before the cold winter, if that original value was close to the optimum.

4.5   Biological causes of variation

4.5.1   Body size

It is an almost trivial finding that body size is the best predictor of FID in interspecific comparative analyses, because it is also the best predictor of life history, anatomy, physiology, behavior, and conservation status (Bennett & Owens 2002). Body size is also the best intraspecific predictor of these characters in species with indeterminate growth, such as fish, amphibians, and reptiles, but not in species with determinate growth such as birds and mammals (Bennett & Owens 2002). Thus a larger flying animal takes longer before take-off (Pennycuick 1989), and I would thus expect longer FID in larger species for this reason alone. Cooke (1980) reported that smaller bird species were more approachable in suburban than in rural areas. Blumstein (2006) found an effect size of 0.21 for 150 species of birds. Møller (2008b) reported an effect size equal to 0.64 for 100 species of European birds and Glover *et al.* (2011) an effect size of 0.77 for 28 species, while Weston *et al.* (2012) reported an effect size of 0.69 for 138 species of Australian birds. The allometry coefficient in Weston *et al.*'s study was 0.29 and in that of Møller (2008b) 0.27, respectively. These coefficients were smaller than isometry (which equals a slope of 1; in the study by Møller 2008b $t = 24.33$, d.f. $= 97$, $P < 0.0001$), implying relatively shorter FIDs for large-sized species. While the previously reported allometry coefficients are not phylogenetically controlled such an analysis showed an even less steep slope of only 0.20 for FID in relation to body mass in European birds (Møller 2008b). Hence FID shows negative allometry (i.e., the allometry coefficient of 0.20 is positive but significantly smaller than one). Thus large species have relatively shorter FID for their body size.

4.5.2   Life history

The decision to flee represents a life history decision because individuals trade foraging efficiency, and hence energy gain, against disturbance and risk of predation. Therefore individuals should optimize their escape behavior relative to their residual reproductive value, which equals the average survival and reproductive output of an individual of a given age (Roff 1992). Thus individuals with low reproductive output or survival prospects (e.g., because they are ill or suffer from parasitism) should take greater risks than healthy conspecifics. Therefore life history components are also expected to correlate with FID.

Old age at first reproduction implies that individuals should take small risks in order not to die before the start of reproduction. Blumstein (2006) showed a small effect size, as did Møller and Garamszegi (2012) for mean and variance in FID.

Clutch size and fecundity were negatively related to mean FID (Blumstein 2006; Møller & Garamszegi 2012). A study investigating the difference in FID and the difference in clutch size between temperate and tropical populations showed a strong effect (Møller & Liang 2013), implying that paired designs that automatically control for confounding variables provide particularly strong effects. Hatching success in curlews (*Numenius arquata*) peaked at intermediate FID (de Jong *et al.* 2013), as would be expected if long FID prevented efficient incubation. A similar line of argument can be used for a study by Seltmann *et al.* (2012), which found longer incubation periods in eiders (*Somateria mollissima*) with long FID. Interspecific studies of developmental periods only showed weakly related to FID with small effect sizes (Blumstein 2006).

Species with short and variable FID suffer less from disturbance and hence reach a state that allows reproduction more readily than individuals belonging to species with long and invariable FID. Accordingly duration of the breeding season decreased with mean FID and increased with the variance in FID (Møller & Garamszegi 2012).

Both juvenile and adult survival rate increased with mean FID and decreased with variance in FID (Møller & Garamszegi 2012), and this effect was mainly due to the vertical component of FID (Møller 2010b). Therefore, I should expect that longevity and rate of senescence should be related to the vertical component in FID. Indeed, rate of senescence decreased with increasing mean and variance in FID, especially for the vertical component of escape (Blumstein 2006; Møller 2010b; Møller & Garamszegi 2012). This means that individuals belonging to species that mainly escape in the vertical dimension age more slowly than individuals belonging to species that mainly escape in the horizontal dimension.

4.5.3   Urbanization

Urbanization often results in a reduction in fearfulness of animals, and this also applies to FID (Blumstein 2014; Møller 2014a). Cooke (1980) described strong differences in FID between suburban and rural populations of birds, and similar reports exist in the older urbanization literature (Tomialojc 1970; Klausnitzer 1985). Müller *et al.* (2013) recently discovered in analyses of candidate genes in 12 paired populations of blackbirds

(*Turdus merula*) that a gene involved in harm avoidance differed strongly between urban and rural populations. This implies that there has been divergence between populations due to selection.

Flight initiation distance has been known to relate to urbanization for more than 30 years (Cooke 1980). The magnitude of the difference in FID between urban and rural populations is directly linked to time since urbanization (Møller 2008a). Two studies suggest that both mean and variance in FID relate to urbanization, apparently because a higher variance implies a greater diversity of phenotypes and hence more different behavioral phenotypes (or personalities) (Møller 2010a; Carrete & Tella 2011a,b; Møller & Garamszegi 2012). Urban populations also had shorter FID than rural populations of the same species in a study of patterns of FID across Europe (Díaz *et al.* 2013). The difference in FID between rural and urban populations decreased with increasing latitude, paralleling trends in raptor abundance. The latitudinal trend also reflects the fact that the history of urbanization of birds is much older in southern than in northern Europe.

Flight initiation distance may play a crucial role in urbanization of birds because relatively short FID will allow birds to coexist in the proximity of humans as shown in a paired comparison of urbanized and closely related non-urbanized species of birds (Møller 2009a). If only a portion of the phenotypes in the ancestral rural population with specific behavior first colonized urban areas, we should expect an initial reduction in variance in FID, because some phenotypes did not enter cities. This should be followed by an increase in variance in FID as more different behavioral phenotypes develop in novel urban habitats to which urban birds only have adapted recently. These scenarios were supported by independent studies comparing rural and urban birds in Europe and South America (Møller 2010a; Carrete & Tella 2011a,b).

Valcarcel and Fernández-Juricic (2009) tested the safe habitat hypothesis and found a strong relationship between FID and habitat. There is also indirect evidence of predators affecting FID of prey in urban areas because many birds seek refuge near human habitation where raptors are rare. In fact, there was a negative relationship between reduction in flight distance between rural and urban habitats and difference in FID between predators and prey (effect size = 0.37) (Møller 2012). The difference in FID between prey species and that of their predator increased with the preference of prey species by sparrowhawks (*Accipiter nisus*) relative to their abundance (effect size = 0.32) (Møller 2012). Similarly, Guay *et al.* (2013) recently reported that FID was longer when individual black swans (*Cygnus atratus*) were farther from water, which acted as a refuge. These findings fit well with the predominant role of predation in predicting urbanization of birds (Møller 2014b).

4.5.4   Song

Males generally compete more strongly for access to mates than females because females are a limiting resource. Thus we should expect that displaying males have reduced FID compared to non-displaying conspecifics. This hypothesis has been investigated by analyzing FID of singing males and males involved in other activities. Males mainly sing in order to attract mates or repel competitors. A second aspect of display that facilitates success is the height at which individuals display because high display sites facilitate transmission of song, but simultaneously expose individuals to predators.

Singing males took greater risks than males that were not singing by reducing their FID with an effect size that was large (effect size = 0.47, $N = 40$) (Møller *et al.* 2008). The difference in FID between singing and non-singing males was also related to greater song post-exposure with a large effect size (effect size = 0.50, $N = 34$). Such exposed display locations may increase the risk of predation. In contrast, sexual dichromatism was only weakly correlated with mean FID in singing males, with a small effect size (effect size = 0.05, $N = 32$) (Møller *et al.* 2008).

4.5.5   Hormones and FID

Testosterone is the primary sex hormone in male vertebrates affecting sexual behavior. Therefore high testosterone levels imply an increase in adoption of risky behavior. We might expect that FID would decrease in males relative to females during the breeding season, particularly so in species with high testosterone levels. In a comparative analysis of European birds, P. Tryjanowski and A. P. Møller (unpublished data) found that mean FID decreased with increasing testosterone level (effect size = 0.45). The sex difference in FID was positively correlated with testosterone level (effect size = 0.54, $N = 16$). Finally, males are expected to have greater variance in FID than females because males should take greater mean risks, but also greater variance in risk than females due to more intense competition for access to mates (Daly & Wilson 1983). Indeed, the sex difference in variance in FID was negatively related to testosterone (effect size = 0.53, $N = 18$) in a model that included the sex difference in body mass.

These endocrinological findings may also suggest that other hormones, such as corticosterone, could be involved in regulating FID. Indeed, Seltmann *et al.* (2012) showed a positive correlation between FID and corticosterone levels in incubating eiders. And studies of blackbirds have found lower testosterone and corticosterone levels in urban compared to rural individuals (Partecke *et al.* 2005, 2006), which is consistent with the hypothesis that hormones modulate risk taking and FID.

4.5.6   Hunting and disturbance

There is an extensive literature on FID and hunting that shows that hunted birds take flight earlier when approached by humans (Madsen 1995, 1998a, b; Madsen & Fox 1995; Weston *et al.* 2012). For example, Laursen *et al.* (2005) showed a large effect (0.49) of hunting on FID across 19 species of waterbirds in Denmark. However, this literature is not homogeneous. For example, Møller (2008a) found no significant difference in FID between hunted and other species in an analysis of 55 species of birds from Denmark during the hunting season in a model that controlled for body mass (hunting effect size = 0.004). Likewise, there was little difference in FID between inhabited and uninhabited areas in tropical China in an area with relatively little hunting (Møller & Liang 2013).

4.5.7   Diet

There are only a couple of studies of FID and diet. Carnivorous and omnivorous species of birds were more likely to be flighty than species with other diets (Blumstein 2006). Blumstein suggests that this may reflect a carry-over effect; species that eat live prey may be more generally attuned to movement and may detect threats at a greater distance. Møller and Erritzøe (2010, 2014) did not find evidence for species eating mobile prey having different FIDs than species consuming immobile food.

4.5.8   Sociality

Stankowich and Blumstein (2005) conducted a meta-analysis of risk assessment in animals and found an intermediate-sized effect in most studies. Cooperative breeders were more flighty than species with other breeding systems (Blumstein 2006). Laursen *et al.* (2005) reported intermediate to large effect sizes for intraspecific relationships between FID and flock size in different species of waterbirds with FID being longer for larger flocks. These findings are inconsistent with dilution effects, because if each individual enjoyed a smaller risk we should then expect a shorter FID in larger flocks. In contrast, the results are consistent with effects of many eyes scanning for the presence of a predator, although differences in phenotypic composition of differently sized flocks may be an alternative explanation. Finally, effect sizes for the interspecific relationship between FID and coloniality were all small (Møller 2008a).

4.5.9   Predation

Flight initiation distance was negatively related to susceptibility to predation by sparrowhawks (Møller *et al.* 2008). The difference in FID between urban and rural habitats was correlated with susceptibility to sparrowhawk predation, supporting the previously mentioned safe-habitat hypothesis (Møller 2008a). An intraspecific study that used playback of predator calls showed a strong positive effect of predator calls on increasing FID (Zanette *et al.* 2011). Likewise, another study showed that the abundance of mammalian predators has an intermediate positive effect on FID in plover species (St. Clair *et al.* 2012). Hearing the call of a predator caused crimson rosellas (*Platycercus elegans*) to reduce their FID (Adams *et al.* 2006). Finally, a study showed a relationship between perch exposure and FID (Boyer *et al.* 2006).

4.5.10   Parasitism

Flight initiation distance decreased both with diversity and prevalence of blood parasites in birds, showing a small to intermediate effect. The difference in FID between singing and non-singing males increased strongly with prevalence of *Plasmodium* that causes malaria (Møller *et al.* 2008). Independently, the difference in FID between singing and non-singing males increased strongly with the concentration of natural antibodies (Møller *et al.* 2008). Martín *et al.* (2006) showed for chinstrap penguins (*Pygoscelis antarctica*) that FID decreased with strength of T-cell response, which reflects superior body condition.

4.5.11   Habitat

Most studies have shown intermediate to large effects of the relationship between FID and habitat openness and habitat diversity, although Blumstein (2006) found a small effect. In particular, variance in FID was related to being a habitat generalist. This finding is expected because a greater diversity of behavioral phenotypes can exploit more different habitats (Møller & Garamszegi 2012). Moreover, the horizontal component of FID was more strongly related to habitat openness than the vertical component (Møller & Garamszegi 2012).

4.5.12   Range and population size

Flight initiation distance decreased with increasing latitude (Díaz *et al.* 2013; Møller & Liang 2013). That was particularly the case in paired comparisons investigating the difference in FID between temperate and tropical populations showing large effect sizes for both mean and variance in FID (Møller & Liang 2013). These differences were linked to latitudinal differences in abundance or diversity of predators.

Mean FID decreased and variance in FID increased with increasing range size (Møller & Garamszegi 2012). Thus species with short and variable FIDs have large breeding ranges because these characteristics allow high rates of reproduction and colonization of many different habitats.

Mean FID decreased and variance in FID increased with population size (Møller & Garamszegi 2012). Population density showed quantitatively similar patterns (Lin *et al.* 2012; Møller & Garamszegi 2012).

4.5.13   Dispersal

Mean FID increased with natal dispersal distance. Variance in FID increased with dispersal distance in one study (Lin *et al.* 2012), but decreased with variance in FID in another (Møller & Garamszegi 2012).

4.5.14   Overall assessment of effect sizes for different categories of studies

Effect sizes for bivariate associations between FID and other variables were generally adjusted for allometry effects by the inclusion of body mass as an additional predictor. Effect sizes were also generally adjusted for similarity in phenotype among species due to common phylogenetic descent, as reported in the original publications. However, some studies did not remove effects of alert distance and starting distance. This was because AD was not studied due to difficulties of estimating this parameter without error. Starting distance was controlled statistically in many studies, or it was controlled experimentally by keeping SD fixed at approximately 30 m. I analyzed all effect sizes reported in the electronic supplementary material using random effects meta-analysis that relies on Q-statistics that have F-distributions with numerator and denominator degrees of freedom as in analyses of variance (Rosenberg *et al.* 2000). The 186 effect size estimates varied considerably from -0.81 to $+0.90$ (see electronic supplementary material) with a mean effect size of 0.30 (95% confidence intervals = 0.26, 0.34) in a random effects meta-analysis weighted by sample. Thus the mean effect size was of an intermediate magnitude, as is the common pattern in biology (Møller & Jennions 2002). Variation in individual effect sizes was slightly larger than expected due to sampling error ($Q_{total} = 242.10$, df = 206, $P = 0.0.043$). The robustness of mean effects can be estimated from the number of null results required to eliminate the statistical significance of the mean effect size, the so-called fail-safe number (Rosenberg *et al.* 2000). Rosenthal's fail-safe number of 21,793 unpublished studies means that the significant mean effect size could not readily be eliminated by unpublished studies. There was significant heterogeneity among categories of effect sizes (Table 4.1; $Q = 58.79$, df = 12, 194, $P = 0.001$). Nine out of 13 categories of effects were statistically significant by deviating from zero (Table 4.1). These were urbanization, body mass, predation, range, sociality, parasitism, disturbance, life history, and habitat. Effect sizes were large for urbanization and body mass, explaining more than 25% of the variance. Range size, sociality, parasitism, disturbance, life history, and habitat had intermediate effects, while dispersal, sexual display, and brain size accounted for non-significant, but intermediate to small effects. There was no significant heterogeneity when comparing intraspecific and interspecific studies ($Q = 0.72$, df = 1, 205, $P = 0.73$). Likewise, there was no significant heterogeneity when comparing effects sizes based on mean FID and variance in FID ($Q = 0.40$, df = 1, 205, $P = 0.56$).

In a meta-regression weighted by sample size I found a significant model that accounted for 23% of the variance as estimated from the pseudo R^2 ($F = 5.64$, df = 13, 193, $P < 0.0001$). This model fitted the data ($F = 1.09$, df = 7, 186, $P = 0.37$). Significant predictors of effect size were category of effect (Table 4.2; $F = 5.98$, df = 12, 193, $P < 0.0001$) and marginally whether the study was intraspecific or interspecific ($F = 2.68$, df = 1, 193, $P = 0.10$; mean (SE) for intraspecific studies = 0.19 (0.05), interspecific studies = 0.26 (0.04)). Thus effect sizes differed among categories of characters and interspecific studies had larger effects than intraspecific studies.

4.6   Assumptions

4.6.1   FID reflects predation risk

An inherent assumption underlying the estimation of risk-taking from FID is that shorter FID translates into a greater risk of predation. While this assumption may intuitively appear likely, there are few tests of this assumption. The assumption can be tested at both the level of individual risk and average risk across populations or species. Møller (2014a) recorded FID for 2067 adult barn swallows from 1983 to 2012. Of these

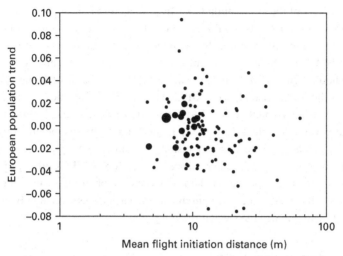

Figure 4.2   Population trend of 115 different species of European breeding birds in relation to mean flight initiation distance. Size of symbols reflects sample size. The partial effect is $F = 4.80$, d.f. $= 1, 113$, $P = 0.031$). (Adapted from Møller 2008b)

birds, 18 individuals were captured by predators (domestic cats (*Felis catus*) or sparrow-hawks). There was a significantly shorter FID among de-predated individuals than survivors. There is also evidence of mean FID of different species of birds reflecting risk of predation. Møller *et al.* (2008) analyzed susceptibility of 63 species of birds in Denmark to predation by sparrowhawks in relation to mean FID, showing a negative relationship accounting for 13% of the variance after adjusting for body mass and body mass squared (Figure 4.2; effect size = 0.36). Predators prefer prey of intermediate body size because such prey is easier to handle while still providing significant resources, hence explaining the inclusion of polynomial effects of body mass. When mean flight distance for different species increased from 6 to 60 m, susceptibility to sparrowhawk predation decreased by a factor ten.

There are two experimental studies of the effects of perceived predation caused by real predators on FID of birds. Adams *et al.* (2006) showed in playback experiments on crimson rosellas that individuals responded to predator calls. Zanette *et al.* (2011) provided direct experimental evidence for FID being linked to risk of predation by either playing back predator calls or control calls produced by species that are not predators of song sparrows (*Melospiza melodia*). This resulted in almost a tripling of FID in the experimental group compared to controls, yielding a large effect size (0.55). Unfortunately this experiment did not allow for discrimination between phenotypic plasticity and phenotypic sorting as the underlying mechanism because individuals were not tested with both treatments. Furthermore, the experiment did not allow discrimination between effects of nest predation and predation on adults as a cause of the change in FID. However, the experiment provides unequivocal evidence for FID being causally linked to predation risk.

An indirect test of the assumption that FID is related to risk of predation is based on basal metabolic rate (BMR). Basal metabolic rate is the minimal metabolic rate in the zone of thermoneutrality required for maintenance. Although many different factors may affect BMR, the fitness costs and benefits in terms of the ability to respond to predators should affect BMR. In other words, BMR is a cost of being wary toward predators. Møller (2009a) analyzed BMR and FID in 76 bird species and found that this positive relationship accounted for 27% of the variance (after inclusion of body mass as a confounding variable; effect size = 0.52). Inclusion of additional potentially confounding variables did not change this conclusion, nor did similarity in phenotype among species due to common phylogenetic descent. Therefore BMR is positively related to risk-taking behavior, and predation is an important factor in the evolution of BMR. It also suggests that the large energy requirements seen in species with high BMR may lead individuals to take greater risks when foraging.

4.6.2   Morphological adaptations to FID

Locomotor efficiency depends on oxygen uptake and transport, large muscles, and appendages that facilitate flight. Møller *et al.* (2013) predicted that hematocrit, which is a measure of packed red blood cell volume and hence reflects efficiency of oxygen transport, would be the highest in species with short FID. Consistent with this prediction, species with short FID had high hematocrit (effect size = 0.25).

Flight initiation distance could vary with wing and hind limb morphology as they can influence parameters associated with taking-off maneuvers (e.g., acceleration and lift). For instance, in a study on 83 bird species controlling for phylogenetic effects, FID was lower in species with rounded and convex wingtips perhaps due to the greater lift and thrust abilities compared to species with pointed and concave wingtips (Fernández-Juricic *et al.* 2006). However, the length of the femur and tarsus was not significantly correlated with FID (Fernández-Juricic *et al.* 2006). In addition, aspect ratio, which reflects maneuverability during flight, was large in species with long FID (effect size = 0.39; Møller *et al.* 2013). Finally, FID increased with wing area, which reflects low costs of lifting a bird with a given body size (effect size = 0.44). These effects were independent of potentially confounding variables (e.g., body size) and similarity due to common phylogenetic descent. These results suggest that physiological and morphological adaptations to FID have evolved as a means of reducing the costs of flight. Alternatively, species that have evolved adaptations to efficient flight have subsequently evolved specific FID. Either way, this suggests that birds with low costs of flight do not await closer approach by a potential predator to compensate for the costs of flight.

4.6.3   Sense organs

Prey rely on their sense organs for monitoring predators and adjusting antipredator behavior to level of risk. Thus well functioning eyes and ears are crucial for escape behavior. An initial study found no significant relationship between eye size and FID (Blumstein *et al.* 2004), but a more comprehensive analysis by Møller and Erritzøe

(2010) analyzed eye size in 97 species of birds in relation to FID, predicting that species with large eyes (i.e., higher ability to resolve visual details) will have relatively longer FID as mediated by longer ADs. This effect size was intermediate (0.34). Visual acuity arises from an effect of eye size and retinal ganglion cells. However, the ability to focus on a predator will also depend on the size of lenses that is likely to mainly be adapted to efficient foraging. Lens size can be broken down into effects of lens size and shape. Indeed, A. P. Møller and J. Erritzøe (unpublished data) weighed and measured the depth and width of lenses in 84 species of birds, showing that FID increased with the interaction between lens depth and lens diameter independent of eye size and body size. This implies that species with long FID had relatively thick and wide lenses in their eyes independent of eye size.

Just as visual information may be crucial for monitoring the behavior of predators, auditory information may independently of visual information play a significant role in predator–prey interactions. The tympanic membrane is crucial for hearing and a relatively larger tympanic membrane for a given body size implies better hearing ability (A. P. Møller & J. Erritzøe unpublished data). Across 37 species of birds, FID was strongly positively related to the size of the tympanic membrane (effect size = 0.74). Likewise, the relationship between the size of the tympanic membrane and the footplate (the flat portion of the stapes, which is set into the oval window of the medial wall of the inner ear) implies better hearing ability, and again there was a significant positive relationship between FID and tympanic membrane/footplate (effect size = 0.35, $N = 37$). These aspects of sensory ecology for eyes and ears are treated in greater detail in Chapter 12.

4.6.4   Brains and cognition

Brains and cognition should play a role in predator–prey interactions because prey glean information on the whereabouts and predator behavior with sense organs (Chapter 12). Information acquired by the sense organs is processed by the brain, and this information subsequently may change an individual's behavior. A large number of studies have investigated the ecological and evolutionary causes of brain size evolution.

This approach has recently been criticized for being superficial and non-scientific (Healy & Rowe 2007). Like all scientific enquiry this avenue of research is based on carefully recorded observations on brain size or size of component parts of the brain, and numerous attempts to verify the reliability of such data have shown a high degree of consistency, even in comparisons of head volume with brain size (Møller *et al.* 2011). Surprisingly, Healy and Rowe (2007) have not themselves adhered to such approaches in their own research by testing for reliability of their brain size data or adopting rigorous phylogenetic analyses, and they have based their analyses on small and heterogeneous sample sizes.

Guay *et al.* (2013) in an analysis of 27 bird species from Australia found no significant association between brain size and FID. Although a relatively larger brain (corrected for body mass) may allow for longer FID because of faster reaction to a potential predator, a larger brain may also allow assessment of the intentions of the predator and the like-lihood of attack before fleeing. This scenario implies that visual information is gleaned by the eyes, processed by the brain and eventually used for making decisions about FID, with these decisions depending on the relative size of the brain (Møller & Erritzøe 2014). Indeed, in a sample of 107 bird species FID increased with relative eye size (effect size = 0.33), but decreased with relative brain size (effect size = -0.23). In other words, species with relatively larger brains for a given body size stayed put for longer before taking off. Møller and Erritzøe (2014) hypothesized that this relationship came about by species with relatively large brains for a given body size using this "extra" time for monitoring the intentions of the predator before taking off. Furthermore, FID increased independently with size of the cerebellum, which plays an important role in motor control (effect size = 0.37, N = 54). These findings are consistent with cognitive monitoring as an antipredator behavior that does not result in the fastest possible escape, but rather the least expensive escape flight that allows for monitoring of predator behavior. Indeed, attentional monitoring costs have been hypothesized to be one cost of monitoring predators (Blumstein 2010; Cooper & Blumstein 2013; Møller & Erritzøe 2014). Information assessment in the interaction between predators and prey may depend on the behavior of the approaching predator. Birds significantly increased their FID or AD when approaching humans looked directly at them rather than elsewhere, as reported by Eason *et al.* (2006) for American robins (*Turdus migratorius*), Bateman and Fleming (2011) for hadeda ibises (*Bostrychia hagedash*), Clucas *et al.* (2013) for American crows (*Corvus brachyrhynchos*) and Lee *et al.* (2013) for magpies (*Pica pica*). Hadeda ibises in addition reduced the FID when approached quickly rather than slowly by a human (Bateman & Fleming, 2011), although a study of galahs (*Cacatua roseicapilla*) only showed a small effect (effect size = 0.017, N = 50; Cárdenas *et al.* 2005). Thus many bird species can distinguish between potential predators intently looking at a prey individual and those only looking intermittently.

Cars are useful tools for assessing cognitive abilities of birds in relation to risk. Recently, birds were shown to adjust their FID to road speed limits by increasing FID as speed limit increases, while there was no similar effect of the speed of the vehicle as such (Legagneux & Ducatez 2013). This response may reduce the risk of collision and decrease mortality. In a second study, Mukherjee *et al.* (2013) showed that American crows (*Corvus brachyrhynchos*) adjusted their risk-taking behavior to the driving direction of cars in a particular lane. Thus crows in the opposite lane to that used by an approaching vehicle stayed put. Additionally, whereas a fifth of crows walked from the driving lane to the safe opposite lane, none walked in the opposite direction. These observations imply that birds are able to assess driving speed and direction, and use this information to reduce risk of collision.

A different way of assessing the effects of cognitive abilities on FID is to determine FID when birds are either approached directly by a human or approached tangentially at a fixed distance. Geist *et al.* (2005), Fernández-Juricic *et al.* (2005), Heil *et al.* (2007) and Bateman and Fleming (2011) showed that birds could distinguish these two kinds of approaches. Møller and Tryjanowski (2014) collected similar data for a large number of bird species in paired populations of rural and urban species. Birds were better able to assess the direction of approach by humans in rural than in urban habitats, apparently because rural birds are more often confronted with human disturbance even at long distances between humans and birds. Thus birds in urban habitats already have very short FID, making it less beneficial to distinguish between direct and tangential approaches.

While prey usually flee in the opposite direction of an approaching predator, there is considerable variation in flight direction among individuals, with some even directly approaching the predator (Domenici *et al.* 2011a, b). Møller (unpublished manuscript) estimated the angle of flight when recording FID, showing considerable more escapes around directions of 90° and 270° than expected by chance. Such escapes are basically escapes from the direction at which a potential predator (in this case a human) is approaching, resulting in energy savings by the bird. The proportion of individuals escaping at angles of 90° and 270° in 84 species of birds increased with brain size (effect size = 0.25), decreased with body mass (effect size = 0.38) and increased with urbanization (effect size = 0.46). A different way of adjusting flight to disturbance is to run away rather than fly. Rodriguez-Prieto *et al.* (2008a) showed for blackbirds (*Turdus merula*) exposed to frequent disturbance by humans fled on foot, rather than engaging in potentially expensive flight.

4.7   Population consequences

The individual consequences of frequent disturbance and the resulting flights to evade risk of predation are not well known. However, the high metabolic cost of short flights can be considerable. Tatner and Bryant (1986) measured costs of short flights typical for human disturbance of the European robin (*Erithacus rubecula*) using doubly labeled water. This species is common in forests, but also in urban habitats including gardens throughout Europe, and hence humans disturb robins at a high rate. The flight costs were extremely high at 23 times basal metabolic rate, implying that they could have consequences for reproduction and during cold spells even survival. Because robins typically have short FIDs (mean = 5.9 m, SD = 2.9 m, N = 247, A. P. Møller unpublished data), the flight costs estimated by Tatner and Bryant (1986) can be considered biologically relevant. Robins living in urban areas may be disturbed by humans, dogs, and cats numerous times per day with the consequence of significant energetic costs. Therefore it is reasonable to ask whether frequent short FIDs have population consequences. Indeed, some hypotheses predict changes in habitat/patch use based on the frequency of disturbance (e.g., number of disturbance events per day; Fernández-Juricic 2002; Frid & Dill 2002).

Costly defensive strategies can reduce population density of animals through indirect effects (Bolnick & Preisser 2005; Preisser *et al.* 2005). The population consequences of FIDs can be investigated by relying on extensive monitoring efforts by amateur ornithologists across Europe (Møller 2008b), but also in other continents. We may expect species with long FIDs for their body size to show declining population trends because humans disturb such species more often. Among 56 species of European birds, FID accounted for 33% of the variance in population trend with effect sizes ranging from 0.36 to 0.58 in different analyses. Therefore species with long FIDs for their body size had declining populations while species with short FIDs had increasing populations. That was also the case when controlling statistically for potentially confounding effects that are known to account for population trends such as migration distance, latitude, farmland, and brain size. Thaxter *et al.* (2010) analyzed population trends in the UK in relation to predictors, but found no significant effect of FID. The reason for this difference in conclusions between the two studies remains unknown. However, stronger effects of brain size on population trends in birds in North-Western Germany, compared to an area from Eastern Germany to the Czech Republic, have shown that effects can be context dependent (Reif *et al.* 2011). It is possible that bird populations have evolved shorter FIDs in countries with higher human population density, such as in the UK, and that such shorter FIDs reduce the impact of human disturbance. The apparent lack of a significant effect of FID on population trends in the UK also implies that the effect is stronger in other countries since the European population trend is based on trends in different countries weighted by the size of the country. The Thaxter *et al.* (2010) study had some shortcomings: they did not use FID data obtained in the UK, nor did they weight their analyses by sample size, which is required because estimates of FID differ in precision depending on sample size, nor did they report the effect size from their analyses.

A more detailed way of investigating the relationship between population trend and FID is to analyze trend and FID data for different countries. Díaz *et al.* (2013) analyzed 329 populations with information on both variables in the same country and found a strong negative correlation between population trend and FID. That was even the case when confounding variables such as migration distance, body mass, and brain mass were included in the models.

These findings raise the possibility that FID can be a useful tool in conservation including assessment of levels of disturbance and susceptibility to disturbance (Madsen 1995, 1998a, b; Tarlow & Blumstein 2007; Weston *et al.* 2012; see also Chapter 17).

4.8   Future prospects

There are numerous open research questions dealing with the causes and consequences of variation in avian FID. Many predator communities are dynamic with rapid spatial and temporal changes. That is, for example, the case with cyclical populations of predators, population declines caused by DDT and other pesticides, and urban environments being colonized by raptors. Such changes in risk of predation should have predictable consequences for risk-taking behavior and hence FID. Islands are interesting laboratories because communities of animals typically are impoverished, and predators are often rare or even completely absent (Blumstein & Daniel 2005). It would be interesting to compare FID of island and mainland bird populations of the same species. Likewise, it would be interesting to investigate FID on islands without mammalian, but with avian, predators. Such situations could potentially be used to make crosses between populations of prey species with and without predators, thereby testing the prediction that crosses should have intermediate FIDs between those of the two parental populations. Furthermore, there are no studies testing whether FID varies with respect to the location of predator nests or roosts. Is it the case the prey that live close to the nest of a raptor adjust their FID to the presence of predators by behaving more cautiously or more frequently use refuges to reduce the risk of predation? Finally, there is a need for studies of the fitness consequences of FID for banded individuals with a focus on risk of predation and reproductive success.

References

Adams, J. L., Camelio, K. W., Orique, M. J. & Blumstein, D. T. (2006). Does information of predators influence general wariness? *Behavioral Ecology and Sociobiology*, **60**, 742–747.

Atwell, J. W., Cardoso, G. C., Whittaker, D. J. *et al.* (2012). Boldness behavior and stress physiology on a novel urban environment suggest rapid correlated evolutionary adaptation. *Behavioral Ecology*, **23**, 960–969.

Bateman, P. W. & Flemming, P. A. (2011). Who are you looking at? Hadeda ibises use direction of gaze, head orientation and approach speed in their risk assessment of a potential predator. *Journal of Zoology*, **285**, 316–323.

Bennett, P. M. & Owens, I. P. F. (2002). *Evolutionary Ecology of Birds*. Oxford: Oxford University Press.

Blumstein, D. T. (2003). Flight-initiation distance in birds is dependent on intruder starting distance. *Journal of Wildlife Management*, **67**, 852–857.

Blumstein, D. T. (2006). Developing an evolutionary ecology of fear: How life history and natural history traits affect disturbance tolerance in birds. *Animal Behaviour*, **71**, 389–399.

Blumstein, D. T. (2014). Attention, habituation, and anti-predator behaviour: Implications for urban birds. In D. Gil & H. Brumm (eds). *Avian Urban Ecology*. Oxford: Oxford University Press, pp. 41–53.

Blumstein, D. T. & Daniel, J. C. (2005). The loss of anti-predator behaviour following isolation on islands. *Proceedings of the Royal Society of London – Series B*, **272**, 1663–1668.

Blumstein, D. T. & Fernández-Juricic, E. (2010). *A Primer of Conservation Behavior*. Sunderland, MA: Sinauer.

Blumstein, D. T., Anthony, L. L., Harcourt, R. & Ross, G. (2003). Testing a key assumption of buffer zones: Is flight initiation distance a species-specific trait? *Biological Conservation*, **110**, 97–100.

Blumstein, D. T., Fernández-Juricic, E., LeDee, O. *et al.* (2004). Avian risk assessment: Effects of perching height and detectability. *Ethology*, **110**, 273–285.

Bolnick, D. I. & Preisser, E. L. (2005). Resource competition modifies the strength of trait-mediated predator–prey interactions: A meta-analysis. *Ecology*, **86**, 2771–2779.

Boyer, J. S., Hass, L. L., Lurie, M. H. & Blumstein, D. T. (2006). Effect of visibility on time allocation and escape decisions in crimson rosellas. *Australian Journal of Zoology*, **54**, 363–367.

Burger, J. (1981). The effect of human activity on birds at a coastal bay. *Biological Conservation*, **21**, 231–241.

Burger, J. & Gochfeld, M. (1981). Discrimination of the threat of direct versus tangential approach to the nest by incubating herring and great black-backed gulls. *Journal of Comparative Physiology and Psychology*, **95**, 676–684.

Cárdenas, Y. L., Shen, B., Zung, L. & Blumstein, D. T. (2005). Evaluating temporal and spatial margins of safety in galahs. *Animal Behaviour*, **70**, 1395–1399.

Carrete, M. & Tella, J. L. (2010). Individual consistency in flight initiation distances in burrowing owls: A new hypothesis on disturbance-induced habitat selection. *Biology Letters*, **6**, 167–170.

Carrete, M. & Tella, J. L. (2011a). Inter-individual variability in fear of humans and relative brain size of the species are related to contemporary urban invasions in birds. *Public Library of Science One*, **6**, e18859.

Carrete, M. & Tella, J. L. (2013). High individual consistency in fear of humans throughout the adult lifespan of rural and urban burrowing owls. *Scientific Reports*, **3**, 3524.

Clucas, B., Marzluff, J. M., Mackovjak, D. & Palmquist, I. (2013). Do American crows pay attention to human gaze and facial expressions? *Ethology*, **119**, 1–7.

Cohen, J. (1988). *Statistical Power Analysis for the Behavioral Sciences*. Hillsdale, NJ: Lawrence Erlbaum.

Cooke, A. S. (1980). Observations on how close certain passerine species will tolerate an approaching human in rural and suburban areas. *Biological Conservation*, **18**, 85–88.

Cooper, W. E. & Blumstein, D. T. (2013). Novel effects of monitoring predators on costs of fleeing and not fleeing explain flushing early in economic escape theory. *Behavioral Ecology*, **25**, 44–52.

Daly, M. & Wilson, M. (1983). *Sex, Evolution, and Behavior*, 2nd edn. Boston, MA: Willard Grant.

Darwin, C. (1868). *The Variation of Animals and Plants under Domestication*. London: John Murray.

de Jong, A., Magnhagen, C. & Thulin, C.-G. (2013). Variable flight initiation distance in incubating European curlew. *Behavioral Ecology and Sociobiology*, **67**, 1089–1096.

Díaz, M., Møller, A. P., Flensted-Jensen, E. *et al.* (2013). The geography of fear: A latitudinal gradient in anti-predator escape distances of birds across Europe. *Public Library of Science One*, **8**, e64634.

Domenici, P., Blagburn, J. M. & Bacon, J. P. (2011a). Animal escapology I: Theoretical issues and emerging trends in escape trajectories. *Journal of Experimental Biology*, **214**, 2463–2473.

Domenici, P., Blagburn, J. M. & Bacon, J. P. (2011b). Animal escapology II: Escape trajectory case studies. *Journal of Experimental Biology*, **214**, 2474–2494.

Dumont, F., Pasquaretta, C., Reale, D., Bogliani, G. & von Hardenberg, A.(2012). Flight initiation distance: Biological effect or mathematical artefact? *Ethology*, **118**, 1051–1062.

Eason, P. K., Sherman, P. T., Rankin, O. & Coleman, B. (2006). Factors affecting flight initiation distance in American robins. *Journal of Wildlife Management*, **70**, 1796–1800.

Falconer, D. S. & Mackay, T. F. C. (1996). *Introduction to Quantitative Genetics*, 4th edn. New York, NY: Longman.

Fernández-Juricic, E. (2002). Can human disturbance promote nestedness? A case study with birds in an urban fragmented landscape. *Oecologia*, **131**, 269–278.

Fernández-Juricic, E., Vaca, R. & Schroeder. N. (2004). Spatial and temporal responses of forest birds to human approaches in a protected area and implications for two management strategies. *Biological Conservation*, **117**, 407–416.

Fernández-Juricic, E., Venier, P., Renison, D. & Blumstein, F. T. (2005). Sensitivity of wildlife to spatial patterns of recreationist behavior: a critical assessment of minimum approaching distances and buffer areas for grassland birds. *Biological Conservation*, **125**, 225–235.

Fernández-Juricic, E., Blumstein, D. T., Abrica, G. *et al.* (2006). Relationships of anti-predator escape and post-escape responses with body mass and morphology: A comparative avian study. *Evolutionary Ecology Research*, **8**, 731–752.

Frid, A. & Dill, L. M. (2002). Human-caused disturbance stimuli as a form of predation risk. *Conservation Ecology*, 6, www.consecol.org/Journal/vol6/iss1/art11/print.pdf.

Geist, C., Liao, J., Libby, S. & Blumstein, D. T. (2005). Does intruder group size and orientation affect flight initiation distance in birds? *Animal Biodiversity and Conservation*, **28**, 69–73.

Glover, H. K., Weston, M. A., Maguire, G. S., Miller, K. K. & Christie, B. A. (2011). Towards ecologically meaningful and socially acceptable buffers: Response distances of shorebirds in Victoria, Australia, to human disturbance. *Landscape and Urban Planning*, **103**, 326–334.

Guay, P.-J., Weston, M. A., Symonds, M. R. E. & Glover, H. K. (2013). Brains and bravery: Little evidence of a relationship between brain size and flightiness in shorebirds. *Austral Ecology*, **38**, 516–522.

Healy, S. D. & Rowe, C. (2007). A critique of comparative studies of brain size. *Proceedings of the Royal Society B*, **274**, 453–464.

Hediger, H. (1934). Zur Biologie und Psychologie der Flucht bei Tieren. *Biologisches Zentralblatt*, **54**, 21–40.

Heil, L., Fernández-Juricic, E., Renison, D. *et al.* (2007). Avian responses to tourism in the biogeographically isolated high Córdoba Mountains, Argentina. *Biodiversity and Conservation*, **16**, 1009–1026.

Keyel, A. C., Peck, D. T. & Reed, J. M. (2012). No evidence far individual assortment by temperament relative to patch area or patch openness in the bobolink. *Condor*, **114**, 212–218.

Koricheva, J., Gurevich, J. & Mengersen, K. (2013). *Handbook of Meta-analysis in Ecology and Evolution*. Princeton, NJ: Princeton University Press.

Laursen, K., Kahlert, J. & Frikke, J. (2005). Factors affecting escape distances of staging waterbirds. *Wildlife Biology*, **11**, 13–19.

Lee, S., Hwang, S., Joe, Y. *et al.* (2013). Direct look from a predator shortens the risk-assessment time by prey. *Public Library of Science One*, **8**, e64977.

Legagneux, P. & Ducatez, S. (2013). European birds adjust their flight initiation distance to road speed limits. *Biology Letters*, **9**, 20130417.

Lin, T., Coppack, T., Lin, Q. *et al.* (2012). Does avian flight initiation distance indicate tolerance towards urban disturbance?*Ecological Indicators*, **15**, 30–35.

Madsen, J. (1995). Impacts of disturbance on migratory waterfowl. *Ibis*, **137**, S67–S74.

Madsen, J. (1998a). Experimental refuges for migratory waterfowl in Danish wetlands. I. Baseline assessment of disturbance effects of recreational activities. *Journal of Applied Ecology*, **35**, 386–397.

Madsen, J. (1998b). Experimental refuges for migratory waterfowl in Danish wetlands. II. Tests of hunting disturbance effects. *Journal of Applied Ecology*, **35**, 398–417.

Madsen, J. & Fox, A. D. (1995). Impacts of hunting disturbance on waterbirds: A review. *Wildlife Biology*, **1**, 193–207.

Martín, J., de Neve, L., Polo, V., Fargallo, J. A. & Soler, M. (2006). Health-dependent vulnerability to predation affects escape responses of unguarded chinstrap penguin chicks. *Behavioral Ecology and Sociobiology*, **60**, 778–784.

Møller, A. P. (2008a). Flight distance of urban birds, predation and selection for urban life. *Behavioral Ecology and Sociobiology*, **63**, 63–75.

Møller, A. P. (2008b). Flight distance and population trends in European breeding birds. *Behavioral Ecology*, **19**, 1095–1102.

Møller, A. P. (2009a). Basal metabolic rate and risk taking behavior in birds. *Journal of Evolutionary Biology*, **22**, 2420–2429.

Møller, A. P. (2009b). Successful city dwellers: A comparative study of the ecological characteristics of urban birds in the Western Palearctic. *Oecologia*, **159**, 849–858.

Møller, A. P. (2010a). Interspecific variation in fear responses predicts urbanization in birds. *Behavioral Ecology*, **21**, 365–371.

Møller, A. P. (2010b). Up, up, and away: Relative importance of horizontal and vertical escape from predators for survival and senescence. *Journal of Evolutionary Biology*, **23**, 1689–1698.

Møller, A. P. (2012). Urban areas as refuges from predators and flight distance of prey. *Behavioral Ecology*, **23**, 1030–1035.

Møller, A. P. (2014). Life history, predation and flight initiation distance in a migratory bird. *Journal of Evolutionary Biology*, **27**, 1105–1113.

Møller, A. P. (2014a). Behavioural and ecological predictors of urbanization. In D. Gil and H. Brumm (eds.) *Avian Urban Ecology*. Oxford: Oxford University Press, pp. 54–68

Møller, A. P. (2014b). Urban birds use cheap escape: Variance in escape direction from predators by prey.

Møller, A. P. & Erritzøe, J. (2010). Flight distance and eye size in birds. *Ethology*, **116**, 458–465.

Møller, A. P. & Erritzøe, J. (2014). Predator–prey interactions, flight initiation distance and brain size. *Journal of Evolutionary Biology*, **27**, 34–42.

Møller, A. P. & Garamszegi, L. Z. (2012). Between individual variation in risk taking behavior and its life history consequences. *Behavioral Ecology*, **23**, 843–853.

Møller, A.P. & Jennions, M.D. (2002). How much variance can be explained by ecologists and evolutionary biologists? *Oecologia*, **132**, 492–500.

Møller, A. P. & Liang, W. (2013). Tropical birds take small risks. *Behavioral Ecology*, **24**, 267–272.

Møller, A. P. & Tryjanowski, P. (2014). Direction of approach by predators and flight initiation distance of urban and rural populations of birds. *Behavioral Ecology*, **25**, 960–966.

Møller, A. P., Nielsen, J. T. & Garamszegi, L. Z. (2008). Risk taking by singing males. *Behavioral Ecology*, **19**, 41–53.

Møller, A. P., Bonisoli-Alquati, A., Rudolfsen, G. & Mousseau, T. A. (2011). Chernobyl birds have smaller brains. *Public Library of Science One*, **6**, e16862.

Møller, A. P., Vágási, C. I. & Pap, P. L. (2013). Risk-taking and the evolution of mechanisms for rapid escape from predators. *Journal of Evolutionary Biology*, **26**, 1143–1150.

Mukherjee, S., Ray-Mukherjee, J. & Sarabia, R. (2013). Behaviour of American crows (*Corvus brachyrhynchos*) when encountering an oncoming vehicle. *Canadian Field-Naturalist*, **127**, 229–233.

Müller, J. C., Partecke, J., Hatchwell, B. J., Gaston, K. J. & Evans, K. L. (2013). Candidate gene polymorphisms for behavioural adaptations during urbanization in blackbirds. *Molecular Ecology*, **22**, 3629–3637.

Partecke, J., Schwabl, I. & Gwinner, E. (2006). Stress and the city: urbanisation and its effects on the stress physiology in European blackbirds. *Ecology*, **87**, 1945–1952.

Partecke, J., Van't Hof, T. J. & Gwinner, E. (2005). Underlying physiological control of reproduction and forest-dwelling blackbirds *Turdus merula*. *Journal of Avian Biology*, **36**, 295–305.

Pennycuick, C. J. (1989). *Bird Flight Performance*. Oxford: Oxford University Press.

Preisser, E. L., Bolnick, D. I. & Benard, M. F. (2005). Scared to death? The effects of intimidation and consumption in predator–prey interactions. *Ecology*, **86**, 501–509.

Rand, A. S. (1964). Inverse relationship between temperature and shyness in the lizard *Anolis lineatopus*. *Ecology*, **45**, 863–864.

Reif, J., Böhning-Gaese, K., Flade, M., Schwarz, J. & Schwager, M. (2011). Population trends of birds across the iron curtain: Brain matters. *Biological Conservation*, **144**, 2524–2533.

Rodriguez-Prieto, I., Fernández-Juricic, E. & Martín, J. (2008a). To run or to fly: Low cost versus low risk strategies in blackbirds. *Behaviour*, **125**, 1125–1138.

Roff, D. (1992). *Life History Evolution*. New York, NY: Chapman & Hall.

Rosenthal, R. (1994). Parametric measures of effect size. In Cooper, H. & Hedges, L. V. (eds). *The Handbook of Research Synthesis*. New York, NY: Russel Sage Foundation, pp. 231–244.

Rosenberg, M. S., Adams, D. C. & Gurevitch, J. (2000). *MetaWin: Statistical Software for Meta-analysis. Version 2.1*. Sunderland, MA: Sinauer Associates.

St. Clair, J. J. H., García-Peña, G. E., Woods, R. W. & Székely, T. (2012). Presence of mammalian predators decreases tolerance to human disturbance in a breeding shorebird. *Behavioral Ecology*, **21**, 1285–1292.

Samia, D. S. M., Nomura, F. & Blumstein, D. T. (2013). Do animals generally flush early and avoid the rush? A meta-analysis. *Biology Letters*, **9**, 20130016.

Scales, J., Hyman, J. & Hughes, M. (2011). Behavioral syndromes break down in urban song sparrow populations. *Ethology*, **117**, 1–9.

Seltmann, M. W., Öst, M., Jaatinen, K. *et al.* (2012). Stress responsiveness, age and body condition interactively affect flight initiation distance in breeding female eiders. *Animal Behaviour*, **84**, 889–896.

Smith-Castro, J. R. & Rodewald, A. D. (2010). Behavioral responses of nesting birds to human disturbance along recreational trails. *Journal of Field Ornithology*, **81**, 130–138.

Stankowich, T. & Blumstein, D. T. (2005). Fear in animals: A meta-analysis and review of risk assessment. *Proceedings of the Royal Society of London B*, **272**, 2627–2634.

Tarlow, E. M. & Blumstein, D. T. (2007). Evaluating methods to quantify anthropogenic stressors on wild animals. *Applied Animal Behaviour Science*, **102**, 429–451.

Tatner, P. & Bryant, D. M. (1986). Flight cost of a small passerine measured using doubly labeled water: Implications for energetic studies. *Auk*, **103**, 169–180.

Thaxter, C. B., Joys, A. C., Gregory, R. D., Baillie, S. R. & Noble, D. G. (2010). Hypotheses to explain patterns of population change among breeding bird species in England. *Biological Conservation*, **143**, 2006–2019.

Tomialojc, L. (1970). Quantitative studies on the synanthropic avifauna of Legnica town and its environs. *Acta Ornithologica*, **12**, 293–392.

Valcarcel, A. & Fernández-Juricic, E. (2009). Antipredator strategies of house finches: Are urban habitats safe spots from predators even when humans are around? *Behavioral Ecology and Sociobiology*, **63**, 673–685.

Weston, M. A., McLeod, E. M., Blumstein, D. T. & Guay, P.-J. (2012). A review of flight-initiation distances and their application to managing disturbance to Australian birds. *Emu*, **112**, 269–286.

Wright, S. (1968). *Evolution and the Genetics of Populations. Vol. 1. Genetic and Biometric Foundations*. Chicago, IL: University of Chicago Press.

Zanette, L. T., White, A. F., Allen, M. C. & Clinchy, M. (2011). Perceived predation risk reduces the number of offspring songbirds produce per year. *Science*, **334**, 1398–1401.

5 Reptiles

William E. Cooper, Jr.

5.1 Introduction

Predator–prey encounters matching the scenario of optimal escape theory begin in two ways. Upon detecting an approaching predator, lizards and other reptiles that are moving often stop, presumably reducing the probability of being detected by the predator. Those that are immobile remain still for the same reason as they monitor approaching predators. A large majority of studies of flight initiation distance (FID) and other escape variables have reported effects of predation risk factors, which are important because they affect the cost of not fleeing. Although fewer studies report effects of factors that impose opportunity costs (i.e., costs of not fleeing), much of what is known about these effects has been learned in studies of lizards. Effects of the initial fitness of lizards and other reptiles on escape behavior have been studied only indirectly.

Reptiles are one of the three taxonomic groups in which escape behavior has been studied most extensively, the others being birds and mammals (Stankowich & Blumstein 2005; Chapter 3; Chapter 4). Although advances in our understanding of phylogenetic relationships among major vertebrate taxa has removed crocodilians from Reptilia, and the placement of turtles on the vertebrate phylogenetic tree remains uncertain, the traditional taxonomic categories of reptiles are covered in this chapter, primarily because herpetologists continue to study these groups. Because little is known about escape decisions by turtles, crocodilians, and snakes, most of this chapter presents current knowledge about escape by lizards. Snakes constitute a major lizard clade, but their escape behavior is presented separately because they differ ecologically and morphologically from other lizards.

Factors affecting decisions about when and how far to flee are the main focus, including factors that affect predation risk and cost of fleeing. The direction of fleeing in relation to predators and refuges, and the selection of and entry into refuges are also discussed. Effect sizes are correlation coefficients taken from the original studies or calculated from P values and sample sizes or other statistics using the Meta-Analysis Calculator. Values are mean ± SE. Many citations have been omitted from the text, but are available in the electronic supplementary material (ESM 5.1) along with a table of effects, effect sizes, taxa, and sources (ESM 5.2). These are available at

Escaping From Predators: An Integrative View of Escape Decisions, ed. W. E. Cooper and D. T. Blumstein. Published by Cambridge University Press. © Cambridge University Press 2015.

www.cambridge.org/9781107060548. Information about alternative escape strategies is presented in concluding sections for lizards and snakes.

5.2   Lizards

5.2.1   Predation risk factors that affect escape during approach

5.2.1.1   Position, habitat, and environmental factors
5.2.1.1.1   Distance to refuge, perch height, and direction to refuge
Many lizards escape by running to and entering refuges, most commonly trees, logs, crevices in rocks, and animal burrows (Cooper 1998a). Fleeing lizards may stop on the surface or enter a refuge; many individuals stop very close to a refuge, avoiding costs of refuge use if the predator does not attack. The distance to the nearest refuge and its direction with respect to the approaching predator determine projected arrival times of predator and prey at the refuge (Cooper 1997a; Kramer & Bonenfant 1997). Because arrival time increases as distance to refuge increases, risk of being captured at a particular FID increases as distance to refuge increases. Therefore FID is predicted by economic escape theory to increase as distance to refuge increases. If lizards farther from a refuge are more likely than those adjacent to a refuge to stop before entering a refuge, distance fled (DF) will be shorter than distance to a refuge, but is likely to be longer than for lizards closer to a refuge for two reasons. First, lizards that remain outside a refuge must move far enough from the predator to provide a margin of safety in the event of continued approach. Second, distance fled by lizards close to a refuge must often be less than the margin of safety.

Lizards closer to a refuge initially are expected to permit closer approach before fleeing and are more likely to enter a refuge than those farther from a refuge. The predator's proximity when escape begins implies greater risk of being captured should the prey not enter a refuge. Therefore when distance to a refuge is shorter, the probability of entering a refuge is predicted to be greater.

In all of 17 studies of ten lizard species representing five families, FID increased as distance to refuge increased (Figure 5.1). The effect size ($r = 0.49 \pm 0.06$, range 0.16–0.93) was intermediate. The primary determinant of the effect size is likely to be the degree of variation in distance to refuge among individuals. The influence of distance to refuge on FID may be somewhat stronger than indicated by the mean effect size because the range of distance to refuge was small in some cases (Cooper & Wilson 2007). In some species that occur at highly variable distances from refuge, the effect size is large (*Anolis lineatopus:* $r = 0.93$, Cooper 2006a; *Egernia cunninghami:* $r = 0.90$, Eifler 2001; and *Leiocephalus carinatus:* $r = 0.87$, Cooper 2007a).

Two of the lowest r values were taken from a study in which the method of approach differed from that in all other studies (Bulova 1994). Bulova walked through the habitat in a straight line, and did not stop upon sighting a lizard, but continued on her path. Researchers in the remaining studies walked through the habitat until sighting a lizard,

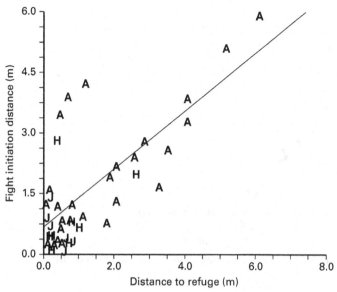

Figure 5.1   As distance to refuge increases, FID increases in *Sceloporus woodi*. (Stiller & McBrayer 2013)

stopped moving, turned toward the lizard, and then walked directly toward it. In the only direct comparison of the effect size for the two methods, the effect sizes for *Callisaurus draconoides* were 0.16 in Bulova's study and 0.47 in Cooper (2010a). Variation in directness of approach using Bulova's method may have affected perceived risk, which is lower for indirect approaches. Because shorter FID is predicted for lower risk, the association between FID and distance to refuge would be weakened by including indirect approaches.

Distance to refuge is positively correlated with distance fled in all of ten studies of species from five families, significantly so in eight of them ($r = 0.49 \pm 0.09$, range 0.12–0.91). Reasons for the large differences in effect size are not entirely clear, but include the difference in method of approach discussed above and interspecific differences in degree of variation in distance from refuge. In the only study to measure the relationship between distance to refuge and the probability of entering refuge when approached, a larger proportion of lizards entered refuge when closer than farther from refuge ($r = 0.56$, Cooper 2007a). The relationships of distance fled and probability of entering refuge to distance to refuge are as predicted by economic escape theory.

For lizards on tree trunks and other surfaces having vertical aspects, perch height strongly affects vulnerability to predation by terrestrial predators. Many species flee up trees to reach heights where they are safe and often flee to and along the side of the tree opposite that of the approaching predator, where their movements are invisible. Therefore perch height is expected to have effects on escape behavior similar to those of distance to refuge. For species that climb upward to escape, predation risk is greatest at perch height (PH) = 0. As a lizard climbs higher, its risk of predation decreases until it attains a height at and above which predation risk is zero and fleeing is unnecessary.

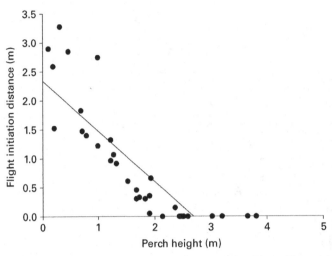

Figure 5.2   As perch height increases, FID decreases in *Anolis graham*. (Cooper 2010b)

Flight initiation distance should therefore decrease as PH increases in the range $0 \leq PH \leq PH_{0risk}$). Distance fled (climbed) should increase as PH decreases in the range $0 \leq PH \leq PH_{0risk}$, but should be unaffected at higher PH. When approached directly, all lizards at risk should flee before the predator reaches the tree.

Fewer species may flee downward from terrestrial or aerial predators. For example, grass-bush anoles (*Anolis spp.*) occupy low bushes that do not permit upward escape from terrestrial predators large enough to reach the tops of the bushes (Williams 1983). These species flee downward, often into low vegetation on the ground (Cooper 2006b, 2012). Other species escape upward when on vertical surfaces that are tall enough to permit escape, but flee downward or onto shorter vertical objects such as fence posts (Schneider *et al.* 2000). When prey flee downward, predation risk is lowest on the ground and increases as PH increases. Economic escape theory predicts that FID increases as PH increases when escape is downward. Distance fled also is expected to increase as PH above ground increases.

Predictions for FID have been confirmed consistently. In all of 13 species that flee upward, including representatives of five families, FID increased as PH decreased (Figure 5.2). The effect size is similar to that of distance to refuge (absolute value of $r = -0.50 \pm 0.07$, range 0.12–0.88). For three species of *Anolis* that fled downward, FID increased as PH increased ($r = 0.36 \pm 0.13$, range 0.27–0.50). Although the absolute magnitudes of the effect sizes for lizards that escape upward and downward are similar, the effects are in opposite directions. The escape responses of lizards that fled upward differed from those of species that escaped by fleeing downward (Fisher exact test, $p = 0.0036$, two-tailed). Distance fled decreased as PH increased in the sole species studied, which escaped upward. However, the relationship was weak and not significant. The range of PH in which some individuals flee and others do not presumably reveals individual differences in boldness or wariness (López *et al.* 2005).

Prey sometimes flee to nearby refuges that may be in any direction, including in the direction of the predator. When a prey flees toward an approaching predator, it has less time to reach refuge ahead of the predator than when it flees away (Kramer & Bonenfant 1997). In one lizard species both FID ($r = 0.55$) and DF ($r = 0.54$) are longer when a prey flees to a refuge toward rather than away from the predator. The finding for FID matches the prediction based on greater risk of fleeing toward a predator. The longer DF for prey approaching predators suggests that the lizards may flee longer distances to reach secure refuges, flee all the way to refuge, or a higher proportion of the distance to refuge, when fleeing toward versus away from the predator, or that they flee toward the predator when alternative refuges are unavailable nearby. In another species when the predator is between the prey and refuge, FID is longer when the prey flees away from the predator ($r = 0.62$); lizards delay fleeing when the refuge is blocked, often fleeing toward, but around the predator at an acute angle (Cooper 1999a).

5.2.1.1.2 *Microhabitat*

Escape behavior may differ among microhabitats for multiple reasons, including differences in distance to refuge, detectability, and effects of substrate on running speed. Lizards that escape by climbing typically have a shorter distance to flee to safety when on trees than on other substrates, and are therefore predicted to have shorter FID and shorter DF. In the skink *Plestiodon laticeps* FID ($r = 0.57 \pm 0.05$) and DF ($r = 0.35 \pm 0.03$, range 0.32–0.37) were longer and likelihood of entering refuge was lower ($r = 0.46 \pm 0.02$, range 0.44 – 0.48) for lizards on rocks and ground than on trees (r values for two studies each) (Cooper 1998a). Similar effects were observed in the phrynosomatid *Sceloporus virgatus* (Cooper & Wilson 2007), for which FID ($r = 0.79 \pm .13$, range = 0.65–0.92) and DF ($r = 0.35 \pm 0.09$, range 0.26–0.45) were shorter for lizards on trees than on ground or rocks (two studies each). These findings are in part an extension of the results for perch height to situations in which prey must flee to a tree to attain zero PH.

5.2.1.1.3 *Habitat openness and exposure*

In habitats or microhabitats where lizards are more detectable or more vulnerable to attack, lizards are expected to be warier, which may be expressed by longer FID and DF, increased tendency to flee, and/or increased likelihood of entering refuge. Such effects have been investigated by comparing escape by lizards in habitats that differ in vegetative cover, when individuals in the same habitat are exposed versus partially concealed, in circumstances that affect their conspicuousness due to background matching and movement, and in microhabitats that differ in safety.

In open, sparsely vegetated habitats, prey may have longer FID and DF because they tend to be farther from refuges and are more detectable. Flight initiation distance was longer in open than densely vegetated habitats in four species; in two other species, FID was longer in open habitats in one of two studies. For all comparisons combined, the effect size is modest (0.37 ± 0.12), but quite variable (range 0.00–0.93), with only two values above 0.33.

Lizards fled longer distances in more open habitats in five of six comparisons in four species; in one of these species no effect was observed in one of two comparisons. The effect size for all comparisons was small ($r = 0.25 \pm 0.07$). In a comparative study of 25 species of *Liolaemus*, DF was longer in more open than less open habitats (Schulte *et al.* 2004).

In all of six species from four families, FID was shorter for partially concealed than fully exposed lizards. The importance of partial concealment for risk assessment is suggested by the large effect size ($r = 0.73 \pm 0.05$, range 0.54–0.85). In two species exposed lizards were more likely to flee than were partially concealed lizards ($r = 0.57 \pm 0.14$, range 0.43–0.71).

5.2.1.1.4 *Temperature*

Body temperature strongly affects running speed in lizards (Huey 1982). At cold temperatures they are immobilized or move very slowly, but running speed increases as body temperature increases until high speed is maintained over a range of body temperatures near the preferred body temperature (Huey 1982). Because escape ability improves and risk when a predator is at a given distance decreases as running speed increases, prey are predicted to have shorter FID as body temperature increases. However, if cooler lizards stay closer to refuge or rely more on immobility to avoid being detected, FID might increase as body temperature increases or be unaffected by body temperature if the effects of temperature on speed and distance to refuge and/or crypsis via immobility counteract each other.

Few studies have reported effects of body temperature on escape behavior because lizards must be captured immediately after fleeing to measure body temperature, whereas air temperature and substrate temperature are easy to measure. Body temperature is more highly correlated with substrate temperature than with air temperature. Due to the weaker correlation of air and substrate temperature than body temperature with running speed (Hertz *et al.* 1983), predictions are less clear than for body temperature.

Flight initiation distance increased as body temperature decreased (Figure 5.3) in three species ($r = 0.52 \pm 0.10$, range 0.39–0.72) and increased as body temperature increased in two other species ($r = 0.44 \pm 0.11$). In two species the proportion of lizards that fled increased as body temperature increased ($r = 0.92 \pm 0.04$, range 0.88–0.97). Flight initiation distance increased as substrate temperature increased in two studies of one species ($r = 0.63 \pm 0.09$, range 0.54–0.72) and decreased as substrate temperature increased in another species ($r = 0.39$). Substrate temperature was uncorrelated with distance fled in two species.

Air temperature, being weakly related to body temperature, is often unrelated or weakly related to escape variables. In four species FID was unrelated to air temperature. In two species FID increased as air temperature increased ($r = 0.16 \pm 0.00$, range 0.16–0.17), and in four species FID decreased as air temperature increased ($r = 0.35 \pm 0.09$, range 0.21–0.57). In five of seven species, distance fled was unrelated to air temperature; in the other two species distance fled increased as air temperature increased ($r = 0.22 \pm 0.06$, range 0.16–0.27). The proportion of lizards that fled increased at air

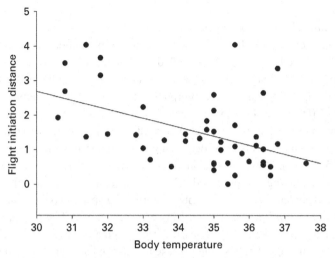

Figure 5.3 As body temperature increases, FID decreases in *Sceloporus virgatus*. (Cooper 2011c)

temperature increased in a single species ($r = 0.79$). The proportion of individuals that entered refuge decreased as air temperature increased in all four studies of three species ($r = 0.65 \pm 0.15$, range 0.28–1.0).

As expected, effect sizes for air temperature were smaller than for body temperature and substrate temperature. Temperature profoundly affects many aspects of behavior in ectotherms such as lizards, including all four escape variables examined. As suggested above, differences among species in the direction of the relationships of temperature to FID and DF may indicate that some species may stay closer to refuges when cool, whereas others do not adjust distance to refuge to current temperatures.

5.2.1.1.5 Wind speed

Bulova (1994) reasoned that high wind speed reduces body temperature, which in turn reduces running speed. She predicted that FID and DF would increase as wind speed increased to compensate for slower running. In one of two species in her study, FID decreased as wind speed increased ($r = -0.13$), but wind speed did not affect DF. In the other species FID was unrelated to wind speed, but DF increased as wind speed increased ($r = 0.26$). These small effects might be indirect effects of environmental correlates of wind speed. That the direction of the effect of wind speed on FID was opposite to that predicted hints that lizards might be harder to detect in windy conditions.

5.2.1.1.6 Time of day and season

Time of day affected neither FID nor DF in the agamid *Lophognathus temporalis* (Blamires 1999). Presumably, behavioral thermoregulation suffices to maintain body temperature in a narrow range throughout the day, obviating any effect of diel variation in temperature on running speed.

5.2.1.2   Prey traits

5.2.1.2.1   *Prey speed, morphology, and body condition*

Because faster prey can reach refuge sooner or outrun predators, FID is predicted to decrease as prey speed increases. Distance fled is predicted to increase as running speed increases provided that lizards often flee without entering refuge and running speed does not affect duration of fleeing. Using morphological correlates of running speed, the prediction for FID was verified for one test and contradicted for another test in the same species (Hawlena *et al.* 2009). That FID increased as tail length decreased ($r = 0.34$) is readily interpretable as an effect of decreasing running speed as tail length decreases (see section 5.2.1.2.4). However, FID increased as relative hind limb length increased ($r = 0.48$), contradicting the predicted effect of longer hind limb length to increase running speed. Hawlena *et al.* (2009) noted that running speed may be unimportant for escape by *Podarcis lilfordi*, which historically experienced very low predation pressure before human beings arrived in the Balearic Archipelago and currently experience very little predation in the population studied. These lizards typically stay close to vegetation that provides cover. Additional studies are needed to directly examine the effect of running speed on FID in lizard populations subject to higher levels of predation.

Morphological correlates of running speed and stride length were examined by Losos *et al.* (2002) in 17 cordylid species. Distance fled increased as femur length increased ($r = 0.76$) and as spine length increased ($r = 0.75$). These large interspecific effects are consistent with the prediction that DF increases as running speed increases.

Prey in better body condition have greater expected fitness than those in poorer condition. The asset protection principle states that prey with larger assets will be more cautious in their defense (Clark 1994). Escape theory therefore predicts that prey having better body condition have longer FID. In a single species FID increased as body condition improved ($r = 0.57$), as predicted. This test confirms the prediction for initial fitness, one of the three major components that determine FID in optimal escape theory (Cooper & Frederick 2007). Further tests of indicators of fitness are needed to assess the general validity of the prediction.

5.2.1.2.2   *Habituation*

When potential predators are present frequently or for long periods, but do not attack, prey may assess the threat of predation to be low, i.e., they may become habituated. Lizards in populations frequently exposed to people are predicted to have shorter FIDs than in populations infrequently exposed. Even if predation risk is high, prey that are constantly exposed to predators must accept greater risk if they are to perform essential activities such as foraging and social behavior. Both risk allocation (Lima & Bednekoff 1999) and habituation predict that FID will be shorter where predators are frequently or constantly present. Nevertheless, habituation is the likely explanation for decreased FID when the predators rarely or never attack because predation risk is very low, which is not the case under the risk allocation hypothesis, and because some prey become so habituated that they allow themselves to be touched (Cooper, personal observations).

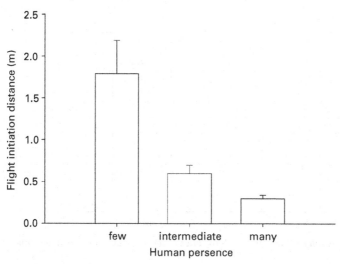

Figure 5.4 In *Anolis lineatopus*, FID is shorter where lizards are habituated to human presence. (Cooper 2010b)

In all of eleven lizard species from six families, FID was shorter in habituated than unhabituated populations (Figure 5.4). The effect size of habituation was substantial ($r = 0.50 \pm 0.06$) and variable (range 0.16–0.73). It is expected to vary with the difference in degree of exposure to human beings among pairs of populations. All findings are consistent with the interpretation that FID is shorter in populations where lizards are habituated to people.

5.2.1.2.3 *Prey sex, age, and body size*

Economic escape theory makes no general predictions about sex differences. However, if ecological or morphological differences between sexes affect predation risk, the sex at greater risk is predicted to be warier. Flight initiation distance has been reported separately for the sexes in 38 species from eight families. Flight initiation distance was longer in males than females in eight species and in one of three populations in a ninth ($r = 0.30 \pm 0.08$, range 0.20–0.42 for cases in which a difference was detected), whereas FID was longer in females than males in three species and in one of six populations of a fourth species ($r = 0.22 \pm 0.06$, range 0.08–0.35). Males had longer FID than females in all three lacertid species studied (Figure 5.5), but no other relationships between families and occurrence of sex differences in FID are apparent. In 66% of 38 species, no sex difference in FID was observed.

Distance fled did not differ between sexes in 21 species, and was longer in males than females in one species ($r = 0.29$) plus one of three populations of a second species ($r = 0.42$). In no case was DF longer for females than males. The proportion of individuals that entered refuges did not differ between sexes in five species. Males were more likely than females to enter refuges in one species and one of three populations of another ($r = 0.39 \pm 0.04$); in no cases were females more likely to enter refuges.

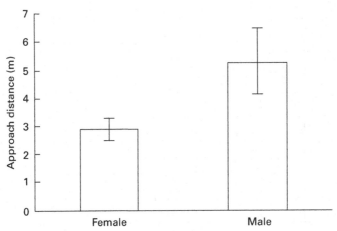

Figure 5.5   In *Platysaurus intermedius*, approach distance (FID) is longer in males than females. (Lailvaux *et al.* 2003)

The sexes of most lizards do not differ substantially in FID, DF, or refuge entry, but when sex differences occur, males seem more likely than females to be the warier sex, perhaps due to greater predation risk associated with some combinations of bright coloration, territorial patrolling and defense, and courtship behavior. However, social costs of fleeing may have countervailing effects (section 5.2.2.2), suggesting that greater wariness by males than females may occur when males are more active and exposed, but not in contexts in which fleeing imposes social opportunity costs. Greater wariness by females could be related to body size differences and slowing due to gravidity or pregnancy (Shine 1980; Cooper *et al.* 1990; Olsson *et al.* 2000). The effect of clutch or litter mass on escape behavior is less clear because gravid females may compensate by remaining closer to refuge or may rely more on crypsis due to immobility to avoid being detected (Cooper *et al.* 1990), which may explain the shorter FID of gravid than non-gravid *Eulamprus tympanum* (Schwartzkopf & Shine 1992).

Relationships between predator and prey sizes and predation risk are variable. As hatchlings grow, they may become too large to be prey of small predators. In such cases, hatchlings might be warier than larger, older individuals. For larger predators, lizards may become increasingly attractive prey as they grow larger. Furthermore, bright tail coloration in juveniles affects both detectability and escape ability (Cooper & Vitt 1985). The balance of these opposing effects may determine the relationship between body size and wariness (Cooper 2011a). Therefore information on such factors is needed to predict the relationships between size/age and wariness.

In studies with a limited range of lizard body size, neither FID (three species) nor DF (two species) was correlated with snout-vent length. However, prey size is important when a wider range of size is included. Larger lizards had longer FID for ten of eleven species belonging to five lizard families ($r = 0.40 \pm 0.09$). In one of these ten species, *Amblyrhynchus cristatus*, a second study reported that FID is longer in juveniles than in either hatchlings or adults ($r = 0.16$), hinting that in this population, juveniles may remain attractive as prey to small predators and have become larger enough to be attractive to larger predators. Given the preponderance of cases in which FID is longer in older, larger, lizards, assessed risk when approached by a large predator appears to be greater for larger lizards. In the sole remaining species, FID did not differ among age/size categories.

For distance fled and refuge entry, age/size relationships to FID are variable. In three species no age/size differences were detected in DF. Of the two other species tested, DF was longer in adults than juveniles in one ($r = 0.56$) and longer in juveniles than adults in the other ($r = 0.67$). The proportion of lizards that entered refuge did not differ among age/size groups in one species; in two species it was greater for larger lizards ($r = 0.49 \pm 0.19$) and in one species it was greater for hatchlings than adults ($r = 0.10$). The relationships of the escape variables DF and refuge entry with age and size may be affected by relationships of age/size with conspicuousness, vulnerability, and distance to refuge, but these factors remain to be investigated.

5.2.1.2.4   *Autotomy and tail condition*

Caudal autotomy (voluntary severing of the tail) often permits lizards to escape when contacted by a predator (Congdon *et al.* 1974; Cooper & Vitt 1985, 1991). Depending on how much of the tail is lost, the ability to use autotomy to escape in future encounters is diminished or lost until the tail regenerates. Running speed decreases after autotomy in most species (Bateman & Fleming 2009; Cooper *et al.* 2009a). Recently autotomized lizards are at greater risk when approached, and are predicted to adjust their behavior to reduce risk. One way of doing so is to increase FID. Additional possibilities are staying closer to refuge and entering refuge.

Effects of recent experimentally induced autotomy have been studied in the field in three species. In *Cordylus melanotus* autotomy did not affect FID or DF, but autotomy also did not affect running speed (McConnachie & Whiting 2003). In *Holbrookia propinqua*, FID was not affected by autotomy, but autotomized lizards stayed closer to refuges ($r = 0.49$) and males, but not females, fled shorter distances than intact lizards ($r = 0.39$; Cooper 2003). In *Sceloporus virgatus* autotomized individuals had longer FID ($r = 0.58$) and were more likely to enter refuges ($r = 0.45$) than individuals having intact tails (Cooper 2007b; Cooper & Wilson 2008).

Effects of autotomy on escape behavior are expected to wane over time as regeneration proceeds, but may persist longer if lizards have adjusted escape strategy to reduce the heightened risk. In observational studies some tail breaks have occurred recently, but others may have occurred weeks or months before observations. In such studies of six species from four families, FID was shorter in autotomized than intact lizards in four species ($r = 0.40 \pm 0.02$), and in larger, but not smaller individuals in a fifth species ($r = 0.68$; Kelt *et al.* 2002). In the remaining species, intact and autotomized lizards had similar FIDs. This suggests that the long-term effect of autotomy on FID may be more consistent across taxa than the short-term effect. The long-term effect may be a consequence of staying closer to refuge or increased reliance on immobility to avoid detection.

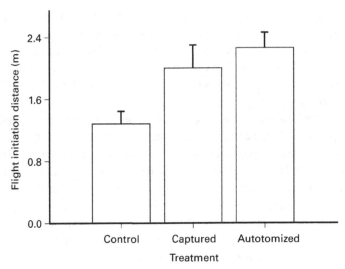

The FID in *Sceloporus virgatus* is longer after the tail is lost by autotomy that in lizards having intact tails. (Cooper 2007b)

Initial and prolonged effects of autotomy may differ. In *Sceloporus virgatus* FID is longer in recently autotomized than intact lizards (Cooper 2007b: Figure 5.6), but shorter when observations are made at longer intervals after autotomy. The initial effect may occur before adjustments in escape strategy occur.

5.2.1.2.5 *Female reproductive condition*

Female lizards run slower when gravid or pregnant than at other times because their mass is increased by eggs or due to changes in physiology while gravid (Shine 1980; Cooper *et al.* 1990; Olsson *et al.* 2000). Because predation risk is greater for slower prey, gravid females are predicted to have longer FID unless they stay closer to refuge or rely more on crypsis conferred by immobility to avoid being detected. Flight inititation distance was shorter for gravid than non-gravid females in three species ($r = 0.30 \pm 0.06$, range 0.18–0.36). In a fourth species FID did not differ between gravid and non-gravid females. Distance fled was shorter for gravid than non-gravid females in one species ($r = 0.23$); in two other species gravidity did not affect DF. Two of the species for which neither FID nor DF was related to gravidity are ecologically similar congeners that usually remain near refuges (Smith 1996; Cooper 2011a). In one of those two species, the proportion of lizards that entered refuge also did not differ between gravid and non-gravid females. That FID was shortened in gravid females in three species and DF in one species suggests that compensatory changes in behavior during gravidity outweighed any increase in risk due to slower running speed. Where no significant differences were detected for FID or DF, gravid females may not have been greatly slowed or any increase in risk was balanced by changes in behavior that reduce risk.

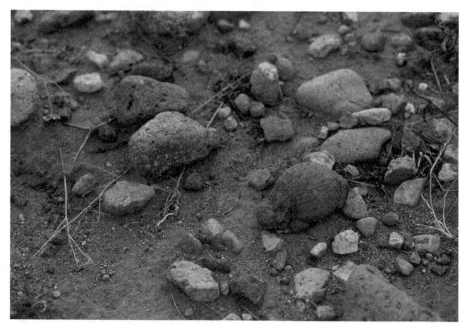

Figure 5.7   The round-tailed horned lizard, *Phrynosoma modestum*, adopts a posture that makes it resemble a small rock. (Cooper & Sherbrooke 2010)

5.2.1.2.6 *Conspicuousness*

Prey that are camouflaged, employ special resemblance to objects, or use cryptic postures (Figure 5.7) are predicted to permit closer approach than more conspicuous lizards. Because movement makes prey highly detectable, prey are predicted to have longer FID after recently moving than after prolonged immobility. Flight initiation distance was shorter where lizards matched backgrounds or objects (Figure 5.8) in two species ($r = 0.56 \pm 0.00$). The horned lizard *Phrynosoma modestum* had longer FID after recent movement than after prolonged immobility ($r = 0.82$; Cooper & Sherbrooke 2010) and when standing than when lying flat on the ground because the contours of the lizard blend into the substrate when lying flat ($r = 0.80$; Cooper & Sherbrooke 2012). In *Callisaurus draconoides* FID and DF were longer after recent movement than immobility (Cooper & Sherbrooke 2013a). These are large effects that deserve further investigation as potentially important cues for risk assessment.

5.2.1.2.7 *Pursuit-deterrent signaling*

Because a predator that has received pursuit-deterrent signals is less likely to attack (Holley 1993; Ruxton *et al.* 2004), predation risk is reduced. In *Callisaurus draconoides*, FID of lizards that have performed a tail-waving display is shorter than in those that have not ($r = 0.57$, Cooper 2011b). This finding confirms the prediction that signaling decreases assessed risk based on the assumption that signaling must be somewhat effective to be maintained by natural selection.

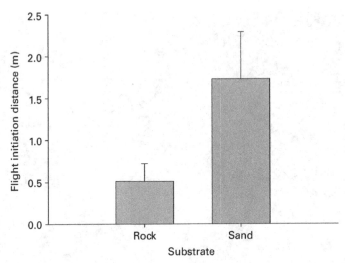

Figure 5.8   When among small rocks *P. modestum* permits closer approach before fleeing than when resting on open sand.

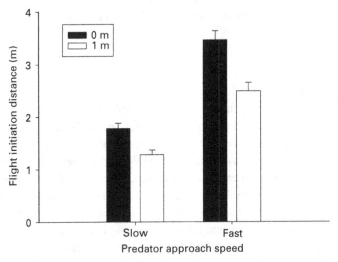

Figure 5.9   In *Sceloporus jarrovii*, FID is longer for direct approaches (0 m) at both slow and fast approach speeds than for indirect approaches that bypass the lizards by 1 m. (Cooper & Avalos 2010)

5.2.1.3   Predator and approach factors

5.2.1.3.1   *Predator approach speed*

The predator's approach speed strongly affects FID. Flight initiation distance was longer for faster than slower approach speed (Figure 5.9) in all seventeen studies of thirteen species representing eight families ($r = 0.72 \pm 0.04$, range 0.30–0.94). These findings emphatically confirm the prediction of economic escape theory that FID increases as predation risk increases. When a predator approaches slowly, lizards allow closer approach because they have more time to reach a refuge than if a predator approaches more rapidly. Even for prey that flee across ground and use refuges infrequently, faster approach speed requires earlier fleeing to attain high escape speed before being overtaken.

Distance fled in two studies was longer when approach was faster ($r = 0.57 \pm 0.19$). The proportion of lizards that entered refuge before ceasing to flee was greater for faster than slower approaches in two studies ($r = 0.65 \pm 0.02$). For both DF and refuge entry, economic predictions are affected by the lizard's distance from refuge. For individuals that flee into refuge or stop by the refuge's entry point, DF is greater for lizards that are farther from the refuge prior to fleeing. The strength of the relationship between distance to refuge and distance fled must increase as the proportion of individuals that enter refuge increases.

Lizards adjacent to refuges are likely to enter upon fleeing, but many individuals at longer distances from refuge flee towards them, but stop fleeing before entering it. This is a consequence of the method of approach used in lizard studies: the approaching researcher stops moving as soon as a lizard begins to flee. After the predator stops, some prey stop before reaching refuge, thereby avoiding costs of refuge use. Lizards farther from refuge are more likely to stop fleeing without entering than lizards closer to refuges, resulting in a decrease in proportion of individuals that enter refuge as initial distance from refuge increases. Therefore the probability of entering refuge decreases as distance to refuge increases, whereas DF increases as distance to refuge increases (section 5.2.1.1.1).

Because FID and DF increase with distance to refuge, studies of effects of approach speed and other risk factors must avoid bias caused by differences in distance to refuge. In typical experimental studies, distance to refuge varies among individual prey, but average distance to refuge is not expected to vary among groups. The effect of variation in distance to refuge is to increase error variance, but not to bias results. This error variance can be reduced by restricting observations to a limited range of distance to refuge. Another way to detect an effect of approach speed is to statistically account for the effect of distance to refuge using multiple regression or by using distance to refuge as a covariate.

5.2.1.3.2 *Directness of approach*

A predator approaching indirectly, i.e., along a path that will not contact the prey, poses less threat than a predator approach directly along a line that intersects the prey's position. An indirectly approaching predator is more likely than one approaching directly to have not yet detected and to fail to detect the prey before the prey passes out of the predator's visual field. A directly approaching predator that has detected the prey is more likely to be approaching to attack, whereas an indirectly approaching predator is more likely to be searching for prey or passing through the area for other reasons.

The main variable used to indicate directness of approach is minimum bypass distance, the predator–prey distance when the predator reaches the closest point to the prey on its path. Minimum bypass distance is zero for direct approaches and is progressively longer as approach becomes less direct. For a fixed minimum bypass distance in such tangential approaches, the angle between the direct and indirect approach paths increases as starting distance decreases. It is important to use a fixed SD across trials unless the goal is to discern an effect of the angle of approach from that of the minimum bypass distance. To my knowledge, no studies have been done to make this potentially important distinction. Several studies have employed the same SD for direct approaches and relatively small minimum bypass distances. They have necessarily used longer SDs to permit longer minimum bypass distances. Reported effect of directness of approach may be a combination of effects of minimum bypass distance and approach angle.

Because risk is predicted to increase as approach becomes more direct, FID is expected to be longest for direct approach and to decrease when approach is less direct. This poses an experimental problem because when the minimum bypass distance exceeds the FID observed for direct approach, lizards do not flee. The minimum bypass distance for lizards that do not flee is therefore not useful as a maximum estimate of FID. For each species, pilot trials must be conducted to determine FIDs for direct approaches and a shorter minimum bypass distance must be chosen for study. Bypass distances longer than the FID for direct approach may be useful in studies of probability of fleeing, but are irrelevant for study of the effect of directness of approach on FID. Due to the effect on assessed risk, DF and probability of fleeing also are predicted to increase as directness of approach increases.

For all of eighteen species of lizards from nine families, FID was longer during direct than indirect approaches (Figure 5.9) using short minimum bypass distances (1–3 m). The longer minimum bypass distances were used for larger or warier species. The effect size was $r = 0.44 \pm 0.06$, range $0.16 - 0.93$).

The proportion of individuals that fled was greater for direct than indirect approaches in all of ten species ($r = 0.70 \pm 0.04$, range 0.19–0.74). During indirect approaches, most individuals that fled did so only when the predator reached the minimum bypass distance (Cooper 1997b). One interpretation is that fleeing frequently occurs at the minimum bypass distance as the risk is greater at that distance than at any other distance. Between the starting point of approach and the point of minimum bypass distance, risk increases should the predator change direction and attack. Probability of fleeing should increase as the predator approaches the point closest to the predator. This presumably accounts for some variance in FID and probability of fleeing. However, the high frequency of fleeing only at the minimum bypass distance suggests another factor. Once the predator passes the closest point to the prey, risk diminishes so that fleeing is not necessary. The prey passes out of a human investigator's line of sight at the minimum bypass distance. Therefore prey that flee at the minimum bypass distance may have delayed escape while the predator was close and could attack upon observing the prey's movements. Once the predator cannot see a prey, the prey can safely withdraw to a nearby refuge (Cooper 1997b).

Little is known about the effect of directness of approach on DF, but DF was longer during direct than indirect approach in two studies. The effect size of directness on DF ($r = 0.35 \pm 0.07$, range 0.28–0.42) was only half as large at its effect on refuge entry. The smaller effect on DF may be a consequence of proximity to refuge of numerous individuals in these studies.

Flight initiation distance, distance fled, and proportion of individuals that fled increase as the directness of approach increases, as predicted. For approaches with longer minimum bypass distances, probability of fleeing decreases to zero as minimum bypass increases. For minimum bypass distances greater than or equal to that for which no lizards flee, FID and DF also equal zero.

5.2.1.3.3 *Predator turn direction*

A predator that has stopped moving near a prey poses a threat that is reflected in the effect of standing distance on latency to flee (Chapter 2). If the predator's body is oriented parallel to the prey's body rather than facing it at a right angle, the predator may turn toward or away from the prey. When the predator rapidly turns toward the prey, assessed risk is expected to increase because the turn may indicate that the predator has detected the prey and is attacking. When a predator turns away from the prey, assessed risk may decrease because the predator may be paying attention to something else.

Risk while the predator is immobile increases as predator–prey distance decreases. When a predator begins to turn rapidly, the assessed risk is expected to increase. At long predator–prey distances, assessed risk will be too low to elicit flight regardless of the direction turned by the predator. When the predator is standing so close that risk is very high if it attacks, the prey may flee regardless of turn direction because it must react immediately to the movement without taking time to ascertain the direction of turning to the movement if it is to escape. It flees even if the predator turns away. The most interesting case occurs at intermediate predator–prey distances that allow the prey enough time to recognize the turn direction. In this range of distances, it may be predicted that the prey is more likely to flee when the predator turns toward than away from it.

These predictions have been verified consistently. At the shortest standing distances virtually all lizards flee immediately regardless of turn direction; at very long standing distances almost no lizards flee regardless of turn direction. Here the results are reported only for intermediate distances where turn direction affects probability of fleeing. For each species it is necessary to conduct pilot tests to determine the appropriate range of distances.

For each of ten lizard species from five families, the proportion of individuals that fled at the intermediate standing distance was greater when the predator turned toward than away from the prey ($r = 0.64 \pm 0.06$, range 0.40–1.00; Figure 5.10). Clearly, lizards assess risk as being greater when a predator turns toward them than away. Two studies reported that the probability of fleeing, regardless of turn direction, increases as distance between the prey and immobile predator decreases ($r = 0.69 \pm 0.22$). These findings confirm the predictions that the proportion of individuals that flee increases as the predator's standing distance decreases and is greater when the predator turns toward the prey in an intermediate range of distances.

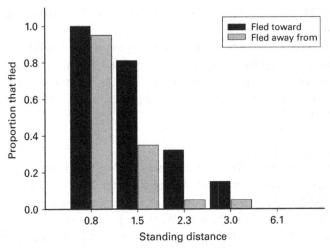

Figure 5.10   When a predator standing nearby suddenly turns, the proportion of *Holbrookia propinqua* that flee does not differ with turn direction for the shortest and longest standing distances, but is higher when the predator turns toward than away from the prey at intermediate distances. (Cooper 1998c)

5.2.1.3.4   *Approach elevation and sidedness*

When prey are situated on slopes, predators may attack from above or below. If lizards interpret attack from above by a researcher as an aerial attack, they might assess risk as being greater due to the high expected speed of aerial predators. They also might be more vulnerable when attacked from above because lizards can escape by running up slopes where larger predators and investigators may be slowed. In a skink and a lacertid, FID was greater for approaches from above than below ($r = 0.35 \pm 0.10$, range 0.26–0.45). Distance fled was greater for approaches from above in the lacertid ($r = 0.24$), but did not differ in the skink. The proportion of lizards that entered refuge did not differ between approached from above and below in the lacertid.

Because many species have side preferences (lateralization) and associated differences in reaction time (Ward & Hopkins 1993; Bisazza *et al.* 1998), escape responses might differ when lizards are approached from the left or right. However, in the sole study of this possibility, FID, DF, and refuge entry were unaffected by the side from which a predator approached (Cooper & Pérez-Mellado 2011).

5.2.1.3.5   *Repeated approach and previous captures*

If a predator approaches, the prey flees successfully, but the predator approaches again after a brief interval, the predator's persistence indicates that it may pose an ongoing threat associated with greater risk of predation than a predator that approaches once and then desists. Therefore economic escape theory predicts that repeated approach should elicit longer FID; its extensions predict that DF and probability of entering refuge are less for initial than subsequent approaches.

In twelve species from four families, FID was longer for the second of two approaches (Figure 5.11). This difference was significant in 11 of 12 species with substantial effect

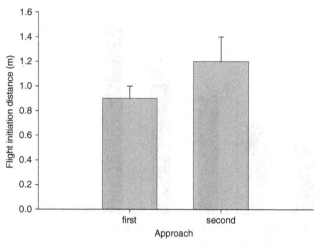

Figure 5.11   In *Sceloporus virgatus* FID is longer for the second of two successive approaches at a fast, but not a slow, approach speed. (Based on data from Cooper 2009c)

size ($r = 0.60 \pm 0.04$, range 0.00–0.84). Distance fled was greater in three species from three families ($r = 0.55 \pm 0.04$, range 0.47–0.61). The proportion of individuals that entered refuge in three species from two families was greater for second than first approaches ($r = 0.55 \pm 0.09$, range 0.47–0.72). All three predictions have been verified, demonstrating that prey update their assessment of predation risk to account for ongoing aspects of predator behavior during encounters.

Lizards that have been captured previously by researchers are expected to assess approach as riskier and to exhibit longer FID and DF. In three species FID increased as number of previous captures increased or was greater for previously captured than naïve prey ($r = 0.37 \pm 0.02$, range 0.34–0.40). Distance fled was longer in one species for lizards that had been captured previously than had not ($r = 0.34$), but the proportion of individuals that entered refuge was not affected by previous capture.

5.2.1.3.6   Starting distance

Because the distance and duration moved by a predator during its approach can be a cue to increasing risk and can affect the ability of prey to obtain benefits while monitoring the predator, FID is predicted to increase as SD increases (Chapter 2; Cooper & Blumstein 2014). In birds and mammals FID typically increases as SD increases (Blumstein 2003; Stankowich & Coss 2007; Williams *et al.* 2014) as predicted, but findings for lizards have been mixed.

The relationship between SD and FID have been studied in seven species from five families. Among these are five species of ambush foragers that have very low rates of spontaneous movement and low cost of monitoring because feeding attempts are infrequent. When these lizards were approached at a slow walking speed, FID was not correlated with SD. When approached at a faster walking speed, FID increased as SD

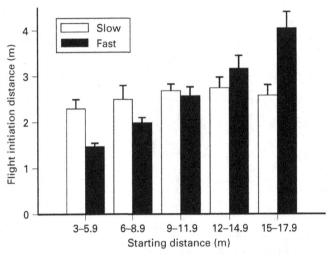

Figure 5.12 At fast, but not slow, approach speed, FID by *Podarcis lilfordi* increases as SD of the predator's approach increases. (Cooper *et al.* 2009b)

increased in one species ($r = 0.50$), but not another. The other two species are active foragers that have higher rates of spontaneous movement and spend a longer proportion of the time moving (Cooper 2007c). Of these, FID increased as SD increased at a fast, but not a slow, approach speed in the lacertid *Podarcis lilfordi* (Cooper *et al.* 2009b; Figure 5.12); it increased as SD increased at a slow approach speed in the teiid *Aspidoscelis exsanguis* ($r = 0.42$; Cooper 2008). These limited data suggest that the FID–SD relationship is stronger when predation risk is higher (at faster approach speed). This is consistent with (1) a dynamic increase in assessed risk related to distance approached by the predator that only occurs at a rapid approach speed in some species and (2) a stronger relationship exists between FID and SD in active foragers than ambush foragers. One reason for the latter effect may be that it is more costly for active than ambush foragers to remain motionless, which prevents active foraging, implying that the cost of monitoring may be greater (Cooper & Blumstein 2014) for active foragers. Starting distance was unrelated to DF in two species and to probability of entering refuge in one.

5.2.1.3.7 Sudden shadowing

A shadow that suddenly passes overhead may be a strong cue to attack by a predator, especially an aerial or large predator. Immediate escape is predicted when a shadow rapidly covers a lizard, and the effect on escape frequency should be greater when the shadow falls directly on a lizard than nearby, greater when the shadow's speed is greater, and greater when a lizard is oriented horizontally where it is more vulnerable to attack from above than when oriented vertically (Cooper 2009a). When shadows were cast by a human hand, the proportion of lizards that fled was greater when the shadow fell directly on lizards than nearby (Figure 5.13) in three species ($r = 0.76 \pm 0.09$, range 0.58–0.89).

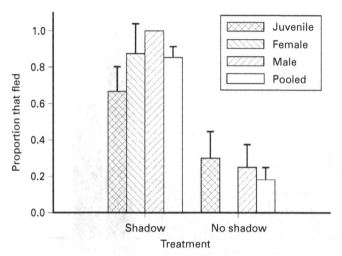

Figure 5.13 The proportion of individuals that flee in *Sceloporus virgatus* is higher when a shadow suddenly passes over them than when it falls nearby. (Cooper 2009a)

In single experiments the proportion of lizards that fled was greater when shadow speed was faster ($r = 0.77$) and when lizards were horizontally rather than vertically oriented ($r = 0.82$). Rapid shadowing appears to be a major cue to immediate threat of predation.

5.2.1.3.8 *Predation pressure*

Prey in populations exposed to higher predation pressure may become warier through experience and via natural selection. In studies of seven species in three families, FID was longer for populations having higher predation pressure in six species. In the seventh species, FID was longer where predation pressure was higher in a study limited to two populations of *Podarcis lilfordi* (Cooper *et al.* 2009c), but was unrelated to FID in a study of seven populations (Cooper & Pérez-Mellado 2012). For the six species in which FID increased as predation pressure increased, the effect size of predation pressure was large ($r = 0.67 \pm 0.08$). Even with the species lacking an effect added, $r = 0.58 \pm 0.12$ (range 0.00–0.86).

In four species, DF was longer where predation pressure was higher ($r = 0.61 \pm 0.21$; Figure 5.14), but DF and predation pressure were unrelated in two species. Overall, the effect size was intermediate ($r = 0.41 \pm 0.18$, range 0.00–0.98). Very large effect sizes ($r \geq 0.96$) occurred for two lacertid species in the Balearic Islands that typically escape without entering refuge in some populations. The proportion of individuals that entered refuges were higher where predation pressure was greater in all of three studies ($r = 0.47 \pm 0.21$, range 0.13–0.84), with a single large effect size in a species that relies heavily on refuges.

Collectively, the findings confirm the predictions of economic escape theory that FID, DF, and refuge entry increase as risk represented by predation pressure increases. The findings for habituation and predation pressure together suggest that lizard populations adjust FID to frequency of past attacks.

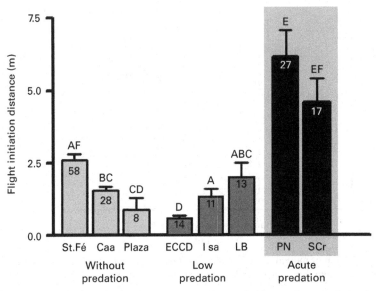

Figure 5.14 In the marine iguana *Amblyrhynchus cristatus*, FID is longer where predation intensity is greater. (Berger *et al.* 2007)

5.2.1.3.9 *Predator size and number*

Potential prey may be too little to be profitable for predators too large to be overcome (Owen-Smith & Mills 2008). Predation risk increases as the prey's size brings it into the range favored by the predator. Within the preferred prey size range, the prey's risk may increase as the size of the predator relative to that of the prey increases. In two lizard species, the proportion of individuals that fled ($r = 0.98 \pm 0.08$, range 0.97–0.99) and FID increased as the size of small predator models increased (Cooper & Stankowich 2010). These findings match predictions based on increase in assessed risk with increase in predator size.

The number of predators approaching simultaneously might also affect FID if the total risk of being captured is greater when more predators approach. In tests at slow approach speed, neither FID nor DF differed for approaches by one predator or two predators side by side; in the same species in using a faster approach speed, FID was longer for approaches by two than one predator, but DF was not affected by number of predators (Cooper *et al.* 2007). The number of predators was important only at the higher risk level associated with faster approach, but more information is needed on responses of additional prey species.

5.2.1.3.10 *Predator facial exposure, direction of gaze, and eye size*

Facial exposure of the predator to the prey may indicate that the predator's field of view includes the prey, and eye contact indicated by directness of gaze is a cue that a predator may have detected the prey. Finally large eye size may indicate high visual acuity and be associated with dangerous predators such as raptors. These factors are expected to increase assessed risk and lengthen FID and DF.

When the predator's face was exposed to *Ctenosaura similis*, FID ($r = 0.58$) and DF ($r = 0.52$) were longer than when its face was hidden (Burger & Gochfeld 1993). In the same species, FID was longer for direct than averted gaze ($r = 0.18$), but DF did not differ between direct and averted gaze (Burger *et al.* 1992). In a different species the proportion of lizards that fled during indirect approaches was much greater as soon as the predator reached a point where the prey passed out of its field of view than at any other point on its approach path ($r = 0.98$; Cooper 1997b). When escape occurred, the predator's face was still visible to the prey, but the eyes were not. During indirect approaches, the proportion of lizards that fled, FID, and DF did not differ when the predator looked directly at the lizard or gazed directly ahead along its path (Cooper 2011c). Directness of gaze may be unimportant during indirect approach that would not lead to contact with the prey. Finally, FID ($r = 0.37$) and DF ($r = 0.18$) were longer when eye size was artificially increased (Burger *et al.* 1991).

Lizards use features of the predator's face and eyes as indicators of the degree of predation risk, but the effects of eye size and directness of gazed were relatively small compared to facial exposure and visibility of eyes. More studies are needed to determine the importance of direct gaze as a predation risk factor.

5.2.2   Cost of fleeing factors that affect FID, DF, and related variables

5.2.2.1   Foraging

Prey in the presence of food must give up a feeding opportunity to flee, which is especially costly when opportunities are limited. Economic escape theory predicts that lizards presented with insects or other food have shorter FID and DF, and that the shortening will be more pronounced as the amount of food present increases. In four species representing four families, FID was shorter when food was present than absent ($r = 0.73 \pm 0.04$, range 0.60–0.81; Figure 5.15). As the number of food items presented to *Podarcis lilfordi* increased, FID became progressively shorter in ($r = 0.93$) and DF decreased ($r = 0.33$; Cooper *et al.* 2006). Loss of feeding opportunities is a major cost of fleeing. In addition to the above findings, FID and DF were shorter above ground on inflorescences where *Podarcis lilfordi* licks nectar than on the ground even though lizards above ground had farther to flee ($r = 0.40$ each; Pérez-Cembranos *et al.* 2013).

5.2.2.2   Social costs of fleeing

If a prey may lose a social opportunity by fleeing, its fitness may be impacted through loss of fertilizations or other social benefits. Males have been the focus of almost all studies of social cost of fleeing, but it may affect females too. Male territory holders are predicted to have shorter FID and DF than other males. In the presence of a female, a territorial male is also expected to be less likely than a non-territorial floater male to enter refuge. In species in which males guard females rather than territories, guarding males are predicted to have shorter FID and DF than non-guarding males. If conspecifics are experimentally introduced, males are predicted to have shorter FID because unfamiliar females may be courted and possibly fertilized, whereas introduced males may be rivals.

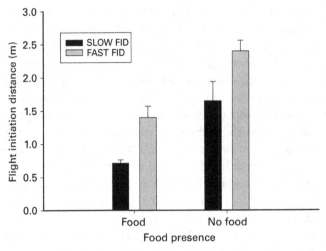

Figure 5.15   Presence of food reduces FID at slow and fast predator approach speeds in *Cnemidophorus murinus*. (Cooper *et al.* 2003)

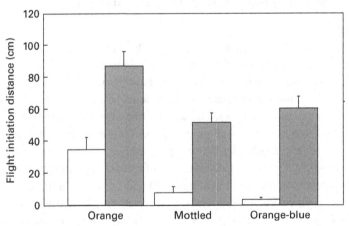

Figure 5.16   In *Urosaurus ornatus* FID is shorter in territorial males with orange-blue than non-territorial males having orange throat coloration. (Thaker *et al.* 2009)

Territorial males are less likely to enter refuge than are floater males ($r = 072$; Stapley & Keogh 2004). In another species males have shorter FID when on than off their territories ($r = 0.56$; Shallenberger 1970). In a third species, *Urosaurus ornatus*, males having orange-blue throat coloration are territorial, whereas those having the orange throat color morph are non-territorial (Thaker *et al.* 2009). For this species, FID is shorter for the territorial orange-blue than orange males ($r = 0.52$; Figure 5.16).

In two species, guarding males had shorter FID than non-guarding males ($r = 0.38 \pm 0.14$, range 0.24–0.52; Figure 5.17), the effect size being larger for a skink than a

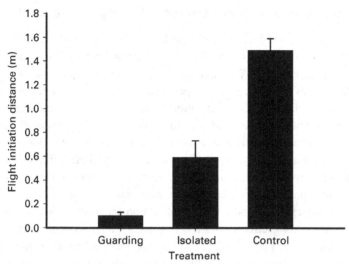

Figure 5.17   Approach distance (FID) in *Plestiodon laticeps* when a female is introduced is shorter for males guarding females than for solitary males; it is also shorter in solitary males when a female rather than a control stimulus is introduced. (Cooper 1999b)

lacertid. Mate guarding did not affect DF in the sole species studied. In the skink, guarding males had shorter FID than guarded females ($r = 0.54$; Cooper 1999b), consistent with the greater cost of fleeing for guarding males. In the lacertid being guarded did not affect FID by females (Martín & López 1999).

When conspecifics are experimentally introduced, FID is consistently affected, but the direction of the effect depends on the sex and circumstances of the focal and introduced lizards. In three species from three families, FID of males was shorter when males rather than control stimuli were introduced ($r = 0.57 \pm 0.15$, range 0.40–0.88). In one of these, the effect of female presence overrode that of approach speed ($r = 0.79$). Male FID in two species was shorter when females rather than control stimuli were introduced ($r = 0.73 \pm 0.14$, range = 0.60–0.88). In one species, FID of guarding males was longer than that of isolated males when a female was introduced ($r = 0.30$), which was interpreted as indicating greater potential gain for the isolated male because guarders would have to relax guarding to court an introduced female.

The FID of females in a territorial phrynosomatid species, *Sceloporus virgatus*, is shorter when a conspecific female rather than a control is introduced ($r = 0.72$, Cooper 2009b). Such females aggressively reject courtship by males. Failure to do so may be costly, resulting in shorter FID. In a study that did not identify sexes of *Phrynosoma modestum*, FID was shorter in the presence of a conspecific than when the focal lizard was alone ($r = 0.62$; Cooper & Sherbrooke 2010).

Collectively, the findings for social costs show that presence of conspecific males or females may impose large costs of fleeing on territorial and mate-guarding males. These costs are reflected in shortened FID as predicted.

5.2.3   Importance of costs of not fleeing and costs of fleeing: relative effect sizes

From the foregoing, it is apparent that FID by lizards is affected by many factors that influence the cost of not fleeing and the cost of fleeing. Effect sizes are highly variable within and between factors. Within a single factor, variation may occur due to inter-specific differences or differences in experimental procedures that affect assessed risk and cost of fleeing. Between-factor variation in effect size may indicate which factors are more important, but caution is needed in such interpretations because effects of all but one or two factors are typically held constant in experiments and factors may interact.

With these provisos in mind, some factors clearly have large effects on FID. Here I mention these factors that have been found to have consistent effects in at least four studies. Among predation risk factors, predator traits appear to have the strongest effects, especially approach speed and repeated approach. Habitat factors and prey traits also have fairly strong effects on FID, especially partial concealment of the prey. Distance from refuge, perch height, body temperature, habituation, the prey's body size, tail loss, conspicuousness, and directness of approach all have substantial effect sizes of 0.40 to 0.56. Foraging and social costs of fleeing also have large effect sizes. These findings indicate that many factors affect escape decisions by lizards. Because effect sizes are affected by levels of other cost of not fleeing and cost of fleeing factors, the effect sizes given cannot be used to rank the importance of the factors. Many factors appear to strongly affect FID, but their relative importance may vary with other risk and cost-of-fleeing factors, as well as with the prey's fitness when the encounter begins.

5.2.4   Escape strategy

Brief allusions to changes in escape strategy have been made while interpreting effects of predation risk factors. A substantial literature documents differences in escape strategy, but this material is too extensive to be covered here. Selected topics are presented (see Chapter 8).

One way prey can decrease the likelihood of being captured is to decrease the predict-ability of their escape behavior. Five species of *Aspidoscelis* fled to diverse microhabitats, exhibited differences in length and linearity of escape runs, and varied in refuge use (Schall & Pianka 1980). The authors argued that escape diversity should increase among conspecific populations as predation pressure increases and should diverge among similar sympatric species having the same predators, but these ideas remain untested.

Locomotor capacities of lizards are related to habitat and escape strategies. Lacertid species occupying more open habitats are faster sprinters having lower endurance and shorter FID than species occupying more vegetated sites; species that use vertical structures tend to be faster climbers (Schulte *et al.* 2004). Eight scincid species differed in diversity of escape behavior, which was related to differences in microhabitats and locomotor specializations (Melville & Swain 2003). Four species had specialized locomotor abilities and escape behaviors; two species that use a range of microhabitats used more diverse escape behaviors requiring different locomotor skills such as sprint-ing, jumping, and climbing (Melville & Swain 2003).

Anolis lizards often escape by running along branches or trunks. As branch diameter decreases, running speed decreases and lizards may switch from running to jumping (Losos & Irschick 1996). Because running speed decreases as the angle at branch points increases, anoles prefer escape paths with small angles at branch points (Mattingly & Jayne 2005).

Destinations and types of escape behavior often vary with circumstances. In *Uta stansburiana* individuals near a cliff fled to it and escaped downward; those located more than 15 m from the cliff fled in circles or non-directionally, perhaps to avoid leaving familiar ground or intruding on territories of conspecifics (Zani *et al.* 2009). *Liolaemus multimaculatus* escape by fleeing into patches of grass or burying themselves rapidly in sand. Burying frequency increased as distance to a patch of grass increased (Kacoliris *et al.* 2009). Differences in escape behavior related to location, habitat structure, and environmental conditions are presumably widespread.

Some lizards undergo ontogenetic color changes and associated changes in escape behavior. Many lizards have brightly colored tails as juveniles that deflect attacks of predators away from the body, permitting escape by caudal autotomy (Cooper & Vitt 1985, 1991). Bright tail coloration increases detectability, but increases escape ability. As lizards grow, they may be less subject to attack by small predators, but more subject to attack by larger, more efficient predators, accounting for ontogenetic loss of bright tail coloration. Another hypothesis, not mutually exclusive, is that hatchlings with brightly colored tails are more active and occupy sites more exposed to predation than adults (Hawlena *et al.* 2006). In *Acanthodactylus beershebensis* hatchlings with bright tails were more active in more open locations than older lizards lacking bright tail coloration; they performed deflective tail displays not used by older lizards (Hawlena *et al.* 2006). Deflective tail displays are much more frequent in juvenile skinks, *Plestiodon laticeps*, having blue tails than in adults having tan tails (Cooper 1998b).

5.2.5 Latency to flee

When a predator is immobile near a prey that is immobile and aware of the predator, latency to flee is predicted to decrease as cost of not fleeing increases and latency to move is predicted to decrease as opportunity cost of remaining immobile increases (Cooper *et al.* 2012; Chapter 2). These predictions have been uniformly verified in three studies. Latency to flee was shorter for high risk represented by prior chasing of the prey than for low risk in which the predator had not previously approached ($r = 0.50$). Latency to flee is shorter when the predator's approach speed before stopping is faster ($r = 0.70 \pm 0.04$, $n = 3$); when the predator approaches less directly ($r = 0.64 \pm 0.03$, $n = 3$); and for the second of two successive approaches ($r = 0.50 \pm 0.02$, $n = 2$); when the predator maintains eye contact with the prey rather averts its gaze by 30° ($r = 0.35$, $n = 1$); and when the predator stands closer to the prey ($r = 0.72 \pm 0.06$, $n = 6$; Martín *et al.* 2009; Cooper *et al.* 2012; Cooper & Sherbrooke 2013b; Figure 5.18). Latency to move is shorter when food is present than absent ($r = 0.74 \pm 0.12$, $n = 2$) and for males in the presence than absence of females ($r = 0.87$, $n = 1$) (Cooper & Sherbrooke 2013b).

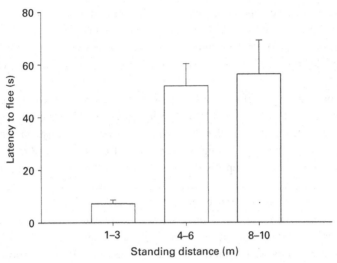

Figure 5.18   Latency to flee in *Podarcis lilfordi* increases as standing distance increases. (Cooper *et al.* 2012)

5.3   Snakes

5.3.1   FID, distance fled, and probability of fleeing

Much less is known about escape decisions by snakes than other lizards. Many snakes permit close approach without moving, relying on crypsis to avoid being detected and/or on envenomation as a defense. Decisions about FID and related variables have been studied for few species (Table 5.1). All but one of these are natricine colubrids, which often occur at high density. For the material below, see Table 5.1 for citations.

Few predation risk factors are known to influence escape decisions by snakes (Table 5.1). As starting distance increased, FID increased. The likelihood of fleeing was greater for snakes in sparser than denser cover, and was longer for moving than immobile snakes (Table 5.1), consistent with predictions of escape theory. Some risk factors have variable effects on FID. No effect was observed for air or water temperature, but FID increased as body temperature increased in *Regina septemvitta*. Because body temperature affects locomotor capacity, it is more closely related to escape than air or substrate temperature. In one study of *Nerodia sipedon*, FID decreased as perch height increased, as in lizards, but in another study PH of basking individuals did not affect FID. Differences in distance from shore and availability of refuges might explain differences in the effect of PH.

Sex differences in FID and probability of fleeing were observed in one of four species. Female *N. sipedon* had longer FID than males, perhaps due to differences in body size or pregnancy. Age and body length did not affect FID in three natricines, but probability of fleeing was greater in juvenile than adult *Pseudonaja textilis*, which often defend themselves aggressively. One reason for lack of effect of age in natricines may be that hatchlings and juveniles were absent or scarce in the samples.

Table 5.1 Factors affecting costs of not fleeing (risk) and of fleeing influence escape decisions by snakes.

Family/species	Risk or cost	Factor	Metric	Effect	Source
Colubridae					
Nerodia sipedon	risk	water temperature	FID	no effect	1
Nerodia sipedon	risk	perch height	FID	↑ as PH ↓	1
Nerodia sipedon	risk	starting distance	FID	↑ as SD ↑	2
Nerodia sipedon	risk	sex	FID	F > M	2
Nerodia sipedon	risk?	age	FID	no effect	2
Nerodia sipedon	risk?	air temperature	FID	no effect	2
Nerodia sipedon	risk	perch height	FID	no effect	2
Regina septemvittata	risk	body temperature	FID	↑ as BT ↑	3
Regina septemvittata	risk?	sex	FID	no effect	3
Regina septemvittata	risk?	body length	FID	no effect	3
Thamnophis sirtalis	risk (cost?)	den vs dispersing	FID	dispersing > den	4
Tropidonophis mairii	risk	pregnancy	FID	↑	5
Tropidonophis mairii	cost	male breeding state	FID	NR ↑ R	5
Tropidonophis mairii	risk?	age	FID	no effect	5
Tropidonophis mairii	risk?	sex	FID	no effect	5
Tropidonophis mairii	risk?	body length	FID	no effect	5
Tropidonophis mairii	risk?	season	FID	no effect	5
Tropidonophis mairii	risk?	air temperature	FID	no effect	5
Tropidonophis mairii	risk?	previous capture	FID	no effect	5
Tropidonophis mairii	risk?	relative humidity	FID	no effect	5
Tropidonophis mairii	risk?	moonlight	FID	no effect	5
Elapidae					
Pseudonaja textilis	risk?	approach speed	FID	no effect	6
Pseudonaja textilis	risk	snake motion	FID	moving > still	6
Pseudonaja textilis	risk	adult vs. juvenile	PF	J > A	6
Pseudonaja textilis	risk?	sex	PF	no effect	6
Pseudonaja textilis	risk?	wind speed	FID	no effect	6
Pseudonaja textilis	risk	cover	FID	sparse > dense	6
Pseudonaja textilis	risk	cover	PF	sparse > dense	6
Pseudonaja textilis	risk	time of day	PF	1001–1800 h > other	6

?: tested, but not shown to have an effect; A: adult; BT: body temperature; F: female; FID: flight initiation distance; J: juvenile; NR: non-reproductive; PF: probability of fleeing = proportion of individuals that fled; M: male; PH: perch height; R: reproductive; SD: starting distance.1: Weatherhead & Robertson 1992; 2: Cooper *et al.* 2008; 3: Layne & Ford 1984; 4: Shine *et al.* 2003a; 5: Brown & Shine 2004; 6: Whitaker & Shine: 1999.

Several differences in escape between snakes and lizards are known. A finding unique to snakes is that FID is longer for *Thamnophis sirtalis* while dispersing from hibernacula than at the dens despite similar body size and temperature (Shine *et al.* 2003a). Several factors might contribute to this result. While dispersing snakes are more likely to be moving and alone. Any risk dilution provided by conspecifics at densely populated dens is lost during dispersal. Because reproduction occurs at dens, snakes there may exhibit shorter FID due to greater cost of fleeing.

Being gravid or pregnant increases body mass and reduces locomotor speed of squamate reptiles (Shine 1980; Cooper *et al.* 1990). Lizards exhibit shorter FID when gravid because gravid females may change their escape strategies, relying more or crypsis to avoid being detected or staying closer to refuges (section 5.2.1.5). In the natricine *T. mairii*, FID is longer in pregnant than non-pregnant females, matching the prediction of escape theory for prey that are slowed, but do not alter escape strategy, when pregnant.

That male *T. mairii* have shorter FID when in reproductive condition than not (Brown & Shine 2004) is also unique among squamates. In lizards, breeding males in the presence of unfamiliar females or guarding mates have shorter FID because fleeing may cost them fertilizations. Although male *T. mairii* were not guarding mates, fleeing might have reduced the probability of mating with undetected females nearby. However, it is not certain that the effect of reproductive condition is mediated by mating opportunity. Other possible differences in the ecology of breeding and non-breeding males, such as frequency of feeding and associated cost of fleeing or differences in movement or microhabitat use that might affect predation risk, might account for the observed difference.

In the elapid *Pseudonaja textilis*, approach speed did not affect FID. This lack of relationship does not contradict the prediction of escape theory because *P. textilis* is a dangerously venomous species that defends itself aggressively when it is likely to be overtaken.

Another way in which escape decisions by snakes may differ from those typical for lizards is that previous capture did not affect FID in *Tropidonophis mairii*. However, this difference may be a consequence of differences in methods of study. In studies of lizards, initial and subsequent captures occurred within a few days, but *T. mairii* were collected in a mark–recapture study and the mean intercapture interval was 229 days, obscuring any effect of being captured recently.

Possible effects of several environmental factors that have no readily predictable effect on escape by snakes have been investigated. No effects were shown for time of day, season, relative humidity, moonlight, or wind speed in one species each (see table in the electronic supplementary material). However, season and time of day might have effects mediated by temperature, vegetative cover, and reproductive condition.

Intraspecific variation in FID was pronounced among populations of *T. sirtalis* from four dens located within 20 m of each other. It is unclear whether the differences reflect genetic variation, differences in exposure to predation, or other factors. In the only comparative study of snakes, FID was longer in *N. sipedon* than in *Thamnopis sauritus*;

it was intermediate in *T. sirtalis*, but did not differ in the other two species (Scribner & Weatherhead 1995). Distance fled was longer in *N. sipedon* than in the other two species (Scribner & Weatherhead 1995).

5.3.2   Refuge selection and entry

Many species of snakes flee to refuges. They may hide in holes, crevices, or under objects, flee into and dive under water, or climb steep slope or plants, or jump from high in trees or on cliffs to prevent predators from pursuing them. However, refuge selection when pursued has received much more anecdotal attention than systematic study. Interspecific differences occur even among closely related species. In the comparative study of natricine snakes (Scribner & Weatherhead 1995), *T. sirtalis* and *T. sauritus* often fled into dense vegetation, whereas *N. sipedon* often dived and swam underwater. These differences in refuge selection reflect differences in habitats because *N. sipedon* occurred almost exclusively in aquatic habitats, often offshore, whereas the two species of *Thamnophis* occurred along the shore or inland.

5.3.3   Escape strategy

Many venomous snakes do not flee while being approached, relying instead on deterrence by or use of their chemical defenses. For example, the viper *Gloydius shedaoensis*, the elapid *Psuedonaja textilis*, and the laticaudine seasnake (*Laticauda colubrina*) often do not flee even when harassed (Shine *et al.* 2002, 2003c). Similarly, North American crotaline vipers often do not flee when approached (my personal observations for several species of *Crotalus, Agkistrodon piscivorus*, and *A. contortrix*). With the exception of very large constrictors and cryptically colored species, other snakes lacking such defenses are more likely to flee from predators (Fitch 1963, 1965), especially species capable of very rapid crawling, such as whipsnakes (*Masticophis*) and racers (*Coluber*; Fitch 1965).

Color patterns of snakes vary greatly and are related to types of defenses, which were divided into tendency to escape versus defenses other than fleeing (Jackson *et al.* 1976). In a survey of North American snakes north of Mexico, species having longitudinal striped color patterns and uniform or speckled patterns had higher escape speed and are exposed to visual predators longer each day than snakes having regular cross-banded patterns (perpendicular to the longitudinal axis), irregular banding patterns (varying in shape along the length of the body and not always perpendicular to the longitudinal axis), or blotched-spotted patterns (Jackson *et al.* 1976).

Snakes having irregular banding and blotched-spotted color patterns tend to have effective defenses other than fleeing, such as envenomation, feigning death, and bluffing. Snakes that are unicolored or unicolored with speckles have a greater tendency to flee and greater flight capability than snakes having irregular banding or blotched-spotted patterns (Jackson *et al.* 1976). Snakes having striped body patterns exhibit similar traits to those of unicolored or unicolored-speckled snakes, but striped snakes rely to an even greater extent on escape rather than alternative defenses (Jackson *et al.*

1976). In the northern garter snake, *Thamnophis ordinoides*, some snakes are striped and others in the same population are not. When neonates were pursued, color morphs with less striping more frequently performed reversals – evasive maneuvers in which the snake suddenly reverses its direction and becomes immobile (Brodie 1989, 1992). Reversal is believed to provide snakes a chance to re-establish crypsis, but striped snakes that employ reversals lose the advantage of difficulty for predators in following movement conferred by striping (Brodie 1989, 1992).

Regularly banded snakes are intermediate in reliance on escape and escape speed to those having the other color patterns; they tend to escape by submerging and to be active in low illumination (Jackson *et al.* 1976). Jackson *et al.* (1976) discussed hypotheses suggesting that uniform, striped, and regularly banded patterns mislead visually oriented predators about immobility versus movement and speed, and presented circumstantial evidence that regularly banded patterns may appear to be uniform at speeds above the flicker fusion frequency of a predator (Pough 1976). Regularly banded snakes moving fast enough to surpass the critical flicker fusion frequency would gain an advantage of uniform body coloration, making it difficult for a predator to judge its speed.

Because the Jackson *et al.* (1976) study was conducted before currently used statistical methods were developed that take phylogenetic relationships into account, it is possible that correlations of traits within genera and families might have produced inflated estimates of significance. The hypothesized mechanisms by which the color patterns create illusions about a fleeing snake's motion and speed deserve experimental testing.

Snakes that flee in some circumstances may rely on alternate defenses in others. The strategy used varies with temperature, degree of cover, and is likely to vary with other factors that affect escape ability and detectability. Temperature affects probability of fleeing via its effect on locomotor capacity, and other variables. The shorter FID at lower body temperatures in *R. septemvittata* hints that snakes may switch from escape to other defenses when body temperature falls too low for rapid crawling. In the natricine *Thamnopis sirtalis* (Shine *et al.* 2003b) and the African viper *Bitis schneideri* (Maritz 2012), the probability of fleeing is reduced at lower temperatures. Because the data for *B. schneideri* were combined, approach and a 30-s interval during which the snakes' heads were touched five times, it is uncertain whether FID or probability of fleeing were affected by approach alone. The probability of fleeing by *P. textilis* is lower in sparser than denser cover (Whittaker and Shine, 1999). It may be predicted that probability of fleeing is reduced at low levels of illumination.

Ecological differences between species may account for differences in escape behavior in two elapids. *Cryptophis nigrescens* hunts actively in open areas at night, whereas *Hoplocephalus bungaroides* ambush their prey in retreat sites in sun-warmed rocks (Llewelyn *et al.* 2010). Both species relied primarily on fleeing to escape, but the antipredatory behavior of *C. nigrescens*, which is exposed to cool temperatures while foraging in the open, was less sensitive to thermal variation and its use of retaliatory defense was less frequent than that of *H. bungaroiedes* (Llewelyn *et al.* 2010).

5.4 Crocodilians, sphenodontidans, and turtles

Literature searches did not reveal any papers about FID (or its synonyms) for crocodilians, tuataras, or turtles. Alligators and other crocodilians often escape when approached by diving beneath the water surface. Tuataras escape into burrows. Aquatic and semi-aquatic turtles typically escape by diving; such turtles often flee to water if encountered near shore or drop off logs or bushes into water when approached. Many turtles use their shells as refuges when overtaken on land or captured in water. Terrestrial turtles and some semi-aquatic species have shells that permit complete or nearly complete withdrawal of vulnerable body parts and, in some the shells close, effectively blocking access by predators to soft body parts.

As discussed in Chapter 9, when the turtle *Mauremys leprosa* is approached while on land, it attempts to flee to water, but if overtaken withdraws into its shell (Martín *et al.* 2003). In terrestrial turtles, running speed is too slow for escape from typical predators. When a predator draws near, these turtles escape not by fleeing, but by withdrawing their hands and necks, legs, and often tails inside their shells. Aquatic turtles and semi-aquatic turtles in water are more likely than terrestrial turtles to flee.

5.5 Future directions

It is apparent from the foregoing that research on snakes, turtles, tuataras, and crocodilians is needed. Incorporating effects of aspects of reptilian cognition, such as learning local escape routes and refuge sites, in escape studies would also be valuable. Studies of escape by reptiles have focused on effects of costs of not fleeing and costs of fleeing in single species. Only recently have studies been published using the comparative method. As data for more species accumulate, comparative studies should make substantial contributions to our knowledge of topics such as relationships of escape decisions to locomotor capacity, sensory ability, morphological traits, ecology, and phylogeny.

References

Bateman, P. W. & Fleming, P. A. (2009). To cut a long tail short: A review of lizard caudal autotomy studies carried out over the last 20 years. *Journal of Zoology*, 277, 1–14.

Berger, S., Wikelski, M., Romero, L. M., Kalko, E. K. V. & Rödl, T. (2007). Behavioral and physiological adjustments to new predators in an endemic island species, the Galápagos marine iguana. *Hormones and Behavior*, 52, 653–663.

Bisazza, A., Rogers, L. J. & Vallortigarac, G. (1998). The origins of cerebral asymmetry: A review of evidence of behavioural and brain lateralization in fishes, reptiles and amphibians. *Neuroscience and Biobehavioral Reviews*, 22, 411–426.

Blamires, S. J. (1999). Factors influencing the escape response of an arboreal agamid lizard of tropical Australia (*Lophognathus temporalis*) in an urban environment. *Canadian Journal of Zoology*, 77, 1998–2003.

Blumstein, D. T. (2003). Flight-initiation distance in birds is dependent on intruder starting distance. *Journal of Wildlife Management*, **67**, 852–857.

Brodie, E. D., III. (1989). Genetic correlations between morphology and antipredator behavior in natural populations of the garter snake *Thamnophis ordinoides*. *Nature*, **342**, 542–543.

Brodie, E. D., III (1992). Correlational selection for clolor patterns and antipredator behavior in the garter snake *Thamnophis ordinoides*. *Evolution*, **46**, 1284–1298.

Brown, G. P. & Shine, R. (2004). Effects of reproduction on the antipredator tactics of snakes (*Tropidophis mairii, Colubridae*). *Behavioral Ecology and Sociobiology*, **56**, 257–262.

Bulova, S. J. (1994). Ecological correlates of population and individual variation in antipredator behavior of two species of desert lizards. *Copeia*, **1994**, 980–992.

Burger, J. & Gochfeld, M. (1993). The importance of the human face in risk perception by black iguanas, Ctenosaura similis. *Journal of Herpetology*, **27**, 426–430.

Burger, J., Gochfeld, M. & Murray, B. G., Jr. (1991). The role of a predator's eye size in risk perception by basking black iguana, Ctenosaura similis. *Animal Behaviour*, **42**, 471–476.

Burger, J., Gochfeld, M. & Murray, B. B., Jr. (1992). Risk discrimination of eye contact and directness of approach in black iguanas (*Ctenosaura similis*). *Journal of Comparative Psychology*, **106**, 97–101.

Clark, C. W. (1994). Antipredator behavior and the asset-protection principle. *Behavioral Ecology*, **5**, 159–170.

Congdon, J. D., Vitt, L. J. & King, W. W. (1974). Geckos: Adaptive significance and energetics of tail autotomy. *Science*, **184**, 1379–1380.

Cooper, W. E., Jr. (1997a). Escape by a refuging prey, the broad-headed skink (*Eumeces laticeps*). *Canadian Journal of Zoology*, **75**, 943–947.

Cooper, W. E., Jr. (1997b). Threat factors affecting antipredatory behavior in the broad-headed skink (*Eumeces laticeps*): Repeated approach, change in predator path, and predator's field of view. *Copeia*, **1997**, 613–619.

Cooper, W. E., Jr. (1998a). Effects of refuge and conspicuousness on escape behavior by the broad-headed skink (*Eumeces laticeps*). *Amphibia-Reptilia*, **19**, 103–108.

Cooper, W. E., Jr. (1998b). Reactive and anticipatory display to deflect predatory attack to an autotomous lizard tail. *Canandian Journal of Zoology*, **76**, 1507–1510.

Cooper, W. E., Jr. (1998c). Direction of predator turning, a neglected cue to predation risk. *Behaviour*, **135**, 55–64.

Cooper, W. E., Jr. (1999a). Escape behavior by prey blocked from entering the nearest refuge. *Canadian Journal of Zoology*, **77**, 671–674.

Cooper, W. E., Jr. (1999b). Tradeoffs between courtship, fighting, and antipredatory behavior by a lizard, *Eumeces laticeps*. *Behavioral Ecology and Sociobiology*, **47**, 54–59.

Cooper, W. E., Jr. (2003). Shifted balance of risk and cost after autotomy affects use of cover, escape, activity, and foraging in the keeled earless lizard (*Holbrookia propinqua*). *Behavioral Ecology and Sociobiology*, **54**, 179–187.

Cooper, W. E., Jr. (2006a). Dynamic risk assessment: Prey rapidly adjust flight initiation distance to changes in predator approach speed. *Ethology*, **112**, 858–864.

Cooper, W. E., Jr. (2006b). Risk factors affecting escape grahamÿr by Puerto rican *Anolis* lizards. *Canadian Journal of Zoology*, **84**, 495–504.

Cooper, W. E., Jr. (2007a). Escape and its relationship to pursuit-deterrent grahamÿrÿ in the Cuban curly-tailed lizard *Leiocephalus carinatus*. *Herpetologica*, **63**, 144–150.

Cooper, W. E., Jr. (2007b). Compensatory changes in escape and refuge use following autotomy in the lizard *Sceloporus virgatus*. *Canadian Journal of Zoology*, **85**, 99–107.

Cooper, W. E., Jr. (2007c). Foraging modes as suites of coadapted movement traits. *Journal of Zoology*, **272**, 45–56.

Cooper, W. E., Jr. (2008). Strong artifactual effect of starting distance on flight initiation distance in the actively foraging lizard *Aspidoscelis exsanguis*. *Herpetologica*, **64**, 200–206.

Cooper, W. E., Jr. (2009a). Rapid covering by shadow as a cue to predation risk in three lizard species. *Behaviour*, **146**, 1217–1234.

Cooper, W. E., Jr. (2009b). Flight initiation distance decreases during social activity in lizards (*Sceloporus virgatus*). *Behavioral Ecology and Sociobiology*, **63**, 1765–1771.

Cooper, W. E., Jr. (2009c). Fleeing and hiding under simultaneous risks and costs. *Behavioral Ecology*, **20**, 665–671.

Cooper, W. E., Jr. (2010a). Pursuit deterrence varies with predation risks affecting escape behavior in the lizard *Callisaurus draconoides*. *Animal Behaviour*, **80**, 249–256.

Cooper, W. E., Jr. (2010b). Escape tactics and effects of perch height and habituation on flight initiation distance in two Jamaican anoles (*Squamata*: Polychrotidae). *Revista de Biologia Tropical*, **58**, 1199–1209.

Cooper, W. E., Jr. (2011a). Age, sex and escape grahamÿr in the striped plateau lizad (*Sceloporus virgatus*) and the mountain spiny lizard (*Sceloporus jarrovii*), with a review of age and sex effects on escape by lizards. *Behaviour*, **148**, 1215–1238.

Cooper, W. E., Jr. (2011b). Pursuit deterrence, predations risk, and escape in the lizard *Callisaurus draconoides*. *Behavioral Ecology and Sociobiology*, **65**, 1833–1841.

Cooper, W. E., Jr. (2011c). Influence of some potential predation risk factors and interaction between predation risk and cost of fleeing on escape by the lizard *Sceloporus virgatus*. *Ethology*, **117**, 620–629.

Cooper, W. E., Jr. (2012). Risk factors affecting escape behavior by the Jamaican lizard *Anolis lineatopus* (Polychrotidae, Squamata). *Caribbean Journal of Science*, **46**, 1–12.

Cooper, W. E., Jr. & Avalos, A. (2010). Predation risk, escape and refuge use by mountain spiny lizards (*Sceloporus jarrovii*). *Amphibia-Reptilia*, **31**, 363–373.

Cooper, W. E., Jr. & Blumstein, D. T. (2014). Starting distance, alert distance and flushing early challenge economic escape theory: New proposed effects on costs of fleeing and not fleeing. *Behavioral Ecology*, **25**, 44–52.

Cooper, W. E., Jr. & Frederick, W. G. (2007). Optimal flight initiation distance. *Journal of Theoretical Biology*, **244**, 59–67.

Cooper, W. E., Jr. & Pérez-Mellado, V. (2011). Escape by the Balearic lizard (*Podarcis lilfordi*) is affected by elevation of an approaching predator, but not by some other potential predation risk factors. *Acta Herpetologica*, **6**, 247–259.

Cooper, W. E., Jr. & Pérez-Mellado, V. (2012). Historical influence of predation pressure on escape behavior by *Podarcis* lizards in the Balearic islands. *Biological Journal of the Linnaean Society*, **107**, 254–268

Cooper, W. E., Jr. & Sherbrooke, W. C. (2010). Crypsis influences escape decisions in the round-tailed horned lizard (*Phrynosoma modestusm*). *Canadian Journal of Zoology*, **88**, 1003–1010.

Cooper, W. E., Jr. & Sherbrooke, W. C. (2012). Choosing between a rock and a hard place: Camouflage in the round-tailed horned lizard *Phrynosoma modestum*. *Current Zoology*, **58**, 541–548.

Cooper, W. E., Jr. & Sherbrooke, W. C. (2013a). Effects of recent movement, starting distance and other risk factors on escape behaviour by two phrynosomatid lizards. *Behaviour*, **150**, 447–469.

Cooper, W. E., Jr. & Sherbrooke, W. C. (2013b). Risk and cost of immobility in the presence of an immobile predator: effects on latency to flee or approach food or a potential mate. *Behavioral Ecology and Sociobiology*, **67**, 583–592.

Cooper, W. E. & Stankowich, T. (2010). Prey or predator? Body size of an approaching animal affects decisions to attack or escape. *Behavioral Ecology*, **21**, 1278–1284.

Cooper, W. E., Jr. & Vitt, L. J. (1985). Blue tails and autotomy: Enhancement of predation avoidance in juvenile skinks. *Zeitschrift fur Tierpsychologie*, **70**, 265–276.

Cooper, W. E., Jr. & Vitt, L. J. (1991). Influence of detectability and ability to escape on natural selection of conspicuous autotomous defenses. *Canadian Journal of Zoology*, **69**, 757–764.

Cooper, W. E., Jr. & Wilson, D. S. (2007). Beyond optimal escape theory: Microhabitats as well as predation risk affect escape and refuge use by the phrynosomatid lizard *Sceloporus virgatus*. *Behaviour*, **144**, 1235–1254.

Cooper, W. E., Jr. & Wilson, D. S. (2008). How to stay alive after losing your tail. *Behaviour*, **145**, 1085–1089.

Cooper, W. E., Jr., Vitt, L. J., Hedges, R. & Huey, R. B. (1990). Locomotor impairment and defense in gravid lizards (*Eumeces laticeps*): Behavioral shift in activity may offset costs of reproduction in an active forager. *Behavioral Ecology and Sociobiology*, **27**, 153–157.

Cooper, W. E., Jr., Pérez-Mellado, V., Baird, T. *et al.* (2003). Effects of risk, cost, and their interaction on optimal escape by nonrefuging Bonaire whiptail lizards, *Cnemidophorus murinus*. *Behavioral Ecology*, **14**, 288–293.

Cooper, W. E., Jr., Perez-Mellado, V. & Hawlena, D. (2006). Magnitude of food reward affects escape behavior and acceptable risk in Balearic lizards, *Podarcis lilfordi*. *Behavioral Ecology*, **17**, 554–559.

Cooper, W. E., Jr., Perez-Mellado, V. & Hawlena, D. (2007). Number, speeds, and approach paths of predators affect escape behavior by the Balearic lizard, *Podarcis lilfordi*. *Journal of Herpetology*, **41**, 197–204.

Cooper, W. E., Jr., Attum, O. & Kingsbury, B. (2008). Escape behaviors and flight initiation distance in the common water snake *Nerodia sipedon*. *Journal of Herpetology*, **42**, 493–500.

Cooper, W. E., Jr., Wilson, D. S. & Smith, G. R. (2009a). Sex, reproductive status, and cost of tail autotomy via decreased running speed. *Ethology*, **115**, 7–13.

Cooper, W. E., Jr., Hawlena, D. & Pérez-Mellado, V. (2009b). Interactive effect of starting distance and approach speed on escape challenges theory. *Behavioral Ecology*, **20**, 542–546.

Cooper, W. E., Jr., Hawlena, D. & Pérez-Mellado, V. (2009c). Islet tameness: Escape behavior and refuge use in populations of the Balearic lizard (*Podarcis lilfordi*) exposed to differing predation pressure. *Canadian Journal of Zoology*, **87**, 912–919.

Cooper, W. E., Jr., López, P., Martín, J. & Pérez-Mellado, V. (2012). Latency to flee from an immobile predator: Effects of risk and cost of immobility for the prey. *Behavioral Ecology*, **23**, 790–797.

Eifler, D. (2001). *Egernia cunninghami* (Cunningham's skink). Escape behavior. *Herpetological Review*, **32**, 40.

Fitch, H. S. (1963). Natural history of the racer *Coluber constrictor*. *University of Kansas Publications, Museum of Natural History*, **15**, 351–468.

Fitch, H. S. (1965). An ecological study of the garter snake, *Thamnophis sirtalis*. *University of Kansas Publications, Museum of Natural History*, **15**, 493–564.

Hawlena, D., Boochnik, R., Abramsky, Z. & Bouskila, A. (2006). Blue tail and striped body: Why do lizards change their infant costume when growing up? *Behavioral Ecology*, **17**, 889–896.

Hawlena, D., Perez-Mellado, V. & Cooper, W. E., Jr. (2009). Morphological traits affect escape behavior of the Balearic lizards (*Podarcis lilfordi*). *Amphibia-Reptilia*, **30**, 587–592.

Hertz, P. E., Huey, R. B. & Nevo, E. (1983). Homage to Santa Anita: Thermal sensitivity of sprint speed in agamid lizards. *Evolution*, **37**, 1075–1084.

Holley, A. J. F. (1993). Do brown hares signal foxes? *Ethology*, **94**, 21–30.

Huey, R. B. (1982). Temperature, physiology, and the ecology of reptiles. In *Biology of the Reptilia, Vol. 12, Physiology C: Physiological Ecology*. London: Academic Press, pp. 25–91.

Jackson, J. F., Ingram, W., III. & Campbell, H. W. (1976). The dorsal pigmentation as an antipredator strategy: a multivariate approach. *American Naturalist*, **110**, 1029–1053.

Kacoliris, F. P., Gurrero, E., Molinari, A., Moyano, B. & Rafael, A. (2009). Run to shelter or bury into the sand? Factors affecting escape grahamÿr decisions in Argentinian sand dun lizards (*Liolaemus multimaculatus*). *Herpetological Journal*, **19**, 213–216.

Kelt, D. A., Nabors, L. K. & Forister, M. L. (2002). Size-specific differences in tail loss and escape behavior in *Liolaemus nigromaculatus*. *Journal of Herpetology*, **36**, 322–325.

Kramer, D. L. & Bonenfant, M. (1997). Direction of predator approach and the decision to flee to a refuge. *Animal Behaviour*, **54**, 289–295.

Lailvaux, S. P., Alexander, G. J. & Whiting, M. J. (2003). Sex-based differences and similarities in locomotor performance, thermal preferences, and escape behaviour in the lizard *Platysaurus intermedius*. *Physiological and Biochemical Zoology*, **76**, 511–521.

Layne, J. R. & Ford, N. B. (1984). Flight distance of the queen snake, Regina septemvittata. *Journal of Herpetology*, **18**, 496–498.

Lima, S. L. & Bednekoff, P. A. (1999). Temporal variation in danger drives antipredator behavior: The predation risk allocation hypothesis. *American Naturalist*, **153**, 649–659.

Llewelyn, J., Webb, J. K. & Shine, R. (2010). Flexible defense: context-dependent antipredator responses of two species of Australian elapid snakes. *Herpetologica*, **66**, 1–11.

López, P., Hawlena, D., Polo, V., Amo, L. & Martín, J. (2005). Sources of shy–bold variations in antipredator grahamÿr of male Iberian rock lizards. *Animal Behaviour*, **69**, 1–9.

Losos, J. B. & Irschick, D. J. (1996). The effect of perch diameter on escape grahamÿr of *Anolis* lizards: Laboratory predictions and field tests. *Animal Behaviour*, **51**, 593–602.

Losos, J. B., Mouton, P. L. F. N., Bickel, R., Cornelius, I. & Ruddock, L. (2002). The effect of body armature on escape behaviour in cordylid lizards. *Animal Behaviour*, **64**, 313–321.

Maritz, B. (2012). To run or hide? Escape behavior in a cryptic African snake. *African Zoology*, **47**, 270–274.

Martín, J. & López, P. (1999). Nuptial coloration and mate-guarding affect escape decisions of male lizards, *Psammodromus algirus*. *Ethology*, **105**, 439–447.

Martín, J., López, P. & Cooper, W. E., Jr. (2003). When to come out from a refuge: balancing predation risk and foraging opportunities in an alpine lizard. *Ethology*, **109**, 77–87.

Martín, J., Luque-Larena, J. J. & López, P. (2009). When to run from an ambush predator: balancing crypsis benefits with costs of fleeing in lizards. *Animal Behaviour*, **78**, 1011–1018.

Mattingly, W. B. & Jayne, B. C. (2005). The choice of arboreal escape paths and its consequences for the locomotor behaviour of four species of *Anolis* lizards. *Animal Behaviour*, **70**, 1239–1250.

McConnachie, S. & Whiting, M. J. (2003). Costs associated with tail autotomy in an ambush foraging lizard, Cordylus melanotus melanotus. *African Zoology*, **38**, 57–65.

Melville, J. & Swain, R. (2003). Evolutionary correlations between escape behaviour and performance ability in eight species of snow skinks from Tasmania (*Niveoscincus*: Lygosominae). *Journal of Zoology*, **261**, 79–89.

Olsson, M., Shine, R. & Bak-Olsson, E. (2000). Locomotor impairment of gravid lizards: is the burden physiological? *Journal of Evolutionary Biology*, **13**, 263–268.

Owen-Smith, N. & Mills, M. G. L. (2008). Predator–prey size relationships in an African large-mammal food web. *Journal of Animal Ecology*, **77**, 173–183.

Pérez-Cembranos, A., Pérez-Mellado, V. & Cooper, W. E. (2013). Predation risk and opportunity cost of fleeing while foraging on plants influences escape decisions of and insular lizard. *Ethology*, **119**, 522–530.

Pough, F. H. (1976). Multiple cryptic effects of crossbanded and ringed patterns of snakes. *Copeia*, **1976**, 834–836.

Ruxton, G. D., Sheratt, T. N. & Speed, M. (2004). *Avoiding Attack: The Evolutionary Ecology of Crypsis, Warning Signals and Mimicry*. Oxford: Oxford University Press.

Schall, J. J. & Pianka, E. R. (1980). Evolution of escape behavior diversity. *American Naturalist*, **115**, 551–556.

Schneider, K. R., Parmerlee, J. S., Jr. & Powell, R. (2000). Escape behavior of *Anolis* lizards from the Sierra de Baoruco, Hispaniola. *Caribbean Journal of Science*, **36**, 321–323.

Schulte, J. A., Losos, J., Cruz, F. B. & Nunez, H. (2004). The relarionship between morphology, escape behavior and microhabitat occupation in the lizard clade *Liolaemus* (Iguanidae: Tropidurinae: Liolaemini). *Journal of Evolutionary Biology*, **17**, 408–420.

Schwarzkopf, L. & Shine, R. (1992). Costs of reproduction in lizards: escape tactics and susceptibility to predation. *Behavioral Ecology and Sociobiology*, **31**, 17–25.

Scribner, S. J. & Weatherhead, P. J. (1995). Locomotion and antipredator behaviour in three species of aquatic snakes. *Canadian Journal of Zoology*, **73**, 321–329.

Shallenberger, E. W. (1970). *Tameness in Insular Animals: a Comparison of Approach Distances of Insular and Mainland Iguanid Lizards*. Los Angeles: University of California at Los Angeles.

Shine, R. (1980). "Costs" of reproduction in reptiles. *Oecologia*, **46**, 92–100.

Shine, R., Sun, L.-X., Fitzgerald, M. & Kearney, M. (2002). Antipredator responses of free-ranging pit vipers (*Gloydius shedaoensis*, Viperidae). *Copeia*, **2002**, 843–850.

Shine, R., Phillips, B., Waye, H. & Mason, R. T. (2003a). Behavioral shifts associated with reproduction in garter snakes. *Behavioral Ecology*, **14**, 251–256.

Shine, R., Phillips, B., Waye, H. & Mason, R. T. (2003b). Small-scale geographic variation in antipredator tactics of garter snakes. *Herpetologica*, **59**, 333–339.

Shine, R., Bonnett, X. & Cogger, H. C. (2003c). Antipredator tactics of amphibious sea snakes (*Serpentes*, Laticaudidae). *Ethology*, **109**, 533–542.

Smith, G. R. (1996). Correlates of approach distance in the striped plateau lizard (*Sceloporus virgatus*). *Herpetological Journal*, **6**, 56–58.

Stankowich, T. & Blumstein, D. T. (2005). Fear in animals: a meta-analysis and review of risk assessment. *Proceedings of the Royal Society of London, Series B, Biological Sciences*, **272**, 2627–2634.

Stankowich, T. & Coss, R. G. (2007). Effects of risk assessment, predator behavior, and habitat on escape behavior in Columbian black-tailed deer. *Behavioral Ecology*, **18**, 358–367.

Stapley, J. & Keogh, J. S. (2004). Exploratory and antipredator behaviours differ between territorial and nonterritorial male lizards. *Animal Behaviour*, **68**, 841–846.

Stiller, R. B. & McBrayer, L. B. (2013). The ontogeny of escape behavior, locomotor performance, and the hind limb in *Sceloporus woodi*. *Zoology*, **116**, 175–181.

Thaker, M., Lima, S. L. & Hews, D. K. (2009). Alternative antipredatory tactics in tree lizard morphs: hormonal and behavioural responses to a predator encounter. *Animal Behaviour*, **77**, 395–401.

Ward, J. P. & Hopkins, W. D. (1993). Primate laterality: current behavioral evidence of primate asymmetries. New York: Springer-Verlag.

Weatherhead, P. J. & Robertson, I. C. (1992). Thermal constraints on swimming performance and escape response of northern water snakes (*Nerodia sipedon*). *Canadian Journal of Zoology*, **70**, 94–98.

Whitaker, P. B. & Shine, R. (1999). Responses of free-ranging brownsnakes (*Pseudonaja textilis*: Elapidae). *Wildlife Research*, **26**, 689–704.

Williams, E. E. (1983). Ecomorphs, faunas, island size, and diverse end points in island radiations of Anolis. In *Lizard Ecology: Studies of a Model Organism*. Cambridge: Harvard University Press, pp. 326–370.

Williams, D. M., Samia, D. S. M., Cooper, W. E., Jr. & Blumstein, D. T. (2014). The flush early and avoid the rush hypothesis holds after accounting for spontaneous behavior. *Behavioral Ecology*, **25**, 1136–1147.

Zani, P. A., Jones, T. D., Neuhaus, R. A. & Milgrom, J. E. (2009). Effect of refuge distance on escape behavior of side-blotched lizards (*Uta stansburiana*). *Canadian Journal of Zoology*, **87**, 407–414.

6   Fish and amphibians

Patricia A. Fleming and Philip W. Bateman

6.1   Introduction

Although at first glance there seem to be significant differences between fish and amphibians in their habitat and therefore predation risk, they share many similar biological features (particularly fish and larval amphibians, i.e., tadpoles) that govern their escape responses. Although anuran tadpoles fill a similar niche to fish, they have a different body form, with a globose body and compressed, tapered tail (Wassersug 1989). In terms of awareness of their environment, escape locomotion, and modifications of escape behavior, fish and amphibians share responses to the risk of potential predation (Wassersug 1989).

Teleost fish species make up about half of all vertebrate taxa (Volff 2005). This diversity of species means that there is a huge range in traits such as body size, color, presence of body armor, and swimming speed. There are also diverse lifestyles, from pelagic, schooling fish through to solitary benthic species. In addition to their biological differences, fish can also experience a range of environmental conditions (e.g., water turbidity, temperature, dissolved oxygen) that can make it more or less physically or physiologically difficult to detect an approaching threat or escape. All these factors can influence the ability of fish to escape detection and predation (Domenici 2010), and therefore influence their reliance on crypsis vs. swimming.

Perhaps stimulated by this marked diversity among fishes, many predictions of the economic escape model (EEM) have been tested in fish. Fish have also been tested under a wide range of conditions, reflecting their diversity of habitats and body forms.

Amphibians are considerably less diverse than fish in terms of species. However, their dramatic change in lifestyle between tadpoles and adults takes them, in most cases, from a three-dimensional water environment similar to that experienced by fish, to a relatively two-dimensional habitat with substantial gravitational effects, at least for some of the time. Visual acuity, visual range, auditory inputs, and the physical limitations of locomotion therefore change during the ontogeny of amphibians. Furthermore, this change can be accompanied by a change in predation risks. On land, adult amphibians are potential prey of many predators that they did not face as tadpoles. Cryptic coloration, immobility, and crouching serve as primary defenses by helping prevent

Escaping From Predators: An Integrative View of Escape Decisions, ed. W. E. Cooper and D. T. Blumstein. Published by Cambridge University Press. © Cambridge University Press 2015.

detection, but active escape behavior is often needed, particularly in species without toxic skin secretions. There is a relative dearth of escape literature for amphibians, and what there is, is dominated by frogs. In the following chapter, we attempt to synthesize the escape behavior of both fish and, primarily, larval amphibians in the light of the predictions of the EEM (Ydenberg & Dill 1986).

6.2   The methodological challenges of working with fish and amphibians

6.2.1   How fish and amphibians perceive the world

Air and water have very different physical properties, and therefore one of the most significant differences between fish and adult amphibians is the medium in which they live. Light levels are attenuated rapidly in water, and therefore the effects of turbidity and depth have a marked effect on visual perception for these animals (see section 6.3.3.1). Visual cues trigger escape in response to looming and movement (e.g., Dill 1974a; Paglianti & Domenici 2006; Hettyey et al. 2012). Auditory cues are important for fish (reviewed by Popper & Fay 1993) and adult frogs (Cooper 2011 and references therein) and potentially for tadpoles (Hettyey et al. 2012). Olfactory cues (predator scents or cues of predated conspecifics) also modulate escape responses in fish (reviewed by Ferrari et al. 2010) and amphibians (Petranka et al. 1987; Semlitsch & Reyer 1992; Stauffer & Semlitsch 1993; Maag et al. 2012). Chemicals released from the skin in response to being attacked apparently act to alert conspecifics of imminent danger; adding the minced-up skins of conspecifics therefore alerts fish and amphibians to potential danger and increases their responses to predatory cues. Some fish (e.g., cartilaginous fishes) are sensitive to electrical stimuli. Because some of these senses exceed our own, and fish and amphibians have senses we lack, these signals often can be overlooked when studying the escape responses of fish and amphibians. We should, therefore, be aware of our inherent bias toward visual or auditory cues.

6.2.2   Neural control of escape behavior

Because each encounter with a predator is potentially lethal, there is strong selection on efficient and effective escape mechanisms. Fish and amphibians make interesting subjects for investigation, since their escape behavior has arguably been stripped back to the most basic responses. Fish and amphibians have some of the simplest vertebrate brains (they have no neocortex); despite this, there is evidence that fish can modify their escape behaviors based on learning and experience (Brown & Laland 2003; Kelley & Magurran 2003).

Immediate escape responses, e.g., the fast burst escape swimming of teleosts and the escape leap in frogs, have strong selection acting upon them, and consequently have become hard-wired as short reflex response neuronal loops in fish and amphibians that generate optimal behavioral responses; these initial reflexes are involuntary and nearly instantaneous "stereotypic" movements in response to stimulus (Eaton et al. 2001) (Box 6.1). Further aspects of escape (e.g., the distance moved and speed and trajectory of escape) are modified by the environmental context or predator type and approach (reviewed for fish by Domenici 2010), and therefore variability in these responses can be dynamically modified as predicted by the EEM (Ydenberg & Dill 1986; Walker *et al.* 2005; Domenici 2010; Marras *et al.* 2011; Chapter 8).

BOX 6.1 "I'm getting out of here!" Short-burst escape responses in fish and amphibians

Both fish and amphibians show dramatic initial escape responses to threatening stimuli, the kinematics, performance, and physiology of which have been well studied (Domenici & Blake 1997; Eaton *et al.* 2001; Wakeling 2005; Walker *et al.* 2005; Domenici 2010). These brainstem escape networks can be stimulated by sensory input from sound, mechanical vibration, electrical field, or visual cues (Eaton *et al.* 2001).

The Mauthner cells are a single pair of giant, bilateral neurons (one for each half of the body) present in the hindbrains of fish and amphibians that mediate a very fast initial escape reflex, as well as participating in a larger parallel, brainstem escape network (Eaton *et al.* 2001). They have been described as "command neurons" (Eaton *et al.* 2001) which are envisioned as a type of neural decision-making cell that could trigger a complete behavioral act with little or no need for additional input from the command neuron.

In fish, the most extreme response to a threatening stimulus is the "fast start" escape response (Figure 6.1), which is a short burst (less than ~1 s) of high-energy swimming associated with a short latency and high acceleration and speed (Domenici & Blake 1997; Turesson *et al.* 2009). Two main types of fast-starts are recognized, C-starts and S-starts in which the fish is bent into a "C" or "S" shape at the end of the first contraction of the lateral musculature. The C-starts are generally associated with escape responses away from the threat, while the S-starts with prey capture where the fish moves toward prey.

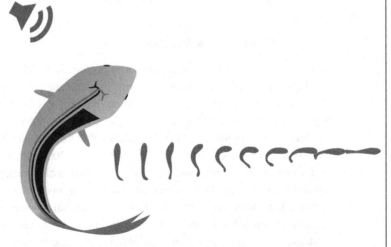

Figure 6.1   Illustration of the fast-start escape response in fish. (Modified from Eaton *et al.* 2001)

Amphibians have a similarly fast escape response system. Tadpoles have a C-start, combined with an extremely flexible tail allowing rapid turning with little or no displacement of their center of mass (Wassersug 1989). In adult frogs, hard-wired stereotyped movement patterns are evident as an explosive long leap (Ingle & Hoff 1990) or diving response (Korn & Faber 2005). In an analogous situation as observed between C-start and S-start responses in fish, frogs also have separate post-tectal pathways stimulated for turning *toward* prey and turning *away* from threat (King & Comer 1996), and both short-term and long-term memories influence jump direction (Ingle & Hoff, 1990). These separate neural control mechanisms may account for why a number of studies reveal independent regulation between predation avoidance and effective foraging (e.g., Horat & Semlitsch 1994).

6.2.3 Logistical issues

One of the major difficulties in comparing these studies is that vastly different stimuli have been used to test the escape responses of different taxa (Figure 6.2). Most studies of small fish and tadpoles have been carried out in small tanks under captive conditions. Larger fish species have principally been examined in the field, e.g., tested for responses to approaching models of predators, humans (i.e., swimmers or wading), or responses to being passed over by a boat. Frog responses have all been tested in response to human approach on foot in the wild.

While it is intuitive to human observers how many vertebrates react to approaching predators or disturbance (e.g., "alert" behavior, cessation of previous behavior, gaze direction, alarm calling), this is less clear for fish and amphibians. It is not obvious when these animals are "alert" to the predator's presence, which means that we need to be very cautious in interpreting "monitoring" or "alert distance" in these animals.

There are also problems with measuring responses of individuals when they are part of a school (reviewed by Krause 1994). Instead, researchers have had to rely on measures such as "responsiveness" (the proportion of a group responding to a stimulus; Blaxter *et al.* 1981), the proportion of animals moving in a particular direction (Domenici & Batty 1997), or "response latency" (the interval of time between stimulus presentation and the first detectable movement of the fish; Domenici & Batty 1997). With some of these measures, it can be difficult to distinguish between prey responses to the approaching predator and responses to conspecifics. As fish group size increases, it appears that both speed and accuracy of decision-making increase when under predatory threat (Ward *et al.* 2011). Tendency of individuals to join shoals is presumed to be a trade-off between predation risk and foraging efficiency. In three-spined sticklebacks *Gasterosteus aculeatus*, bolder individuals tend to be at the front of shoals where both predation risk and foraging opportunities are greater (Ward *et al.* 2004). An individual animal's antipredator behavior is therefore influenced by whether it is approached when alone or in a group of fish (Domenici & Batty 1997).

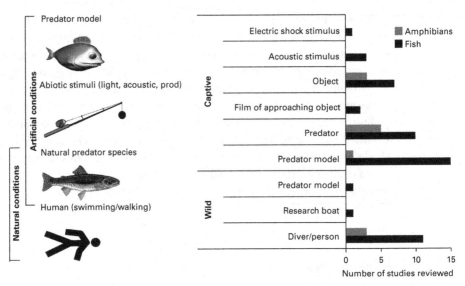

Figure 6.2   A wide range of stimuli have been used to initiate escape responses in fish and amphibians (frogs and tadpoles). The most common method for use in captive studies has been presenting prey with predator models; this has the advantage over real predators of being able to control the speed and type of approach. Under natural conditions, most studies have explored how fish and frogs respond to an approaching person, either swimming, wading or walking toward them.

6.3   Predictions under the Economic Escape Model: 1. Increased risk of capture

Ydenberg and Dill (1986, 234) stated that "If other things are equal, the risk of death in a given encounter with a predator should increase with the approach velocity of the predator and the distance to effective cover; it should decrease with the attainable escape velocity of the prey." Simply (and assuming that other things are equal), we predict that prey should therefore have longer flight initiation distance (FID), longer distance fled (DF), and faster escape speeds ("escape responses") if they face increased risk of capture (Table 6.1). We discuss empirical support for these predictions below.

6.3.1   Prey attributes

6.3.1.1   When prey is slower

Prey locomotion has an effect on predator success. For example, a one standard deviation increase in fast-start performance in guppies *Poecilia reticulata* increases by two- to three-fold the odds of surviving a predation strike by pike cichlid *Crenicichla alta* (Walker *et al.* 2005). Predatory fish (*Micropterus salmoides*) are more likely to abort attacks and less likely to chase prey when their fish prey show higher acceleration performance (Webb 1986).

Table 6.1 Review of the literature for fish and amphibians, showing the predictions of the EEM in terms of flight initiation distance (FID), distance fled (DF), and escape speed (arrows: ↑ increase predicted, ↓ decrease predicted) and the number of studies we located that either supported these predictions (highlighted cells) or did not (non-highlighted cells).

Category	Factor	Flight initiation distance (FID)				Distance fled (FD)				Escape speed			
		Prediction	Decreases	Same	Increases	Prediction	Decreases	Same	Increases	Prediction	Decreases	Same	Increases
1. Increased risk of capture		↑											
if prey is slower		↑											
e.g, environment of prey	O_2 or CO_2 level	↑	1	2–4							4	3	
	pollution	↑		5,6							5		
	parasitism	↑		6									
	osmotic shock	↑					7						
	ammonia in water											8		
	temperature (heat shock)	↑	9										
If prey is	bright and colorful	↑				↑							
	distracted (e.g., foraging, fighting)	↑	10–13			↑							
	experienced (can identify predator)	↑	14		14–18	↑↓			19			16	16,19,20
	is exposed to intensive fishing	↑			21–27	↑							
environment interferes with prey senses or responses	turbidity (decreased visibility)	↑	28–30			↑			31				31
	greater distance to cover	↑		32	25,32–34	↑							34
predator	more predators	↑				↑							
	faster predator	↑	28,35		36	↑				↑			28,36
	persistent predator	↑				↑							

Table 6.1 (cont.)

	Flight initiation distance (FID)				Distance fled (FD)				Escape speed			
	Prediction	Decreases	Same	Increases	Prediction	Decreases	Same	Increases	Prediction	Decreases	Same	Increases
2. Increased cost of fleeing												
prey												
loss of crypsis	→											
body size (large fish – swimming less costly)	↑		37	33,38–40								
injury that increases cost of fleeing	→											
gravid	→											
hungry (leaving food)	→	33										
opportunity costs												
3. Effectiveness of alternative defense tactics												
crypsis	→	41,42	37		→	42,43						
armor (e.g., spines, plates)	→	37			→	44,45				44–46		
poison (frogs only)												
4. Group size												
FID varies according to the fitness benefits attached to group membership of different sizes	↑↓	37,47 48		30,49								

References: 1. Allan et al. (2013); 2. Domenici et al. (2007); 3. Lefrancois & Domenici (2006); 4. Lefrançois et al. (2005); 5. Alvarez et al. (2006); 6. Krause et al. (2010); 7. Handeland et al. (1996); 8. McKenzie et al. (2009); 9. Webb & Zhang (1994); 10. Krause & Godin (1996); 11. Brick (1998); 12. Bohórquez-Herrera et al. (2013); 13. Jakobsson et al. (1995); 14. Healey & Reinhardt (1995); 15. Arai et al. (2007); 16. Dill (1974); 17. Malavasi et al. (2004); 18. D'Anna et al. (2012); 19. Ghalambor et al. (2004); 20. Langerhans et al. (2004); 21. Januchowski-Hartley et al. (2011); 22. Januchowski-Hartley et al. (2012); 23. Kulbicki (1998); 24. Feary et al. (2011); 25. Gotanda et al. (2009); 26. Januchowski-Hartley et al. (2013); 27. Cole (1994); 28. Meager et al. (2006); 29. Miner & Stein (1996); 30. Semeniuk & Dill (2005); 31. Hartman & Abrahams (2000); 32. McLean & Godin (1989); 33. Grant & Noakes (1987); 34. Dill (1990); 35. Fuiman (1993); 36. Dill (1974); 37. Abrahams (1995); 38. Webb (1981); 39. Paglianti & Domenici (2006); 40. Miller et al. (2011); 41. Radabaugh (1989); 42. Cooper et al. (2008); 43. Eterovick et al. (2010); 44. Andraso & Barron (1995); 45. Bergstrom (2002); 46. Andraso (1997); 47. Seghers (1981); 48. Godin & Morgan (1985); 49. Semeniuk & Dill (2006).

Escape speed in tadpoles is influenced by their body form (Dayton *et al.* 2005), as well as environment and previous experience. *Rana dalmatina* tadpoles reared with pursuit predators (sticklebacks) can swim faster (and have longer and deeper tail muscles) than conspecifics raised with ambush predators (dragonfly larvae) or no predators (Teplitsky *et al.* 2005). In a comparison across species, in addition to speed, evasiveness and habitat use also influence risk: *Bufo bufo* tadpoles are highly susceptible to predation by dragonfly larvae due to their constant slow movements, while *Hyla arborea* tadpoles, although slow generally, also showed high evasiveness, while *R. dalmatina* tadpoles were the least susceptible being benthic and immobile but capable of high bursts of speed (Chovanec 1992).

Larger fish may not be targeted by gape-limited predators (Januchowski-Hartley *et al.* 2011), and larger fish can also generally move faster than smaller fish (Videler 1993). We discuss the effects of body size on costs of fleeing in section 6.4.2. However, other factors may substantially affect swimming speed in fish. Water is 800 times denser than air and hence it is more difficult to displace; consequently, movement through water causes more turbulence and drag and requires more energy than moving through air (Denny 1993). Water also has lower oxygen levels than air (Denny 1993). Because escape speed is so important, the physiological state of prey is important in determining whether their escape is successful. Decreased oxygen levels, elevated CO_2 and ammonia in water, pollution, parasitism, being injured or gravid, or subject to physiological shock (e.g., osmotic shock or heat shock) can all contribute to impaired escape in fish, generally due to impaired neural function and locomotion. Under the predictions of the EEM, this decreased mobility would increase risk of capture and should influence FID as fish respond with greater caution on account of their increased vulnerability; however, most empirical findings contradict these predictions. A number of studies have found no difference in FID of fish subject to low oxygen levels (Lefrancois & Domenici 2006; Domenici *et al.* 2007). Similarly, Lefrancois *et al.* (2005) reported no difference in escape speed; while Lefrancois and Domenici (2006) reported an increase in escape speed. Krause *et al.* (2010) report no effect of parasitism on FID. Similarly, Alvarez *et al.* (2006) and Krause *et al.* (2010) found no change in FID for fish exposed to pollution, while Alvarez *et al.* (2006) also found no effect on escape speed. Handeland *et al.* (1996) reported a decrease in escape distance due to osmotic shock, McKenzie *et al.* (2009) reported a decrease in escape speed as a result of ammonia in the water, while Webb and Zhang (1994) report a decrease in FID as a consequence of heat shock. Recent studies investigating the effects of exposure to increased CO_2 levels in water demonstrate reduced responsiveness for prey damselfish *Pomacentrus amboinensis*, although their dottyback *Pseudochromis fuscus* predators also succumb to the effects of increased CO_2 and suffer reduced capture success when similarly exposed (Allan *et al.* 2013).

Since alertness (i.e., visual, auditory etc. responses contribute to FID) and locomotion (escape speed and duration, escape trajectories) are our usual measures of escape responses, the effects of injury and other impairment are confounded with the measures that we are making. Additionally, the predictions of the EEM are clouded in regard to injuries. If risk increases due to injury or other impairment (e.g., survival of tadpoles with tails damaged in previous predatory encounters is reduced; Semlitsch 1990) then FID, DF, etc., should increase, but if the same condition increases the cost of fleeing, then it is likely to decrease responses. If it does both, then it is possible that there are ambiguous escape responses, and the animal may be more likely to resort to changes in habitat use.

6.3.1.2   When prey is bright and colorful

The polymorphic frog *Oophaga granulifera* can rely more on crypsis or aposematism, depending on variation in conspicuousness, and this variation is also reflected in escape behavior, with FID in response to a bird model being higher for more conspicuous red morphs than for cryptic green morphs or intermediate morphs (Willink *et al.* 2013). Despite the diversity of color patterns in fish, we found no studies that tested the effects of prey coloration on their escape responses. It may be that brightly colored fish tend to rely on alternative defenses (e.g., including spines and toxins; section 6.5).

6.3.1.3   When prey is distracted

Prey that are engaged in other activities may be exposed to increased risk due to diverted attention (Chan & Blumstein 2011). The foraging position of guppies influenced their vulnerability to predation since guppies foraging with their heads down were more vulnerable and more likely to be attacked by a cichlid predator. However, guppies foraging with their heads down showed shorter FIDs than animals that were foraging horizontally or those that were not foraging at all (Krause & Godin 1996). Non-foraging guppies reacted sooner, having longer FIDs, and horizontally foraging individuals reacted before downward-foraging individuals (Krause & Godin 1996). Bohórquez-Herrera *et al.* (2013) similarly showed silver-spotted sculpins *Blepsias cirrhosus* had reduced responsiveness during prey handling (compared with non-foraging or fish that were targeting prey).

As another form of "distraction," golden dwarf cichlids *Nannacara anomala* engaged in fights demonstrate a decrease in FID (Jakobsson *et al.* 1995). In the presence of a predator model, fighting males changed their fighting behavior, showing more lateral display and tail beating (presumably behaviors that allow them to simultaneously monitor their environment) in preference over mouth wrestling (Brick 1998).

6.3.1.4   When prey has previous experience

The cognitive abilities of fish are more developed than most might assume (Laland *et al.* 2003). Previous experience with predators can influence subsequent behavior of fish: intensive catch and release of rainbow trout *Oncorhyncus mykiss* by anglers results in a rapid decline in catch rates within seven to ten days, suggesting that caught and released fish learnt to ignore hooks (Askey *et al.* 2006). Guppies learn to avoid trawl nets by escaping through a hole; a skill that was socially transmitted through observing previously trained conspecifics (Reader *et al.* 2003).

Consistent with the predictions of the EEM, as a result of experience with a predator, an increase in FID (Dill 1974b; Healey & Reinhardt 1995; D'Anna *et al.* 2004; Malavasi *et al.* 2004; Arai *et al.* 2007), DF (Ghalambor *et al.* 2004), and escape speed (Dill 1974b; Ghalambor *et al.* 2004; Langerhans *et al.* 2004) have been recorded. Some

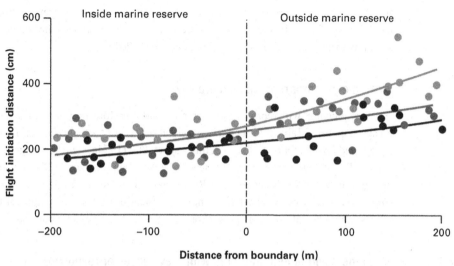

Figure 6.3 Relationship between FID for surgeon fishes (Acanthuridae) and distance from a marine reserve boundary. The different shaded dots represent data from three sites. (Januchowski-Hartley *et al.* 2013)

interesting variations in escape response might suggest species differences as a consequence of previous experience. For example, Healey and Reinhardt (1995) reported changes in FID for experienced coho *Oncorhynchus kisutch* and chinook salmon *O. tshawytscha* over their predator-naïve responses: coho increased their FID (i.e., benefitted from experience and showed more flight behavior), but experienced chinook were more likely to stay immobile. These two species therefore show different tactics in response to the same predator, with coho using "a strategy based on rapid and early flight with, perhaps, a dependence on maneuverability and school cohesion to avoid capture" (Healey & Reinhardt 1995: 621), a strategy that may be more successful in the presence of safe refuge under natural conditions.

Consistent with the predictions of the EEM, a number of studies reveal that there is an increase in FID in response to high levels of fishing compared with marine reserves (Cole 1994; Kulbicki 1998; Gotanda *et al.* 2009; Feary *et al.* 2011; Januchowski-Hartley *et al.* 2011, 2012, 2013; Figure 6.3). This may reflect social learning among individuals that are able to escape, or alternatively, increased FID may simply tell us that we have removed all the less wary (i.e., more curious) individuals from the population (Sutter *et al.* 2012). Fish targeted by spear-fishing also alter their use of refuge as a result of exposure to fishing – at protected reefs, sea breams *Diplodus sargus* and *D. vulgaris* frequently swam into the closest shelters, whereas in fished reefs they mostly escaped in open water (Guidetti *et al.* 2008).

Fish will often show predator inspection behavior, where a prey fish fixates on a predator, and slowly swims toward it (Pitcher *et al.* 1986). While inherently risky, this behavior may allow assessment of predator intent and dissuasion of predation, while also advertising fitness to potential mates (Sutter *et al.* 2012). However, this behavior may make fishes particularly vulnerable to spear fishers, bringing them closer to the fisher, and highlighting the fish as a target. Consequently, differences in responses by various fish families to fishing pressures may reflect differences in longevity, trophic level, availability of and differential use of refuges, or potentially group size (influencing social learning) (Januchowski-Hartley *et al.* 2011, 2013).

6.3.2   When the predator represents more risk

A faster predator will represent greater risk, and therefore prey should show increased escape responses (Table 6.1). There is empirical support of these predictions for fish, but we have found no data for amphibians in this respect. Dill (1974a) reported longer FID in zebra danios (*Brachydanio rerio*) in the presence of a faster approaching model of a predator, but others (Fuiman 1993; Meager *et al.* 2006) reported shorter FID in *Clupea harengus* and *Gadus morhua*, respectively. Interestingly, we found no published empirical tests of the effects of number of predators present or the persistence of predators on escape responses.

6.3.3   When the environment interferes with prey senses or responses

6.3.3.1   Turbidity (decreased visibility)

Conditions that make it harder to detect a predator (and therefore greater risk of the predator approaching while the prey is unaware) should elicit greater responsiveness in potential prey following predictions of the EEM. The problem is how to measure this change in responses. In an environment where visibility is reduced due to turbidity, the distance at which a predator is detected may be reduced below the optimal FID in clear conditions; therefore flight may be instantaneous on detection of a predator, but FID would be decreased. Numerous studies have shown that turbidity is correlated with decreased FID (Miner & Stein 1996; Semeniuk & Dill 2005; Meager *et al.* 2006). Prey therefore have less time to evade the predator in turbid water (Meager *et al.* 2006). There are, however, other ways of reacting to this increased risk. When in turbid water, fathead minnows *Pimephales promelas* display significantly fewer dashes in response to a visual predator stimulus, but fishes moved significantly further and faster in turbid waters (Hartman & Abrahams 2000).

6.3.3.2   Greater distance to cover

Predictions of the EEM suggest that animals show an increase in escape responses with greater distance to cover (Table 6.1). Data for fish indicate an increase in FID with greater distance to cover (Grant & Noakes 1987; McLean & Godin 1989; Dill 1990; Gotanda *et al.* 2009). Dill (1990) recorded no difference in fish escape speed with distance to cover.

6.4   Predictions under the Economic Escape Model: 2. increased cost of fleeing

If fleeing is costly, prey should show shorter FID (Ydenberg & Dill 1986: 237), and shorter DF (Table 6.1). It is possible that escape speed would also be slower. We discuss empirical support for these predictions below.

6.4.1   Loss of crypsis

As soon as an animal starts to move away from an approaching predator, it will forfeit any potential benefit of crypsis (Ydenberg & Dill 1986), and therefore cryptic animals may benefit from not responding immediately to the presence of a predator. Ydenberg and Dill (1986) also cover the effects of crypsis under "alternative strategies" (see section 6.5.1). Cryptic animals should only move away when the benefits of moving outweigh those of remaining stationary. Martín *et al.* (2006) reported decreased FID for green frogs in the absence of vegetation; the frogs presumably allowed an observer to approach closer, remained for long periods immobile and cryptic, due to their green or brown skin coloration.

6.4.2   Body size

The size of a fish may be correlated with measures of fitness such as reproductive value, which may in turn influence risk assessment. Warner (1998) found that female bluehead wrasse *Thallosoma bifasciatum*, which are iteroparous, are relatively risk averse, which may reflect residual reproductive value of individuals. Larger fish can, in general, move faster than smaller fish (Videler 1993). Importantly, however, the methods of swimming vary with body size in fish. In parrotfish, there is a link between body size and type of swimming locomotion (Miller *et al.* 2011). Larger fish are more likely to use less costly but relatively slower escape (paired fin swimming), whereas smaller fish use an energetically more costly, but relatively faster escape (body and caudal fin swimming) (Figure 6.4). Under the EEM, both decreased cost and slower

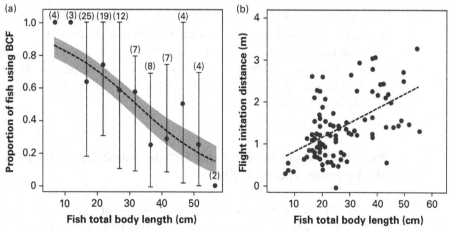

Figure 6.4   (a) In response to being approached by a snorkeler, small parrotfish are more likely to use body and caudal fin swimming (BCF), while large fish are more likely to swim away using slower paired fin swimming. (b) In the same study, there is a positive relationship between FID and body size across 95 parrotfish (three species combined). (Miller *et al.* 2011)

swimming (in larger fish) would predict greater FID. Supporting these predictions, various studies report an increase in FID with body size (Webb 1981; Grant & Noakes 1987; Gotanda *et al.* 2009; Januchowski-Hartley *et al.* 2011; Miller *et al.* 2011)(but see Abrahams 1995; and Feary *et al.* 2011 who report no effect).

In Southern Leopard frogs *Lithobates sphenocephalus*, larger frogs are more likely to hide in cover away from water than smaller ones (Bateman & Fleming 2014). When disturbed, they are more likely to resort to cover on land than smaller frogs, which retreat to water (Bateman & Fleming 2014). Ontogenetic changes in size can also influence escape tactics in tadpoles: *Rana sylvatica* tadpoles swim slowest when they are newly hatched and just prior to metamorphosis, which are also presumed to be the times when they are most susceptible to predation (Brown & Taylor 1995). At these times, they also show the highest propensity to engage in rapid turning behavior and ability to maneuver at sharper angles, which may compensate for decreased speed (Brown & Taylor 1995).

6.4.3   Opportunity costs

Escaping from a stimulus that is not threatening will ensure immediate safety, but incurs high opportunity costs (Chapters 2, 5). Therefore modulating responses is important, ensuring that the animal does not overreact to non-lethal stimuli. Consistent with the EEM, the presence of a food resource caused guppies (horizontally foraging ones only) to delay their flight compared to fish that were not given any food (Krause & Godin 1996). Similarly, unfed brook trout *Salvelinus fontinalis* decrease their FID in the presence of food (Grant & Noakes 1987). Feeding and antipredation behavior may be independently neurally controlled (Blanchard *et al.* 1991; Box 6.1); consequently, it may not be surprising that feeding activities can modulate antipredator responses.

An example of cost due to forfeiting opportunity in amphibians is illustrated in Box 6.2. Developing embryos will hatch prematurely in the presence of an immediate threat, forfeiting the opportunity of additional time developing in terrestrial nests away from aquatic predators.

6.5   Predictions under the Economic Escape Model: 3. Effectiveness of alternative defense tactics

Effective alternative defenses would reduce "the cost of remaining at a given distance from an approaching predator" (Ydenberg & Dill 1986: 239). Therefore prey having such defenses should be less reliant on escape behavior and modify their responses accordingly.

BOX 6.2 When you can't wait around

Tadpole eggs are particularly vulnerable to predation during development and there-fore frogs may preferentially lay eggs in vegetation above waterways to protect the eggs from aquatic predators. However, when approached by terrestrial predators, it is advantageous for these developing eggs to hatch rapidly (Figure 6.5), dropping to the water below and facing increased risk from aquatic predators as an underformed tadpole rather than face certain death (Warkentin, 1995). The eggs are sensitive to vibrations in their substrate, hatching up to 30% earlier than undisturbed nests (Warkentin, 2005).

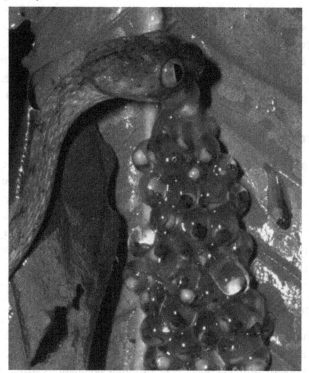

Figure 6.5   Chunk-headed snake *Imantodes inornatus* attacking an egg clutch of the treefrog *Agalychnis callidryas*. (Photo by Karen Warkentin).

6.5.1   Crypsis

Cryptic animals are predicted to be less responsive than more visible prey under the EEM. Several species of fish show counter-shading (Ruxton *et al.* 2004) or cryptic coloration (Donnelly & Dill 1984 and references therein). However, we found only one paper that specifically explored the influence of crypsis on escape behavior. Radabaugh (1989) showed that among male darters *Etheostoma* spp., those which exchanged cryptic colors for bright courtship colors became less likely to "freeze" and more likely to flee when approached by a simulated predatory threat.

To maintain the effect of crypsis, some fish have modified their escape behavior. Three species of nocturnal South American fish (the catfishes *Tetranematichthys quadrifilis* and *Helogenes marmoratus* and the knifefish *Steatogenys duidae*) are camouflaged as leaves: two species even lie on their sides, increasing their resemblance to fallen leaves (Sazima *et al.* 2006). When disturbed, they do not simply swim away; two species drift off like waterlogged leaves, while *H. marmoratus* moves up submerged root tangles, exposing its head and forebody, and looking like a leaf wedged in the roots.

When on substrates that enhance their crypsis, cryptic *Bokermannohyla alvarengai* tadpoles swim only short distances after disturbances and again become immobile (Eterovick *et al.* 2010). In adult frogs, immobility is crucial to maintaining crypsis, and is a major component of behavioral defense against predation. When approached by a human, over 90% of individuals belonging to five *Craugastor* species remained immobile until the predator reached them (Cooper *et al.* 2008).

6.5.2   Alternative defenses: poison

Because some frogs are poisonous, they may rely less on escape due to their aposomatic coloration and learned avoidance responses of predators. Cooper *et al.* (2009) examined the escape responses of poison dart frogs (*Dendrobates auratus* and *Oophaga pumilio*) and recorded low escape reactions: short FID and short DF – essentially the frogs got out of the way of the person's approach and then stopped moving again. Although there are many venomous/poisonous fishes, it is surprising that there are no publications testing the predictions of the EEM in these animals.

6.5.3   Armor: spines and plates

Armor is an effective form of defense in fish (e.g., Lescak & von Hippel 2011). The influence of armor on escape behavior has been examined in fish, comparing the behavior of different species or different populations of the same species that have varying levels of armor (e.g., spines or bony plates). Consistent with the EEM, such studies report a decrease in FID for armored fish (Abrahams 1995), a decrease in escape distance (Andraso & Barron 1995; Bergstrom 2002), and a reduction in escape speed (Andraso & Barron 1995; Andraso 1997; Bergstrom 2002).

6.5.4   Retreat to safer sites

Retreating to cover is an important antipredator response in fish, frogs, and tadpoles. For example, several species of frog retreat to water from land when approached by humans (Martín *et al.* 2005, 2006; Cooper 2011; Bateman & Fleming 2014), which they use as cover (reviewed in Chapter 9).

6.6   Predictions under the Economic Escape Model: 4. Group size

Ydenberg and Dill (1986: 240) predicted that "if risk of predation or foraging efficiency varies with group size, then this will be reflected in flight distances," but did not predict the direction of these changes because group size and membership have many facets that might affect FID, possibly in opposing ways. Because most predators target a single individual, the presence of group members decreases the risk of predation for each individual (risk dilution). The fitness benefits attached to group membership vary among group sizes, locations, food density, and predation regimes (Chapter 2).

Group membership can present an advantage of early warning (the "many eyes" hypothesis). Consequently, alert distance can be greater, and, since AD and FID are correlated, FID would be predicted to be greater for groups than solitary individuals: the whole group flees according to the most reactive individual. This has been tested with small groups of green frogs *Rana perezi* (Martín *et al.* 2006), but there was no difference in FID between solitary individuals and the first (most reactive) individual of small groups of up to four frogs. Similarly, Godin and Morgan (1985) found no difference in FID in response to a fish predator model between solitary and schooling banded killifish *Fundulus diaphranus*, and FID was statistically constant over a wide range of school sizes. However, other studies have found that escape responses vary with group size. Data for stingrays supports the early warning hypothesis (Semeniuk & Dill 2005, 2006) (Box 6.3). Interestingly, Abrahams (1995) showed that FID was shorter in grouped ($n = 3$) than solitary brook sticklebacks *Culea incostans*, suggesting that these animals were more sensitive to the effects of risk dilution than early warning. Because premature, or unwarranted responses to being approached can be costly, it is possible that the effects of group sizes on FID sometimes may only come into play when a minimal proportion of the group responds.

BOX 6.3 Selective stingrays

Consistent with the early warning hypothesis, approaching cowtail stingrays *Pastinachus sephen* with a mock predator model, Semeniuk and Dill (2005) showed greater FID for the first cowtail in a group to flee compared with solitary cowtails. Cowtails will often settle next to reticulate whiprays *Himantura uarnak*, which have longer tails (Figure 6.6), show earlier responses than cowtails to a threat (approaching boat), and were most frequently the first to respond when in a mixed group (Semeniuk & Dill 2006). The whiprays have longer tails and may have an advantage in increased likelihood of predator detection via the mechanoreceptors found along the length of the tail. In 34 mixed-species groups, whiprays responded first 25 times (73%), although they made up only 49% of the membership of these groups. Whiprays could be preferred resting partners under conditions of poor visibility due to differences in predator-response capabilities between these two species. Cowtails also preferentially settle next to artificial ray shapes (unpainted marine plywood decoys) made with a longer tail, inspecting the tails before settling.

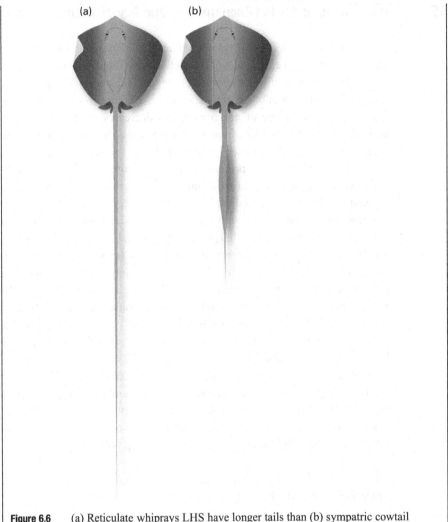

Figure 6.6   (a) Reticulate whiprays LHS have longer tails than (b) sympatric cowtail stingrays RHS.

Another consideration is the effect of group size on DF. If group cohesion is lost while fleeing, then perhaps DF should be shorter in a group. However, it appears that fish cohesion and reaction and response to predatory threat actually improve with increasing group size (Ward *et al.* 2011).

In Cuban tree frog tadpoles *Osteopilus septentrionalis*, fewer tadpoles swam away from a predatory stimulus from above when housed in higher density groups (Bateman & Fleming 2015). Among those that swim away, distance swum is shorter for tadpoles in smaller groups (Bateman & Fleming 2015).

6.7   Conclusions

As we reviewed the literature for this chapter, it became obvious that there is a massive literature on the escape responses of fishes, much of which is largely ignored in the literature of terrestrial taxa. Many key principles of the EEM have been tested in fish species, with varying results. Many studies do not support the simple predictions of the EEM (Table 6.1), either because the animals do not show measurable variation in their responses, or sometimes because they show responses that contradict the direction of our predictions. We have highlighted a few studies where careful examination of the responses of these animals can be explained through physiological effects of their environment, and it is clear that this needs to be considered carefully in terms of escape responses in fishes.

With regard to amphibians, it is surprising how little of the ecology of their anti-predator escape has been explored. Ontogenetic change in antipredator responses as tadpoles metamorphose and move from water to land is an important aspect of the adaptation of frogs to life on land that reflects vulnerability to different suites of predators. Understanding these responses is likely to be an important tool for conservation management of frogs in these days of diminishing amphibian populations worldwide.

Finally, studies of escape behavior may provide information useful as a conservation tool for various taxa (Chapter 17). Escape behavior has been used as a measure of human impact on fish and frogs, and hence may prove useful for conservation of these animals (Blumstein & Fernández-Juricic 2010). For frogs, FID has been used to identify the effects of repeated exposure to human traffic for endangered Iberian frogs *Rana iberica* and to develop setback distances (Rodríguez-Prieto & Fernández-Juricic 2005). Escape behavior has also been widely used as a measure of environmental pollution on animals. For example, fish born of mothers exposed to methyl mercury demonstrate concentration-dependent effects on survival skills, including impairment of escape speeds (Alvarez *et al.* 2006). *Rana blairi* tadpoles exposed to sublethal levels of carbaryl (an insecticide) have reduced swimming performance and activity, which may result in increased predation and generate changes at the local population level (Bridges 1997). Recent observations that increased CO_2 levels in water can impede escape responses (Allan *et al.* 2013) rings warning bells for climate change predictions.

Escape behavior in fishes has been shown to be a powerful indicator of fishing intensity or even occasional poaching (Cole 1994; Gotanda *et al.* 2009; Feary *et al.* 2011; Januchowski-Hartley *et al.* 2011, 2013), and therefore could be used to gauge levels of compliance with no-take regulations of marine reserves. Escape measures are arguably more tractable for studies requiring high levels of replication than other survey methods (Figure 6.7), and are sensitive even to low levels of fishing (Feary *et al.* 2011; Januchowski-Hartley *et al.* 2012).

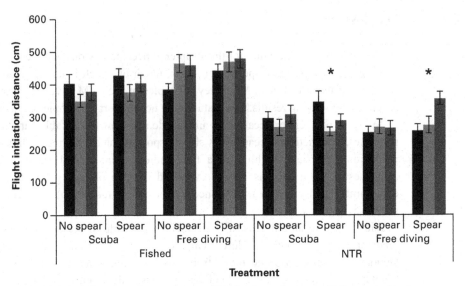

Figure 6.7   Flight initiation distance estimates (mean ± SE) for three observers (different shading) approaching fish in a fished or no-take marine reserve (NTR), using either scuba or free diving, and carrying a fishing spear or not. This study showed minor observer differences in estimates (asterisks) but the main effect was the difference between locations. (Redrawn from Januchowski-Hartley *et al.* 2012)

References

Abrahams, M. V. (1995). The interaction between antipredator behaviour and antipredator morphology: Experiments with fathead minnows and brook sticklebacks. *Canadian Journal of Zoology*, **73**, 2209–2215.

Allan, B. J. M., Domenici, P., Mccormick, M. I., Watson, S.-A. & Munday, P. L. (2013). Elevated CO_2 affects predator–prey interactions through altered performance. *PloS ONE*, **8**, e58520.

Alvarez, M. C., Murphy, C. A., Rose, K. A., Mccarthy, I. D. & Fuiman, L. A. (2006). Maternal body burdens of methylmercury impair survival skills of offspring in Atlantic croaker (*Micropogonias undulatus*). *Aquatic Toxicology*, **80**, 329–337.

Andraso, G. M. (1997). A comparison of startle response in two morphs of the brook stickleback (*Culaea inconstans*): Further evidence for a trade-off between defensive morphology and swimming ability. *Evolutionary Ecology*, **11**, 83–90.

Andraso, G. M. & Barron, J. N.(1995). Evidence for a trade-off between defensive morphology and startle-response performance in the brook stickleback (*Culaea inconstans*). *Canadian Journal of Zoology*, **73**, 1147–1153.

Arai, T., Tominaga, O., Seikai, T. & Masuda, R. (2007). Observational learning improves predator avoidance in hatchery-reared Japanese flounder *Paralichthys olivaceus* juveniles. *Journal of Sea Research*, **58**, 59–64.

Askey, P. J., Richards, S. A., Post, J. R. & Parkinson, E. A. (2006). Linking angling catch rates and fish learning under catch-and-release regulations. *North American Journal of Fisheries Management*, **26**, 1020–1029.

Bateman, P. W. & Fleming, P. A. (2014). Living on the edge: effects of body size, group density and microhabitat selection on escape behaviour of Southern Leopard Frogs (*Lithobates sphenocephalus*). *Current Zoology*, **60**, 712–718.

Bateman, P. W. & Fleming, P. A. (2015). Body size and group size of Cuban tree frogs (*Osteopilus Septentrionalis*) tadpoles influence their escape behaviour. *Acta Ethologica*, doi: 10.1007/s10211-014-0201-9.

Bergstrom, C. (2002). Fast-start swimming performance and reduction in lateral plate number in threespine stickleback. *Canadian Journal of Zoology*, **80**, 207–213.

Blanchard, R. J., Blanchard, D. C., Rodgers, J. & Weiss, S. M. (1991). The characterization and modelling of antipredator defensive behavior. *Neuroscience & Biobehavioral Reviews*, **14**, 463–472.

Blaxter, J., Gray, J. & Denton, E. (1981). Sound and startle responses in herring shoals. *Journal of the Marine Biology Association UK*, **61**, 851–870.

Blumstein, D. T. & Fernández-Juricic, E. (2010). *A Primer on Conservation Behavior.* Sunderland, MA: Sinauer Associates Inc.

Bohórquez-Herrera, J., Kawano, S. M. & Domenici, P.(2013). Foraging behavior delays mechanically-stimulated escape responses in fish. *Integrative and Comparative Biology*, **53**, 780–786.

Brick, O. (1998). Fighting behaviour, vigilance and predation risk in the cichlid fish *Nannacara anomala*. *Animal Behaviour*, **56**, 309–317.

Bridges, C. M. (1997). Tadpole swimming performance and activity affected by acute exposure to sublethal levels of carbaryl. *Environmental Toxicology and Chemistry*, **16**, 1935–1939.

Brown, C. & Laland, K. N. (2003). Social learning in fishes: A review. *Fish and Fisheries*, **4**, 280–288.

Brown, R. M. & Taylor, D. H. (1995). Compensatory escape mode trade-offs between swimming performance and maneuvering behavior through larval ontogeny of the wood frog, *Rana sylvatica*. *Copeia*, 1–7.

Chan, A. A. Y.-H. & Blumstein, D. T. (2011). Attention, noise, and implications for wildlife conservation and management. *Applied Animal Behaviour Science*, **131**, 1–7.

Chovanec, A. (1992). The influence of tadpole swimming behaviour on predation by dragonfly nymphs. *Amphibia-Reptilia*, **13**, 341–349.

Cole, R. (1994). Abundance, size structure, and diver-oriented behaviour of three large benthic carnivorous fishes in a marine reserve in northeastern New Zealand. *Biological Conservation*, **70**, 93–99.

Cooper, W., E Jr. (2011). Escape strategy and vocalization during escape by American bullfrogs (*Lithobates catesbeianus*). *Amphibia-Reptilia*, **32**, 213–221.

Cooper, W. E. Jr., Caldwell, J. P. & Vitt, L. J. (2008). Effective crypsis and its maintenance by immobility in *Craugastor* frogs. *Copeia*, **2008**, 527–532.

Cooper, W. E. Jr., Caldwell, J. P. & Vitt, L. J. (2009). Risk assessment and withdrawal behavior by two species of aposematic poison frogs, *Dendrobates auratus* and *Oophaga pumilio*, on forest trails. *Ethology*, **115**, 311–320.

D'anna, G., Giacalone, V. M., Badalamenti, F. & Pipitone, C.(2004). Releasing of hatchery-reared juveniles of the white seabream *Diplodus sargus* (L., 1758) in the Gulf of Castellammare artificial reef area (NW Sicily). *Aquaculture*, **233**, 251–268.

D'anna, G., Giacalone, V. M., Fernández, T. V. *et al.* (2012). Effects of predator and shelter conditioning on hatchery-reared white seabream *Diplodus sargus* (L., 1758) released at sea. *Aquaculture*, **356–357**, 91–97.

Dayton, G. H., Saenz, D., Baum, K. A., Langerhans, R. B. & Dewitt, T. J. (2005). Body shape, burst speed and escape behavior of larval anurans. *Oikos*, **111**, 582–591.

Denny, M. W. (1993). *Air and Water: The Biology and Physics of Life's Media*. Princeton University Press.

Dill, L. M. (1974a). The escape response of the zebra danio (*Brachydanio rerio*) I. The stimulus for escape. *Animal Behaviour*, **22**, 711–722.

Dill, L. M. (1974b). The escape response of the zebra danio (*Brachydanio rerio*) II. The effect of experience. *Animal Behaviour*, **22**, 723–730.

Dill, L. M. (1990). Distance-to-cover and the escape decisions of an African cichlid fish, *Melanochromis chipokae*. *Environmental Biology of Fishes*, **27**, 147–152.

Domenici, P. (2010). Context-dependent variability in the components of fish escape response: Integrating locomotor performance and behavior. *Journal of Experimental Zoology Part A: Ecological Genetics and Physiology*, **313**, 59–79.

Domenici, P. & Batty, R. S.(1997). Escape behaviour of solitary herring (*Clupea harengus*) and comparisons with schooling individuals. *Marine Biology*, **128**, 29–38.

Domenici, P. & Blake, R. (1997). The kinematics and performance of fish fast-start swimming. *Journal of Experimental Biology*, **200**, 1165–1178.

Domenici, P., Lefrancois, C. & Shingles, A. (2007). Hypoxia and the antipredator behaviours of fishes. *Philosophical Transactions of the Royal Society B: Biological Sciences*, **362**, 2105–2121.

Donnelly, W. A. & Dill, L. M. (1984). Evidence for crypsis in coho salmon, *Oncorhynchus kisutch* (Walbaum), parr: Substrate colour preference and achromatic reflectance. *Journal of Fish Biology*, **25**, 183–195.

Eaton, R. C., Lee, R. K. K. & Foreman, M. B. (2001). The Mauthner cell and other identified neurons of the brainstem escape network of fish. *Progress in Neurobiology*, **63**, 467–485.

Eterovick, P. C., Oliveira, F. F. R. & Tattersall, G. J. (2010). Threatened tadpoles of *Bokermannohyla alvarengai* (Anura: Hylidae) choose backgrounds that enhance crypsis potential. *Biological Journal of the Linnean Society*, **101**, 437–446.

Feary, D. A., Cinner, J. E., Graham, N. A. J. & Januchowski-Hartley, F. A. (2011). Effects of customary marine closures on fish behavior, spear-fishing success, and underwater visual surveys. *Conservation Biology*, **25**, 341–349.

Ferrari, M. C. O., Wisenden, B. D. & Chivers, D. P. (2010). Chemical ecology of predator–prey interactions in aquatic ecosystems: A review and prospectus. *Canadian Journal of Zoology*, **88**, 698–724.

Fuiman, L. A. (1993). Development of predator evasion in Atlantic herring, *Clupea harengus* L. *Animal Behaviour*, **45**, 1101–1116.

Ghalambor, C. K., Reznick, D. N. & Walker, J. A. (2004). Constraints on adaptive evolution: the functional trade-off between reproduction and fast-start swimming performance in the Trinidadian guppy (*Poecilia reticulata*). *The American Naturalist*, **164**, 38–50.

Godin, J.-G. J. & Morgan, M. J. (1985). Predator avoidance and school size in a cyprinodontid fish, the banded killifish (*Fundulus diaphanus* Lesueur). *Behavioral Ecology and Sociobiology*, **16**, 105–110.

Gotanda, K. M., Turgeon, K. & Kramer, D. L. (2009). Body size and reserve protection affect flight initiation distance in parrot fishes. *Behavioral Ecology and Sociobiology*, **63**, 1563–1572.

Grant, J. W. & Noakes, D. L. (1987). Escape behaviour and use of cover by young-of-the-year brook trout, *Salvelinus fontinalis. Canadian Journal of Fisheries and Aquatic Sciences*, **44**, 1390–1396.

Guidetti, P., Vierucci, E. & Bussotti, S. (2008). Differences in escape response of fish in protected and fished Mediterranean rocky reefs. *Journal of the Marine Biological Association of the UK*, **88**, 625–627.

Handeland, S. O., Järvi, T., Fernö, A. & Stefansson, S. O.(1996). Osmotic stress, antipredatory behaviour, and mortality of Atlantic salmon (*Salmo salar*) smolts. *Canadian Journal of Fisheries and Aquatic Sciences*, **53**, 2673–2680.

Hartman, E. J. & Abrahams, M. V. (2000). Sensory compensation and the detection of predators: The interaction between chemical and visual information. *Proceedings of the Royal Society of London. Series B: Biological Sciences*, **267**, 571–575.

Healey, M. C. & Reinhardt, U. (1995). Predator avoidance in naive and experienced juvenile chinook and coho salmon. *Canadian Journal of Fisheries and Aquatic Sciences*, **52**, 614–622.

Hettyey, A., Rölli, F., Thürlimann, N., Zürcher, A.-C. & Buskirk, J. V. (2012). Visual cues contribute to predator detection in anuran larvae. *Biological Journal of the Linnean Society*, **106**, 820–827.

Horat, P. & Semlitsch, R. D. (1994). Effects of predation risk and hunger on the behaviour of two species of tadpoles. *Behavioral Ecology and Sociobiology*, **34**, 393–401.

Ingle, D. J. & Hoff, K. (1990). Visually elicited evasive behavior in frogs. *BioScience*, **40**, 284–291.

Jakobsson, S., Brick, O. & Kullberg, C. (1995). Escalated fighting behaviour incurs increased predation risk. *Animal Behaviour*, **49**, 235–239.

Januchowski-Hartley, F. A., Feary, D., Morove, T. & Cinner, J. (2011). Fear of fishers: Human predation explains behavioral changes in coral reef fishes. *PloS ONE*, doi: 10.1371/journal.pone.0022761.

Januchowski-Hartley, F. A., Graham, N. A. J., Cinner, J. E. & Russ, G. R. (2013). Spillover of fish naïveté from marine reserves. *Ecology Letters*, **16**, 191–197.

Januchowski-Hartley, F. A., Nash, K. L. & Lawton, R. J. (2012). Influence of spear guns, dive gear and observers on estimating fish flight initiation distance on coral reefs. *Marine Ecology Progress Series*, **469**, 113.

Kelley, J. L. & Magurran, A. E. (2003). Learned predator recognition and antipredator responses in fishes. *Fish and Fisheries*, **4**, 216–226.

King, J. R. & Comer, C. (1996). Visually elicited turning behavior in *Rana pipiens*: comparative organization and neural control of escape and prey capture. *Journal of Comparative Physiology A*, **178**, 293–305.

Korn, H. & Faber, D. S. (2005). The Mauthner cell half a century later: a neurobiological model for decision-making? *Neuron*, **47**, 13–28.

Krause, J. (1994). Differential fitness returns in relation to spatial position in groups. *Biological Reviews*, **69**, 187–206.

Krause, J. & Godin, J.-G. J. (1996). Influence of prey foraging posture on flight behavior and predation risk: Predators take advantage of unwary prey. *Behavioral Ecology*, **7**, 264–271.

Krause, R. J., Grant, J. W., Mclaughlin, J. D. & Marcogliese, D. J. (2010). Do infections with parasites and exposure to pollution affect susceptibility to predation in johnny darters (*Etheostoma nigrum*)? *Canadian Journal of Zoology*, **88**, 1218–1225.

Kulbicki, M. (1998). How the acquired behaviour of commercial reef fishes may influence the results obtained from visual censuses. *Journal of Experimental Marine Biology and Ecology*, **222**, 11–30.

Laland, K. N., Brown, C. & Krause, J. (2003). Learning in fishes: From three-second memory to culture. *Fish and Fisheries*, **4**, 199–202.

Langerhans, R. B., Layman, C. A., Shokrollahi, A. & Dewitt, T. J. (2004). Predator-driven phenotypic diversification in *Gambusia affinis*. *Evolution*, **58**, 2305–2318.

Lefrancois, C. & Domenici, P. (2006). Locomotor kinematics and behaviour in the escape response of European sea bass, *Dicentrarchus labrax* L., exposed to hypoxia. *Marine Biology*, **149**, 969–977.

Lefrançois, C., Shingles, A. & Domenici, P. (2005). The effect of hypoxia on locomotor performance and behaviour during escape in *Liza aurata*. *Journal of Fish Biology*, **67**, 1711–1729.

Lescak, E. A. & Von Hippel, F. A. (2011). Selective predation of threespine stickleback by rainbow trout. *Ecology of Freshwater Fish*, **20**, 308–314.

Maag, N., Gehrer, L. & Woodhams, D. C. (2012). Sink or swim: a test of tadpole behavioral responses to predator cues and potential alarm pheromones from skin secretions. *Journal of Comparative Physiology A*, **198**, 841–846.

Malavasi, S., Georgalas, V., Lugli, M., Torricelli, P. & Mainardi, D. (2004). Differences in the pattern of antipredator behaviour between hatchery-reared and wild European sea bass juveniles. *Journal of Fish Biology*, **65**, 143–155.

Marras, S., Killen, S. S., Claireaux, G., Domenici, P. & McKenzie, D. J. (2011). Behavioural and kinematic components of the fast-start escape response in fish: Individual variation and temporal repeatability. *Journal of Experimental Biology*, **214**, 3102–3110.

Martín, J., Luque-Larena, J. J. & López, P. (2005). Factors affecting escape behavior of Iberian green frogs (*Rana perezi*). *Canadian Journal of Zoology*, **83**, 1189–1194.

Martín, J., Luque-Larena, J. J. & López, P. (2006). Collective detection in escape responses of temporary groups of Iberian green frogs. *Behavioral Ecology*, **17**, 222–226.

McKenzie, D. J., Shingles, A., Claireaux, G. & Domenici, P. (2009). Sublethal concentrations of ammonia impair performance of the teleost fast-start escape response. *Physiological and Biochemical Zoology*, **82**, 353–362.

McLean, E. B. & Godin, J.-G. J. (1989). Distance to cover and fleeing from predators in fish with different amounts of defensive armour. *Oikos*, 281–290.

Meager, J. J., Domenici, P., Shingles, A. & Utne-Palm, A. C. (2006). Escape responses in juvenile Atlantic cod *Gadus morhua* L.: The effects of turbidity and predator speed. *Journal of Experimental Biology*, **209**, 4174–4184.

Miller, B. M., Mcdonnell, L. H., Sanders, D. J. *et al.* (2011). Locomotor compensation in the sea: Body size affects escape gait in parrotfish. *Animal Behaviour*, **82**, 1109–1116.

Miner, J. G. & Stein, R. A. (1996). Detection of predators and habitat choice by small bluegills: Effects of turbidity and alternative prey. *Transactions of the American Fisheries Soçiety*, **125**, 97–103.

Paglianti, A. & Domenici, P. (2006). The effect of size on the timing of visually mediated escape behaviour in staghorn sculpin *Leptocottus armatus. Journal of Fish Biology*, **68**, 1177–1191.

Petranka, J. W., Kats, L. B. & Sih, A. (1987). Predator–prey interactions among fish and larval amphibians: Use of chemical cues to detect predatory fish. *Animal Behaviour*, **35**, 420–425.

Pitcher, T. J., Green, D. A. & Magurran, A. E. (1986). Dicing with death: predator inspection behaviour in minnow shoals. *Journal of Fish Biology*, **28**, 439–448.

Popper, A. N. & Fay, R. R. (1993). Sound detection and processing by fish: critical review and major research questions (Part 1 of 2). *Brain, Behavior and Evolution*, **41**, 14–25.

Radabaugh, D. (1989). Seasonal colour changes and shifting antipredator tactics in darters. *Journal of Fish Biology*, **34**, 679–685.

Reader, S. M., Kendal, J. R. & Laland, K. N. (2003). Social learning of foraging sites and escape routes in wild Trinidadian guppies. *Animal Behaviour*, **66**, 729–739.

Rodríguez-Prieto, I. & Fernández-Juricic, E.(2005). Effects of direct human disturbance on the endemic Iberian frog *Rana iberica* at individual and population levels. *Biological Conservation*, **123**, 1–9.

Ruxton, G. D., Speed, M. P. & Kelly, D. J. (2004). What, if anything, is the adaptive function of countershading? *Animal Behaviour*, **68**, 445–451.

Sazima, I., Carvalho, L. N., Mendonça, F. P. & Zuanon, J.(2006). Fallen leaves on the water-bed: Diurnal camouflage of three night active fish species in an Amazonian streamlet. *Neotropical Ichthyology*, **4**, 119–122.

Seghers, B. H. (1981). Facultative schooling behavior in the spottail shiner (*Notropis hudsonius*): Possible costs and benefits. *Environmental Biology of Fishes*, **6**, 21–24.

Semeniuk, C. A. D. & Dill, L. M. (2005). Cost/benefit analysis of group and solitary resting in the cowtail stingray, *Pastinachus sephen. Behavioral Ecology*, **16**, 417–426.

Semeniuk, C. A. D. & Dill, L. M. (2006). Anti-predator benefits of mixed-species groups of cowtail stingrays (*Pastinachus sephen*) and whiprays (*Himantura uarnak*) at rest. *Ethology*, **112**, 33–43.

Semlitsch, R. D. (1990). Effects of body size, sibship, and tail injury on the susceptibility of tadpoles to dragonfly predation. *Canadian Journal of Zoology*, **68**, 1027–1030.

Semlitsch, R. D. & Reyer, H.-U. (1992). Modification of anti-predator behaviour in tadpoles by environmental conditioning. *Journal of Animal Ecology*, 353–360.

Stauffer, H.-P. & Semlitsch, R. D. (1993). Effects of visual, chemical and tactile cues of fish on the behavioural responses of tadpoles. *Animal Behaviour*, **46**, 355–364.

Sutter, D. A. H., Suski, C. D., Philipp, D. P. *et al.* (2012). Recreational fishing selectively captures individuals with the highest fitness potential. *Proceedings of the National Academy of Sciences*, **109**, 20960–20965.

Teplitsky, C., Plénet, S., Léna, J. P. *et al.* (2005). Escape behaviour and ultimate causes of specific induced defences in an anuran tadpole. *Journal of Evolutionary Biology*, **18**, 180–190.

Turesson, H. K., Satta, A. & Domenici, P. (2009). Preparing for escape: Anti-predator posture and fast-start performance in gobies. *Journal of Experimental Biology*, **212**, 2925–2933.

Videler, J. J. (1993). *Fish Swimming*. London: Chapman & Hall.

Volff, J. N. (2005). Genome evolution and biodiversity in teleost fish. *Heredity*, **94**, 280–294.

Wakeling, J. M. (2005). Fast-start mechanics. *Fish Physiology*, **23**, 333–368.

Walker, J. A., Ghalambor, C. K., Griset, O. L., Mckenney, D. & Reznick, D. N. (2005). Do faster starts increase the probability of evading predators? *Functional Ecology*, **19**, 808–815.

Ward, A. J., Herbert-Read, J. E., Sumpter, D. J. & Krause, J. (2011). Fast and accurate decisions through collective vigilance in fish shoals. *Proceedings of the National Academy of Sciences*, **108**, 2312–2315.

Ward, A. J. W., Thomas, P., Hart, P. J. & Krause, J. (2004). Correlates of boldness in three-spined sticklebacks (*Gasterosteus aculeatus*). *Behavioral Ecology and Sociobiology*, **55**, 561–568.

Warkentin, K. M. (1995). Adaptive plasticity in hatching age: a response to predation risk trade-offs. *Proceedings of the National Academy of Sciences*, **92**, 3507–3510.

Warkentin, K. M. (2005). How do embryos assess risk? Vibrational cues in predator-induced hatching of red-eyed treefrogs. *Animal Behaviour*, **70**, 59–71.

Warner, R. R. (1998). The role of extreme iteroparity and risk avoidance in the evolution of mating systems. *Journal of Fish Biology*, **53**, 82–93.

Wassersug, R. J. (1989). Locomotion in amphibian larvae (or "Why aren't tadpoles built like fishes?"). *American Zoologist*, **29**, 65–84.

Webb, P. W. (1981). Responses of northern anchovy, *Engraulis mordax*, larvae to predation by a biting planktivore, *Amphiprion percula*. *Fishery Bulletin*, **79**.

Webb, P. W. (1986). Effect of body form and response threshold on the vulnerability of four species of teleost prey attacked by largemouth bass (*Micropterus salmoides*). *Canadian Journal of Fisheries and Aquatic Sciences*, **43**, 763–771.

Webb, P. W. & Zhang, H. (1994). The relationship between responsiveness and elusiveness of heat-shocked goldfish (*Carassius auratus*) to attacks by rainbow trout (*Oncorhynchus mykiss*). *Canadian Journal of Zoology*, **72**, 423–426.

Willink, B., Brenes-Mora, E., Bolaños, F. & Pröhl, H. (2013). Not everything is black and white: Color and behavioral variation reveal a continuum between cryptic and aposematic strategies in a polymorphic poison frog. *Evolution*, **67**, 2783–2794.

Ydenberg, R. C. & Dill, L. M. (1986). The economics of fleeing from predators. *Advances in the Study of Behavior*, **16**, 229–249.

7 Invertebrates

Philip W. Bateman and Patricia A. Fleming

7.1 Introduction

Invertebrates comprise an estimated 80% of all multicellular animals. Understanding their antipredator responses therefore makes a substantial contribution to our knowledge of animal responses to predators. The diversity of invertebrates, including a range of lifestyles, body forms, and habitat use, means that day to day, they encounter a similarly wide range of risky situations. Surprisingly, however, there are actually few studies that have examined invertebrate escape behavior from the point of view of the Economic Escape Model (EEM). Of the studies carried out, there has been a bias toward decapods (e.g., crabs), with notable contributions from Lepidoptera (particularly moths), Orthoptera (crickets and grasshoppers), and Arachnida (spiders).

It is possible that the paucity of data for invertebrate escape behavior may be due to methodological challenges. Firstly, multicellular invertebrates are generally smaller than vertebrates. Invertebrates might therefore face a wider range of predator sizes than vertebrates, including a higher likelihood of "accidental" predation through events such as being ingested with foliage by herbivores (Ben-Ari & Inbar 2013). Because they are so small in size, we need to be cautious to not overinterpret the responses of invertebrates. While, to human observers, it may be intuitive how vertebrates react to approaching predators or disturbance (e.g., "alert" behavior, cessation of previous behavior, gaze direction, alarm calling), this is less clear for many invertebrates. Secondly, invertebrates perceive their world through a wide range of sensory modalities: in addition to sight and sound, they also respond to chemicals, air pressure, vibration or changes in light level. Locusts, for example, detect potential threats through a wide range of senses (Table 7.1). These different modes of sensitivity to their environment often mean that we have to think "outside the box" when working with invertebrates, to ensure that we correctly assess the stimuli and consequent responses.

Identifying common responses to being approached by a predator can be a challenge in interpreting invertebrate antipredator behavior. However, this is helped by recognizing that their escape behavior can be effectively pared down to the simplest responses to stimuli. A recent review (Card 2012) emphasizes that there are relatively few synapses involved in insect escape behavior, reducing processing time and consequently resulting in remarkably

Escaping From Predators: An Integrative View of Escape Decisions, ed. W. E. Cooper and D. T. Blumstein.
Published by Cambridge University Press. © Cambridge University Press 2015.

Table 7.1 Avoidance behavior of locusts in response to stimuli has been described for several sensory modalities.

Receptors	Responses
Mechanoreceptors	Tactile hair receptors on different regions of the body can elicit specific avoidance responses ranging from simple retraction of a leg to active defense.
	e.g., wind receptors: setae on the dorsal surface of the head, which when stimulated with air currents, cause wing flapping for as long as the wind flows (Camhi 1969).
	Auditory input from ultrasound sources induces avoidance steering.
Chemoreceptors	Chemical cues from leg contact chemoreceptors elicit avoidance by setting the tarsus into a new position.
Thermoreceptors	Heat (infrared radiation) is avoided by flying locusts.
Photoreceptors	Visual cues reliably initiate the aversive reactions of collision avoidance in flying locusts. Expanding shapes elicit steering responses that have been interpreted as collision-avoidance strategies in different flight situations. Several large visual interneurones descending from the brain react to expanding shapes and may therefore contribute to these visually elicited avoidance responses.

(Modified from Hassenstein & Hustert, 1999, and references therein)

rapid responses. However, Card (2012) also points out that even the escape of a fly is a series of "sub-behaviors" that allow adaptive abortion of the process, i.e., it is not a fixed action pattern and is therefore potentially highly flexible.

In addition to their diversity and abundance, invertebrates can also carry evidence of past predatory encounters, which may modify their responses. Many invertebrates undergo autotomy – the voluntary shedding of a limb or other part of the body along a breakage plane (reviewed by Fleming *et al.* 2007). Autotomy happens as a result of entrapment (usually when grabbed by a potential predator), and therefore an autotomized body part directly reflects a successful previous escape. Most invertebrates that have lost a leg have reduced locomotory ability (reviewed by Fleming *et al.* 2007). Animals may also autotomize an appendage that could have been used in self-defense, e.g., the chelipeds of crabs (Juanes & Smith 1995). Autotomy can therefore render an individual more vulnerable to future encounters with a predator (McPeek *et al.* 1996; Stoks 1998, 1999; Gyssels & Stoks 2005; Bateman & Fleming 2006a) and will potentially influence economic escape decisions (Cooper & Frederick 2010).

7.2   Measures of invertebrate escape response

Invertebrates use a diversity of antipredator behavior, including cessation of movement, falling silent, dropping, taking flight (walking, running, or flying), or retreating to cover, as appropriate to their environment, morphology, and ecology (Figure 7.1). In

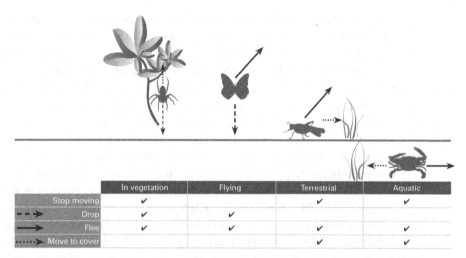

	In vegetation	Flying	Terrestrial	Aquatic
Stop moving	✔		✔	✔
Drop	✔	✔		
Flee	✔	✔	✔	✔
Move to cover			✔	✔

Figure 7.1 A range of behavioral options are available for invertebrates that usually are found within vegetation, fly, or are epigeic. Crypsis is an important primary defense (functioning regardless of whether a predator is present or not; *sensu* Edmunds 1974), but when crypsis fails, invertebrates must resort to a range of secondary defense responses.

this section, we discuss these antipredator responses in terms of the measures that can be made.

7.2.1 Watching and waiting

Measuring predator monitoring in invertebrates can be problematic because, to a human observer, it is not always evident when an invertebrate is "alert" to the predator's presence or has modified its behavior accordingly (i.e., is "monitoring" its environment). Below we discuss where monitoring is evident because animals stop their previous actions, alter their body position, or retreat to cover.

Fiddler crabs *Uca vomeris* visually monitor approaching predatory stimuli until deciding to retreat to their burrows (Hemmi 2005a, b), but also continue to monitor them from the entrance of their burrows before retreating wholly (Hemmi & Pfeil 2010). *Uca pugilator* fiddler crabs retreat to burrows if they see conspecifics reacting to threats, even if they do not see the threat themselves (Wong *et al.* 2005). *Uca pugilator* are therefore monitoring their conspecifics for cues about potential predators.

7.2.1.1 Cessation of movement

Cessation of movement, tonic immobility, or thanatosis (where the organism effectively plays dead) is a first line of defense for several invertebrate species. Stopping moving is typical of cryptic species (e.g., Hatle & Faragher 1998). *Xanthodius sternberghii* crabs disturbed by human activity initially rely on keeping still (which is effective due to their cryptic coloration), but, after a minute, the crabs will either slowly edge for cover or imperceptibly dig themselves into the sand (Robinson *et al.* 1970).

Larvae of the damselfly *Ischnura elegans* that have autotomized lamellae (used for gas exchange and locomotion) through unsuccessful predation events enter thanatosis more frequently when exposed to a predatory stimulus than intact individuals (Gyssels & Stoks 2005). In ponds where these damselfly larvae have only invertebrate predators, this form of defense may be sufficient to avoid predation. However, predatory fish are able to locate larvae whether they are immobile of not, and larvae from ponds with fish predators are less likely to become immobile and stay immobile for shorter lengths of time than are larvae from ponds without fish predators.

Ohno and Miyatake (2007) demonstrated a trade-off (a negative genetic correlation) between different responses (thanatosis and flying ability) to potential predation in bean beetles *Callosobruchus chinensis*. This suggests that, within a population, there may be groups of individuals that are more or less likely to resort to one of these two mutually exclusive antipredator tactics. The propensity of ceasing movement also appears to be influenced by what an individual was doing before being disturbed. Sweet potato beetles *Cylas formicarius* that were moving when disturbed are less likely to enter thanatosis compared with individuals that were already still (Miyatake 2001).

Cessation of movement probably comes with minimal energetic costs, but since we know very little about the mechanisms that cause tonic immobility in invertebrates, it is difficult to assess whether there are any indirect effects of monitoring risk until they recommence movement. The biggest costs to such behavior are likely to be opportunity costs and cost of monitoring the environment.

7.2.1.2   Falling silent

For organisms that signal acoustically, falling silent is another way of enhancing crypsis when a potential predator is detected. Orthopterans that are acoustically signaling cease movement and fall silent when disturbed by a predatory stimulus (Hedrick 2000; Bateman & Fleming 2013b). Male armored ground crickets, *Acanthoplus speiseri*, stridulate both during the day and night. They fall silent and initially rely on crypsis when approached by a human. These crickets use visual cues to recognize the intruder during the day, stopping calling when the person is still some distance away, but at night they can be approached and touched before they fall silent (Bateman & Fleming 2013b).

Animals may then remain silent for varying lengths of time; this latency until the resumption of signaling may be influenced by risk assessment. Their latency to resume signaling is influenced by perceived presence of predators (Zuk & Kolluru 1998; Lewkiewicz & Zuk 2004) but it can also vary according to previous experience with predators: crickets that autotomized a limb in a predatory encounter and thus have reduced locomotory ability (Bateman & Fleming 2005, 2006a) increase and maintain a high latency to begin calling again postdisturbance (Bateman & Fleming 2006b).

7.2.1.3   "Positioning" behavior

Between cessation of moving and active flight away from a predator is a small suite of behavioral actions that we term "positioning behavior." Many grasshoppers perched on vegetation reposition themselves on the other side of a stem or leaf from the approaching predator ("squirreling"). Other positioning/hiding responses include "jerking" (short, lateral movements), "crouching," and small backward motions (Hassenstein & Hustert 1999). Locusts *Locusta migratoria* squirrel around stem perches in response to visual stimuli, i.e., dark, moving, or expanding shapes. Interestingly, they do not respond to acoustic stimuli, although noises prior to a visual stimulus may increase their propensity to hide (Hassenstein & Hustert 1999).

The likelihood of squirreling may be influenced by body condition. Semi-aquatic grasshoppers *Paroxya atlantica* that had autotomized a hind limb show a greater likelihood to squirrel from an approaching observer than intact individuals (Bateman & Fleming 2011). They also perch lower on emergent vegetation than intact individuals, presumably in readiness for escape via water.

This sort of behavior is likely to be energetically inexpensive, is less likely to attract a predator's attention than fleeing, has a lower latency until normal behavior can be resumed, and allows continued monitoring of the predator.

7.2.2   Fleeing

If keeping still and/or silent is not sufficient to avoid detection by a predator, prey have the option to flee. The various forms of fleeing reflect the wide range of prey biology.

7.2.2.1   Dropping

The simplest form of "fleeing," which is common to many arthropods on vegetation or in flight, is to drop vertically toward the ground (aided by gravity), out of the way of the predator or an approaching disturbance. Colonial spiders *Metepeira incrassata* drop out of communal nests into vegetation below when predatory wasps attack the nest (Uetz *et al.* 2002). Caterpillars of the lymantrid moth *Orgyia leucostigma* rely on their coating of bristly hairs, not only as a primary defense of a barrier against attack, but also as sensors (Castellanos *et al.* 2011). Low hair-bending velocity results in the caterpillar walking away from the disturbance, but high hair-bending velocity results in dropping from their perch, presumably as it is interpreted as a higher risk predatory stimulus.

Dropping is an important antipredator response of flying invertebrates. Various insects have evolved the ability to acoustically detect predatory bats and dramatically drop from the air to avoid them. Green lacewings *Chrysopa carnea* fold their wings and nose dive in response to the echolocation calls of bats (Miller & Olesen 1979). Many species of moths, crickets, bush crickets, mantids, and some flies and beetles show similar bat-avoidance behavior (Miller & Surlykke 2001). Female parasitic flies *Ormia ochracea* perform phonotaxis at night to their victims, which are singing male crickets (Rosen *et al.* 2009). Like female crickets performing phonotaxis to the males, these flies also drop from the air in response to bat echolocation calls.

Arthropods also drop from plants even when the disturbance is unintentional. Aphids drop when herbivores feed on the plants they are on (Gish *et al.* 2010, 2011). Up to 14% of pea aphids *Acyrthosiphon pisum* feeding on alfalfa bushes drop to the ground when hemipteran predators are introduced to the bush, and up to 60% of the aphids drop when the highly predatory ladybird *Coccinella septempunctata* is placed on the bush (Losey & Denno 1998). Pea aphids also drop from food plants when they detect alarm pheromones from conspecifics indicating active predation (Dill *et al.* 1990). Both larvae and adults of three coccinellid beetle species drop when mammalian herbivores feed on the plants they are on (Ben-Ari & Inbar 2013). When breathed on by humans, 60 to 80% of the beetles drop, probably reacting to heat and humidity, but they do not drop if the plant is merely shaken (Ben-Ari & Inbar 2013).

Dropping comes with costs, such as cessation of feeding, desiccation (for sap-feeding insects), increased locomotory costs in regaining their position, or greater exposure to animals on the ground. Pea aphids therefore "assess" risk and are less likely to drop when the environment is hot and dry, or when they are feeding on high-quality rather than low-quality host plants (Dill *et al.* 1990). Because dropping is costly, there needs to be good discrimination between reasonably safe situations vs. truly dangerous stimuli. The dogbane tiger moth *Cycnia tenera* can differentiate between the echolocation calls of bats that are flying nearby looking for prey ("early attack") and calls of these bats that have detected prey and are moving into pursuit ("late attack"). When first exposed to bat echolocation calls post-adult molt, moths show equal defensive responses ("startle" calls of ultrasonic clicks and dropping) to both types of call, but soon learn to discriminate between them, and subsequently will continue other behavior in the presence of "early attack" echolocation calls (Ratcliffe *et al.* 2011). Similar differentiation between "early" and "late" echolocation calls has been recorded for the moth *Bertholdia trigona* (Corcoran *et al.* 2013).

7.2.2.2   Taking flight: walking, running, flying, or swimming

When an invertebrate flees from an approaching predator there are various measures that can reveal important information about this response. Measures include FID, DF, angle of flight away from the predator, and the type of flight used (i.e., fast or slow; straight or protean).

7.2.2.2.1   *Flight initiation distance (FID)*

Under predictions of the EEM, FID should increase in the presence of greater risk (Chapter 2). A number of studies apparently support FID as a measure of level of risk in invertebrates (Table 7.2). Cooper (2006) recorded an increase in FID in *Dissosteira carolina* grasshoppers that were approached faster, more directly, or twice in succession, while Hemmi (2005a) showed that fiddler crabs *Uca vomeris* approached by a model seabird showed increased FID when they were further from their burrow.

Other studies, however, have recorded no increase in FID in response to increased risk. Three other grasshopper species show little evidence for an increase in FID when approached repeatedly or for autotomized grasshoppers (other escape tactics are instead evident, including increases in DF, altering angle of escape, or use of crypsis) (Bateman & Fleming 2011, 2014). Autotomy can influence FID as loss of limb may reduce locomotory ability, such that an increased FID would be adaptive, but lower initial fitness after autotomy, encouraging decreased FID (Cooper & Frederick 2010). This relationship needs more study in invertebrates. Orb-weaver spiders *Argiope florida* do not vary their FID in response to varying types of approach (Bateman & Fleming 2013b). Hemmi (2005b) reported that *Uca vomeris* actually show decreased

Table 7.2 Studies of FID in response to varying threat levels to test the EEM in invertebrates.

Prey organism	Stimulus	Treatment	Was there a difference in FID?	Reference
Grasshoppers				
– *Dissosteira carolina*	Person	Approach speed	**Yes** ↑ for faster approach	[1]
		Directness of approach	**Yes** ↑ for direct approach	[1]
		Repeated approach	**Yes** ↑ for 2nd approach	[1]
– *Schistocerca alutacea*	Person	Approached repeatedly	**No**	[2]
– *Psinidia fenestralis*	Person	Approached repeatedly	**No** (Marginally ↑ FID on the second approach, but not for subsequent approaches)	[2]
– *Paroxya atlantica*	Person	Autotomized vs. intact	**No**	[3]
Armored ground crickets *Acanthoplus speiseri*	Person	Calling males, at night and in the day	**Yes** ↓ at night	[4]
Mayfly larvae *Baetis tricaudatus*	Predatory fish and stonefly larvae	High- vs. low-food patches		[5]
– Large larvae			**Yes** ↓ (¼ ×) in high-food patches[a]	
– Small larvae			**No**	
Water strider *Gerris remigis*	Adult water striders approaching juveniles	Group size of juveniles	**Yes** ↑ for larger groups, then ↓ for even larger groups	[6]
Wolf spiders *Hogna carolinensis*	Model lizard	Mass, size, sex, and speed of spiders	**Yes** ↓ for slower individuals	[7].
Colonial spiders *Metepeira incrassata*	Predatory wasp	Position in nest, age of spiders	**Yes** ↑ for adult females in center of nest (furthest from initiation of wasp attack: **No** for immature spiders)	[8]

Table 7.2 (cont.)

Prey organism	Stimulus	Treatment	Was there a difference in FID?	Reference
Orb weaver spiders *Argiope florida*	Person or shape	Person "looming" or small fluttering shape "hovering"	No[b]	[9]
Fiddler crabs *Uca vomeris*	Model seabird	Distance to refuge	**Yes** ↓ FID when closer to refuge	[10]
		Angle of approach (directly or tangentially)	**Yes** ↓ FID when approached directly	[11]
Caribbean hermit crabs *Coenobita clypeatus*	Person or shape	Silent or noisy approach	**Yes** ↓ "FID" (withdrawing into shell) when distracted by noise	[12]

[a] FID through drift in the stream flow.

[b] Only effect was height of web from the ground, which could reflect differences in visual contrast from the vegetation.

References: [1]: Cooper, 2006; [2]: Bateman & Fleming, 2014; [3]: Bateman & Fleming, 2011; [4]: Bateman & Fleming, 2013b; [5]: Scrimgeour, et al., 1994; [6]: Dill & Ydenberg, 1987; [7]: Nelson & Formanowicz, 2005; [8]: Uetz *et al.* 2002; [9]: Bateman & Fleming, 2013a; [10]: Hemmi, 2005a; [11]: Hemmi, 2005b; [12]: Chan, *et al.* 2010.

FID when approached directly (rather than tangentially), and Caribbean hermit crabs *Coenobita clypeatus* similarly show decreased hiding initiation distance (i.e., when they withdraw into their shell) when disturbed by noise (Chan *et al.* 2010).

We need to be cautious not to overinterpret the results of FID experiments in invertebrates, since the physiological limitations of the animals may contribute to responses. Flight initiation distance may simply vary as a consequence of visual acuity (Box 7.1), or depth perception, or speed of cognitive processing (e.g., Dukas 1998; Bateman & Fleming 2013a; Lee *et al.* 2013), and individuals may therefore show limited plasticity in FID. Consequently, we might not predict variation in FID *within* individuals and populations, but we might expect variation *between* populations that vary in predation intensity that might, for example, select for individuals with a lower response threshold.

Fleeing will result in opportunity costs as well as metabolic costs. Interestingly, flight in many invertebrates is particularly efficient, such that the metabolic costs of flight may be fairly minimal. The tracheal system of invertebrates such as a grasshopper is particularly efficient in ensuring oxygen availability to metabolically active tissue, and consequently (unlike vertebrates, which will readily resort to anaerobic respiration during sprint escapes) they are unlikely to have to rely on anaerobic respiration (Weyel & Wegener 1996). Lack of oxygen is rare for such invertebrates (although it can certainly apply to aquatic invertebrates that may encounter hypoxic zones) and, unlike many mammals and birds, they can maintain high metabolic rates and ATP synthesis (Weyel & Wegener 1996). Notably, however, "injury" through autotomy of a limb can increase costs of locomotion and decrease stamina in field crickets (Fleming & Bateman 2007).

7.2.2.2.2   *Distance fled (DF)*
In a high-risk situation (e.g., when approached by a fast, persistent predator), it would be beneficial to increase DF. *Dissosteira carolina* grasshoppers approached quickly

---

BOX 7.1 Vision in arthropods

The compound eyes of arthropods come in a number of general patterns. Both simple (or single chambered) and compound (or multifaceted) eyes split up incoming light according to its direction and origin. Compound eyes are of two distinct and optically different kinds. In apposition eyes (most diurnal insects), each cluster of receptors has their own lens. In superposition eyes, such as in Lepidoptera, the image at any point on the retina is the product of many lenses.

Flight responses are triggered by a threshold size and/or speed of a "looming" image on the retina (Rind & Simmons 1992; Javůrková *et al.* 2012). When the image reaches a threshold size (i.e., number of ommatadia neurons firing), then the escape response will be triggered (Figure 7.2). For example, hiding responses (squirreling to the other side of a branch from the approaching object) in locusts *Locusta migratoria*, stimulated by expanding shapes, occur only after the expanding image has exceeded a threshold visual angle of 8 to 9.5° (Hassenstein & Hustert 1999).

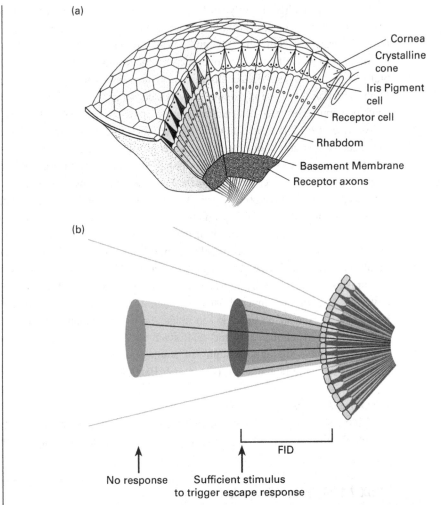

(a)

Cornea
Crystalline cone
Iris Pigment cell
Receptor cell
Rhabdom
Basement Membrane
Receptor axons

(b)

FID

No response   Sufficient stimulus
to trigger escape response

Figure 7.2   (a) Basic structure of an appositon compound eye found in most diurnal insect species, showing its construction from ommatidial elements. (b) A looming shape will cause an escape response when a threshold angle (i.e., number of ommatidia stimulated) are triggered. The distance from the eye when this occurs will therefore determine the FID for the animal.

by a human observer showed greater FID than individuals approached more slowly, but also fled further (Cooper 2006). In response to being approached repeatedly, *Schistocerca alutacea* grasshoppers did not increase FID but fled farther, such that the pursuer failed to keep up with them (Bateman & Fleming 2014). *Gryllus bimaculatus* crickets can be stimulated to flee by a puff of air on the cerci from behind. A single puff causes a short run, but a continuous sequence of puffs causes sustained escape running and turning away from the stimulus source (Gras & Hörner 1992). Mosquito pupae *Culex pipiens* close to the surface of the water are presumably more at risk of aerial predation than ones that are deeper in the water column. When exposed to a simulated attack from above, they flee farther than ones that are initially deeper (Rodríguez-Prieto *et al.* 2006).

Increasing the DF comes with costs, since it removes the prey animal farther from its original position, which may have been optimal for the individual. Increasing DF must also come at a metabolic cost, and the energy used for locomotion will need to be later replaced through increased foraging.

7.2.2.2.3 Flight behavior

Flight can be augmented as an effective escape tactic by varying the angle of flight (Chapter 8). Assassin bugs *Triatoma infestans* consistently escape away from a stimulus at approximately 120°, which corresponds to the limits of their visual zone, thereby maximizing distance from the predator while still allowing the assassin bug to track it (Lazzari & Varjú 1990). However, repeatedly fleeing away from a predator on a set trajectory may result in anticipation of this escape response by the predator while, in some cases, completely random-direction fleeing may sometimes result in fleeing toward a predator (Card 2012).

Unpredictable, changing, flight patterns (termed "protean" behavior) can therefore be advantageous (Humphries & Driver 1970; Jones *et al.* 2011; Chapter 8). Cockroaches *Periplaneta americana* choose from a variety of escape trajectories that are at angles away from the threat (Domenici *et al.* 2008). On the approach of a predator model, ocean skaters *Halobates robustus* not only increase escape speed but also the frequency of turns on the water's surface, performing protean turning and moving (Treherne & Foster 1981).

The grasshopper *Psinidia fenestralis* shows a bimodal pattern of escape trajectories, leaping either directly away from or at right angles to the observer's approach path (Bateman & Fleming 2014) (Figure 7.3). When approached repeatedly, however, the grasshoppers more consistently use lateral escape routes. Protean flight and flight lateral to the predator's trajectory may be farther enhanced by wing coloration in oedipodine grasshoppers (e.g., *Dissosteira carolina*, Cooper 2006; *Oedipoda caerulescens*, Kral 2010; *Psinidia fenestralis*, Bateman & Fleming 2014): the rapid disappearance of their colorful underwings upon landing may enhance subsequent crypsis. Performing "hook" landings (e.g., *Oedipoda caerulescens*; Kral 2010), such that they face back the way they came, makes it more difficult for predators to shift to a different kind of search image to find their prey, and also improves monitoring of the approaching predator. Interestingly, the cyrtacanthridine grasshopper *S. alutacea*, which has non-contrasting under-wings, tends to shift away from use of lateral escape paths with persistent pursuit, and rely more on longer escape flights directly away from the observer (Bateman & Fleming 2014). *Paroxya atlantica* grasshoppers that have undergone autotomy of a limb always escape from a disturbance laterally (Bateman & Fleming 2011).

7.2.2.3 Retreating to cover

Some organisms that flee have the option of hiding in refuges (Chapter 9). Among invertebrates, some of the best studied taxa for this behavior are fiddler crabs that

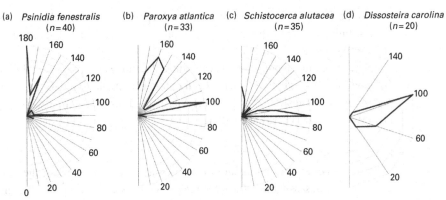

Figure 7.3   Movement of four grasshopper species in relation to the trajectory of an approaching human observer. Angles of 180° indicate the animals moved directly away from the observer, angles around 90° indicate they moved away perpendicularly to the observer's approach path; escapes to the left- and right-hand side of the approach path have been pooled. Each circular line shows one individual. Data for (a) to (c) clearly show a bimodal distribution of escape angles. Data for (b) to (d) were for the first approach of these individuals. (Bateman & Fleming 2011; 2014; we calculated (d) from Cooper, 2006)

retire toward self-constructed burrows when approached by predatory stimuli (e.g., Hemmi 2005a,b; Wong *et al.* 2005; Hemmi & Pfeil 2010). Having entered a refuge, a prey organism must make an economic decision on when to emerge (Hugie 2003; Martín 2014).

Boldness in emerging from shelter can vary between and among populations and individuals (Chapter 15), and is influenced by risk assessment (Sih 1986). Fiddler crabs *Uca mjoebergi* show a correlation between "boldness" (indicated by emerging sooner) and higher aggression in other interactions, and bold and aggressive males ultimately have higher mating success (Reaney & Backwell 2007). *Gryllus integer* cricket males vary in calling-bout lengths, and males with longer, more conspicuous songs take longer to emerge from a shelter in a novel environment than do males with shorter songs (Hedrick 2000). Male *G. bimaculatus* that have undergone a simulated predatory encounter resulting in autotomy of a hind limb also show more caution in emerging from a shelter than do intact conspecifics (Bateman & Fleming 2014). The spider *Agelenopsis aperta* retreats down the funnel of its web when disturbed by large-amplitude vibrations of the web consistent with disturbance by a bird predator; latency to re-emergence to a foraging position on the web is greater in sites with higher risk of predation by birds (Riechert & Hedrick 1990).

Hermit crabs carry shells of other organisms into which they can retreat. Alternatively, they can flee. *Pagurus acadianus* spends a longer time hiding in its shell when it has been handled by predatory lobsters (Scarratt & Godin 1992). The type of shell used by hermit crabs can also influence economic decisions: exposure to the odor of a crushed conspecific had no effect on the choice of either of two host shells (one of which was more robust than the other) in *P. filholi*, but the presence of a predatory crab induced a preference for the more robust host shell (Mima *et al.* 2003). Additionally, although hermit crabs spent longer in the more robust shells than the more vulnerable shells, they reduced time spent in the both shells overall and resorted to fleeing from a predator stimulus in the presence of the predatory crab. Hermit crabs also seem to be able to assess their conspicuousness: *P. bernhardus* that have been induced to inhabit shells that are conspicuous against the substrate show much longer hiding times in these shells after disturbance than when in shells that are cryptic against the substrate (Briffa & Twyman 2011).

Although sessile organisms cannot flee, but only retreat to shelter, they will still face the economic decision of how long to remain in the refuge before re-emerging to feed. The polychaete worm *Serpula vermicularis* filter-feeds from the entrance of its self-constructed calcareous tube. As food in the water column tends to come in "pulses" rather than uniformly, time spent hiding in the tube can be costly. Variation in latency to emerge after a predatory stimulus (a mechanical shock) is, then, a relatively elaborate result of tracking short-term changes in food availability (even changes in food availability on a relative basis) through comparing current feeding conditions to those previously experienced (Dill & Fraser 1997). Similarly, the barnacle *Balanus glandula*, when induced to hide by a shadow simulating a predator, hid longer if they had been feeding prior to hiding (Dill & Gillett 1991).

Major costs of retreating to shelter are the cost of monitoring the environment to ensure it is safe before re-emerging (see also section 7.2.1; Chapter 9) and the cost of suspending other activities, particularly foraging. Once an organism has descended into a burrow, it cannot effectively monitor the predator: over 70% of *Uca vomeris* crabs approached tangentially by a dummy predator remain on the surface and monitor the predator, despite having retreated toward their burrows, and only descend into the burrow when the predatory stimulus approaches directly (Hemmi & Pfeil 2010).

Monitoring can potentially be disrupted by other stimuli. The hermit crab *Coenobita clypeatus* withdraws into its shell when a black object (the "predator" stimulus) looms toward it. If the crabs are exposed to the noise of a motor boat engine at the same time, they allow the looming stimulus to approach closer before withdrawing, implying that the noise obscures the stimulus or "distracts" the prey and ultimately makes it more vulnerable to predation (Chan *et al.* 2010).

7.3 Factors that influence invertebrate escape response

The EEM predicts that animals should vary their responses according to the risk presented by the situation, balancing the benefits of moving away with the costs incurred (Chapter 2). In this section, we discuss the moderating effects of certain intrinsic and extrinsic variables on escape behavior.

7.3.1   Food handling

In addition to the examples for sessile organisms (section 7.2.2.3), food handling can also influence the escape behavior of mobile invertebrates. In captivity, crayfish *Procambarus clarkii* that are manipulating large, immobile pieces of food have shorter FID and are less likely to try to escape from an approaching fish net than if they are feeding on small, portable pieces of food (Bellman & Krasne 1983). This finding is consistent with the prediction by the EEM that FID is greater for larger food items because the cost of fleeing increases as the amount of food left behind increases. Alternatively, it is possible that the net is not perceived as a "predatory stimulus," but may actually be inducing behavior typical for crayfish avoiding competition with conspecifics, i.e., staying to guard immobile sources of food. By comparison, in a similar situation, FID of hermit crabs *Pagurus acadianus* (stimulated with real and model predatory lobsters) was not influenced by mass of a food item, but the crabs moved further away when they were carrying lighter food items (Scarratt & Godin 1992).

7.3.2   Group living

The drivers of group living in invertebrates may be much the same as in vertebrates, including enhanced predator detection through higher cumulative vigilance via the "many-eyes" effect, dilution of predation risk, and increased predator defense through behaviors such as bunching (Krause & Ruxton 2002). Group size is therefore likely to influence the economics of FID decisions.

Juvenile water striders *Gerris remigis* show an increase in FID with increasing group size when approached by potentially cannibalistic adults, which appears to support the "many-eyes" hypothesis (Dill & Ydenberg 1987). However, when the group size continues to increase, FID decreases. Although Dill and Ydenberg (1987) proposed that this response suggested a trade-off between fleeing and risk dilution as a factor of increased group size, predator detection might also be compromised in larger groups.

As their colony increases in size, colonial-dwelling spiders *Metepeira incrassata* have a reduced chance of falling victim to predatory wasps that attack a series of spiders in each raid, mainly through an "early-warning" effect due to web vibrations caused by the wasps (Uetz *et al.* 2002). The likelihood of spiders dropping from the nest increased later in the attack run of the wasps' raid. Consequently, adult female spiders at the center of the nest had longer FID than did those on the edge of the nest due to this "early warning." Interestingly, immature spiders (which are less preferred prey for the wasps) showed no difference in FID among positions in the colony.

Ocean skaters *Halobates robustus* approached by a predatory stimulus swiftly transmit avoidance behavior (speeding up and increasing frequency of turns) through their groups. This transmission is faster even than the speed of the approaching stimulus (Treherne & Foster 1981).

7.3.3   Effects of body size and age on escape behavior

Body size of prey in relation to the predator may influence escape responses for two reasons. Firstly, larger individuals may more effectively protect themselves by using other defenses (e.g., kicking, biting, struggling, faster running; Bateman & Fleming 2008). Secondly, performance traits may be related to size: e.g., jumping spiders *Servaea incana* can run and climb faster as body size increases, but endurance decreases, suggesting an evolutionary trade-off (McGinley *et al.* 2013). Additionally, changes in body size may influence more fundamental features, such as the suite of predators a prey species faces.

Consequently, we should predict ontogenetic differences in escape behavior. Following a puff of air (intended to simulate a predatory spider), juvenile wood crickets *Nemobius sylvestris* are more likely to jump than are adults, and juveniles also flee proportionally farther (Arai *et al.* 2007). Mayfly larvae *Baetis tricaudatus* that have detected predatory fish or stonefly larvae reduce their foraging activity and increase the likelihood of drifting out of dangerous patches (Scrimgeour & Culp 1994); the likelihood of drift in the presence of the dace was, however, reduced in large larvae, which could reflect higher risk assessment by smaller individuals (Scrimgeour *et al.* 1994). Smaller barnacles *Balanus glandula* hide longer than larger ones after a disturbance (Dill & Gillett 1991), possibly reflecting higher risk for smaller individuals.

7.3.4   Effects of temperature on escape behavior

Temperature influences all biochemical processes and therefore fundamentally influences the physiological responses of ectotherms. Rates of processes rise with increasing temperature before stabilizing and then falling as temperatures increase beyond thermal tolerance limits (Hochachka & Somero 2002). The contractile frequency and power output of muscle tissues depend greatly on temperature: the minimum flight temperature for the thoracic muscles of locusts to generate enough power for sustained flight is ~20°C (Chappell & Whitman 1990 and references therein). Under higher temperatures, tonic immobility in water scorpions *Ranatra* sp. is reduced (Holmes 1906). Scallops escape by jet propulsion of water through a valve and the clapping of the bivalve shell by the muscular mantle; higher temperatures generally result in higher valve contraction, and muscle contractile properties also increase (Guderley & Tremblay 2013). Indeed, the scallop *Argopecten colbecki* cannot swim at all at 2°C (Peck *et al.* 2004).

Crustaceans actively avoid and exit temperature zones that approach their tolerance limits and, when in the middle of their optimum range, they show reduced movement, which ensures remaining in the zone (Lagerspetz & Vainio 2006). Outside this zone, many species of crustacean show reduced ability to carry out reproductive behavior, perform phototactic behavior, right themselves, or show efficient escape reflexes; in some cases they even have reduced walking ability (see Lagerspetz & Vainio 2006 for a review). Barnacles withdraw their cirrae when the predatory stimulus of a shadow falls across them and this response is temperature dependent, occurring faster in the center of the optimum temperature range (Lagerspetz & Kivivuori 1970).

7.4   Conclusions and future research

Although there is a growing body of research that explores the economic decisions of escape behavior with invertebrate models, there are still many taxa that have not been examined. Each taxon promises its own unique insight into the costs and benefits of escape behavior according to the particular set of circumstances it faces. In particular, the different modes of communication (visual, acoustic, tactile, and chemical) are each likely to have different influences on antipredation behavior.

Despite the fact that one of the first empirical papers to explore the predictions of the EEM was on water striders (Dill & Ydenberg 1987), invertebrates are underrepresented in the literature since then. Given their great diversity, we encourage more researchers to consider invertebrates as model taxa for studies of escape behavior; they can be very useful for such studies, particularly considering the ease of manipulating them, the effects of autotomy and ontogenetic stages, and the ease of obtaining large sample sizes.

References

Arai, T., Tominaga, O., Seikai, T. & Masuda, R. (2007). Observational learning improves predator avoidance in hatchery-reared Japanese flounder *Paralichthys olivaceus* juveniles. *Journal of Sea Research*, **58**, 59–64.

Bateman, P. W. & Fleming, P. A. (2005). Direct and indirect costs of limb autotomy in field crickets *Gryllus bimaculatus*. *Animal Behaviour*, **69**, 151–159.

Bateman, P. W. & Fleming, P. A. (2006a). Increased susceptibility to predation for autotomized house crickets (*Acheta domestica*). *Ethology*, **112**, 670–677.

Bateman, P. W. & Fleming, P. A. (2006b). Sex, intimidation and severed limbs: The effect of simulated predator attack and limb autotomy on calling behavior and level of caution in the field cricket *Gryllus bimaculatus*. *Behavioral Ecology and Sociobiology*, **59**, 674–681.

Bateman, P. W. & Fleming, P. A. (2008). An intra-and inter-specific study of body size and autotomy as a defense in Orthoptera. *Journal of Orthoptera Research*, **17**, 315–320.

Bateman, P. W. & Fleming, P. A. (2011). Failure to launch? The influence of limb autotomy on the escape behavior of a semiaquatic grasshopper *Paroxya atlantica* (Acrididae). *Behavioral Ecology*, **22**, 763–768.

Bateman, P. W. & Fleming, P. A. (2013a). The influence of web silk decorations on fleeing behaviour of Florida orb weaver spiders, *Argiope florida* (Araneaidae). *Canadian Journal of Zoology*, **91**, 468–472.

Bateman, P. W. & Fleming, P. A. (2013b). Signaling or not-signaling: variation in vulnerability and defense tactics of armored ground crickets (*Acanthoplus speiseri*: Orthoptera, Tettigoniidae, Hetrodinae). *Journal of Insect Behavior*, **26**, 14–22.

Bateman, P. W. & Fleming, P. A. (2014). Switching to Plan B: changes in the escape tactics of two grasshopper species (Acrididae: Orthoptera) under repeated predatory approaches. *Behavioral Ecology and Sociobiology*, **68**, 457–465.

Bellman, K. L. & Krasne, F. B. (1983). Adaptive complexity of interactions between feeding and escape in crayfish. *Science*, **221**, 779–781.

Ben-Ari, M. & Inbar, M.(2013). When herbivores eat predators: Predatory insects effectively avoid incidental ingestion by mammalian herbivores. *PloS ONE*, **8**, e56748.

Briffa, M. & Twyman, C. (2011). Do I stand out or blend in? Conspicuousness awareness and consistent behavioural differences in hermit crabs. *Biology Letters*, **7**, 330–332.

Camhi, J. M. (1969). Locust wind receptors I. Transducer mechanics and sensory response. *Journal of Experimental Biology*, **50**, 335–348.

Card, G. M. (2012). Escape behaviors in insects. *Current Opinion in Neurobiology*, **22**, 180–186.

Castellanos, I., Barbosa, P., Zuria, I., Tammaru, T. & Christman, M. C. (2011). Contact with caterpillar hairs triggers predator-specific defensive responses. *Behavioral Ecology*, **22**, 1020–1025.

Chan, A. A. Y.-H., Giraldo-Perez, P., Smith, S. & Blumstein, D. T. (2010). Anthropogenic noise affects risk assessment and attention: The distracted prey hypothesis. *Biology Letters*, **6**, 458–461.

Chappell, M. A. & Whitman, D. W. (1990). Grasshopper thermoregulation. In Chapman, R. F. & Joern, A. (eds.) *Biology of Grasshoppers*. New York: Wiley.

Cooper, W. E., Jr. (2006). Risk factors and escape strategy in the grasshopper *Dissosteira carolina*. *Behaviour*, **143**, 1201–1218.

Cooper, W. E., Jr. & Frederick, W. G. (2010). Predator lethality, optimal escape behavior, and autotomy. *Behavioral Ecology*, **21**, 91–96.

Corcoran, A. J., Wagner, R. D. & Conner, W. E. (2013). Optimal predator risk assessment by the sonar-jamming Arctiine moth *Bertholdia trigona*. *PloS one*, **8**, e63609.

Dill, L. & Fraser, A. (1997). The worm re-turns: Hiding behaviour a tube-dwelling marine polychaete, *Serpula vermicularis*. *Behavioral Ecology*, **8**, 186–193.

Dill, L. M. & Gillett, J. F. (1991). The economic logic of barnacle *Balanus glandula* (Darwin) hiding behavior. *Journal of Experimental Marine Biology and Ecology*, **153**, 115–127.

Dill, L. M. & Ydenberg, R. C. (1987). The group size-flight distance relationship in water striders (*Gerris remigis*). *Canadian Journal of Zoology*, **65**, 223–226.

Dill, L. M., Fraser, A. H. G. & Roitberg, B. D. (1990). The economics of escape behaviour in the pea aphid, *Acyrthosiphon pisum*. *Oecologia*, **83**, 473–478.

Domenici, P., Booth, D., Blagburn, J. M. & Bacon, J. P. (2008). Cockroaches keep predators guessing by using preferred escape trajectories. *Current Biology*, **18**, 1792–1796.

Dukas, R. (1998). *Cognitive Ecology: The Evolutionary Ecology of Information Processing and Decision Making*. University of Chicago Press.

Edmunds, M. (1974). *Defence in Animals: A Survey of Anti-predatory Defences*. Burnt Mill, Harlow: Longman.

Fleming, P. A. & Bateman, P. W. (2007). Just drop it and run: The effect of limb autotomy on running distance and locomotion energetics of field crickets (*Gryllus bimaculatus*). *Journal of Experimental Biology*, **210**, 1446–1454.

Fleming, P. A., Muller, D. L. & Bateman, P. W. (2007). Leave it all behind: A taxonomic perspective of autotomy in invertebrates. *Biological Reviews*, **82**, 481–510.

Gish, M., Dafni, A. & Inbar, M. (2010). Mammalian herbivore breath alerts aphids to flee host plant. *Current Biology*, **20**, R628–R629.

Gish, M., Dafni, A. & Inbar, M. (2011). Avoiding incidental predation by mammalian herbivores: Accurate detection and efficient response in aphids. *Naturwissenschaften*, **98**, 731–738.

Gras, H. & Hörner, M. (1992). Wind-evoked escape running of the cricket, *Gryllus bimaculatus*. I. Behavioural analysis. *Journal of Experimental Biology*, **171**, 189–214.

Guderley, H. & Tremblay, I. (2013). Escape responses by jet propulsion in scallops. *Canadian Journal of Zoology*, **91**, 420–430.

Gyssels, F. G. M. & Stoks, R. (2005). Threat-sensitive responses to predator attacks in a damselfly. *Ethology*, **111**, 411–423.

Hassenstein, B. & Hustert, R. (1999). Hiding responses of locusts to approaching objects. *Journal of Experimental Biology*, **202**, 1701–1710.

Hatle, J. D. & Faragher, S. G. (1998). Slow movement increases the survivorship of a chemically defended grasshopper in predatory encounters. *Oecologia*, **115**, 260–267.

Hedrick, A. V. (2000). Crickets with extravagant mating songs compensate for predation risk with extra caution. *Proceedings of the Royal Society of London Series B-Biological Sciences*, **267**, 671–675.

Hemmi, J. M. (2005a). Predator avoidance in fiddler crabs: 1. Escape decisions in relation to the risk of predation. *Animal Behaviour*, **69**, 603–614.

Hemmi, J. M. (2005b). Predator avoidance in fiddler crabs: 2. The visual cues. *Animal Behaviour*, **69**, 615–625.

Hemmi, J. M. & Pfeil, A.(2010). A multi-stage anti-predator response increases information on predation risk. *Journal of Experimental Biology*, **213**, 1484–1489.

Hochachka, P. W. & Somero, G. N.(2002). *Biochemical Adaptation: Mechanism and Process in Physiological Evolution*. New York: Oxford University Press.

Holmes, S. J. (1906). Death-feigning in *Ranatra. Journal of Comparative Neurology and Psychology*, **16**, 200–216.

Hugie, D. M. (2003). The waiting game: a "battle of waits" between predator and prey. *Behavioral Ecology*, **14**, 807–817.

Humphries, D. A. & Driver, P. M. (1970). Protean defence by prey animals. *Oecologia*, **5**, 285–302.

Javůrková, V., Šizling, A. L., Kreisinger, J. & Albrecht, T. (2012). An alternative theoretical approach to escape decision-making: the role of visual cues. *PloS one*, **7**, e32522.

Jones, K. A., Jackson, A. L. & Ruxton, G. D. (2011). Prey jitters; protean behaviour in grouped prey. *Behavioral Ecology*, **22**, 831–836.

Juanes, F. & Smith, L. (1995). The ecological consequences of limb damage and loss in decapod crustaceans: A review and prospectus. *Journal of Experimental Marine Biology and Ecology*, **193**, 197–223.

Kral, K. (2010). Escape behaviour in blue-winged grasshoppers, *Oedipoda caerulescens. Physiological Entomology*, **35**, 240–248.

Krause, J. & Ruxton, G. D. (2002). *Living in Groups*. Oxford University Press.

Lagerspetz, K. Y. & Vainio, L. A.(2006). Thermal behaviour of crustaceans. *Biological Reviews*, **81**, 237–258.

Lagerspetz, K. Y. H. & Kivivuori, L.(1970). The rate and retention of the habituation of the shadow reflex in *Balanus improvisus* (Cirripedia). *Animal Behaviour*, **18**, 616–620.

Lazzari, C. & Varjú, D. (1990). Visual lateral fixation and tracking in the haematophagous bug *Triatoma infestans*. *Journal of Comparative Physiology A*, **167**, 527–531.

Lee, S.-I., Hwang, S., Joe, Y.-E. *et al.* (2013). Direct look from a predator shortens the risk-assessment time by prey. *PloS ONE*, **8**, e64977.

Lewkiewicz, D. A. & Zuk, M. (2004). Latency to resume calling after disturbance in the field cricket, *Teleogryllus oceanicus*, corresponds to population-level differences in parasitism risk. *Behavioral Ecology and Sociobiology*, **55**, 569–573.

Losey, J. E. & Denno, R. F. (1998). The escape response of pea aphids to foliar-foraging predators: Factors affecting dropping behaviour. *Ecological Entomology*, **23**, 53–61.

Martín, J. & Pilar, L. (2014). Hiding time in refuge. In Cooper, W. E., Jr. & Blumstein, D. T. (eds.) *Escaping from Predators: An Integrative View of Escape Decisions.* Chapter 9.

McGinley, R. H., Prenter, J. & Taylor, P. W. (2013). Whole-organism performance in a jumping spider, *Servaea incana* (Araneae: Salticidae): Links with morphology and between performance traits. *Biological Journal of the Linnean Society*, **110**, 644–657.

McPeek, M. A., Schrot, A. K. & Brown, J. M. (1996). Adaptation to predators in a new community: Swimming performance and predator avoidance in damselflies. *Ecology*, **77**, 617–629.

Miller, L. A. & Olesen, J. (1979). Avoidance behavior in green lacewings. *Journal of Comparative Physiology*, **131**, 113–120.

Miller, L. A. & Surlykke, A. (2001). How some insects detect and avoid being eaten by bats: Tactics and countertactics of prey and predator. *BioScience*, **51**, 570–581.

Mima, A., Wada, S. & Goshima, S. (2003). Antipredator defence of the hermit crab *Pagurus filholi* induced by predatory crabs. *Oikos*, **102**, 104–110.

Miyatake, T. (2001). Diurnal periodicity of death-feigning in *Cylas formicarius* (Coleoptera: Brentidae). *Journal of Insect Behavior*, **14**, 421–432.

Nelson, M. K. & Formanowicz, D. R., Jr. (2005). Relationship between escape speed and flight distance in a wolf spider, *Hogna carolinensis* (Walckenaer 1805). *Journal of Arachnology*, **33**, 153–158.

Ohno, T. & Miyatake, T. (2007). Drop or fly? Negative genetic correlation between death-feigning intensity and flying ability as alternative anti-predator strategies. *Proceedings of the Royal Society B: Biological Sciences*, **274**, 555–560.

Peck, L. S., Webb, K. E. & Bailey, D. M. (2004). Extreme sensitivity of biological function to temperature in Antarctic marine species. *Functional Ecology*, **18**, 625–630.

Ratcliffe, J. M., Fullard, J. H., Arthur, B. J. & Hoy, R. R. (2011). Adaptive auditory risk assessment in the dogbane tiger moth when pursued by bats. *Proceedings of the Royal Society B: Biological Sciences*, **278**, 364–370.

Reaney, L. T. & Backwell, P. R. Y. (2007). Risk-taking behavior predicts aggression and mating success in a fiddler crab. *Behavioral Ecology*, **18**, 521–525.

Riechert, S. E. & Hedrick, A. V. (1990). Levels of predation and genetically based anti-predator behaviour in the spider, *Agelenopsis aperta*. *Animal Behaviour*, **40**, 679–687.

Rind, F. C. & Simmons, P. J. (1992). Orthopteran DCMD neuron: a reevaluation of responses to moving objects. I. Selective responses to approaching objects. *Journal of Neurophysiology*, **68**, 1654–1666.

Robinson, M. H., Abele, L. G. & Robinson, B.(1970). Attack autotomy: A defence against predators. *Science*, **169**, 301–302.

Rodríguez-Prieto, I., Fernández-Juricic, E. & Martín, J. (2006). Anti-predator behavioral responses of mosquito pupae to aerial predation risk. *Journal of Insect Behavior*, **19**, 373–381.

Rosen, M. J., Levin, E. C. & Hoy, R. R. (2009). The cost of assuming the life history of a host: acoustic startle in the parasitoid fly *Ormia ochracea*. *Journal of Experimental Biology*, **212**, 4056–4064.

Scarratt, A. M. & Godin, J.-G. J. (1992). Foraging and antipredator decisions in the hermit crab *Pagurus acadianus* (Benedict). *Journal of Experimental Marine Biology and Ecology*, **156**, 225–238.

Scrimgeour, G. J. & Culp, J. M. (1994). Foraging and evading predators: The effect of predator species on a behavioural trade-off by a lotic mayfly. *Oikos*, 71–79.

Scrimgeour, G. J., Culp, J. M. & Wrona, F. J. (1994). Feeding while avoiding predators: evidence for a size-specific trade-off by a lotic mayfly. *Journal of the North American Benthological Society*, 368–378.

Sih, A. (1986). Antipredator responses and the perception of danger by mosquito larvae. *Ecology*, 434–441.

Stoks, R. (1998). Effect of lamellae autotomy on survival and foraging success of the damselfly *Lestes sponsa* (Odonata: Lestidae). *Oecologia*, **117**, 443–448.

Stoks, R. (1999). Autotomy shapes the trade-off between seeking cover and foraging in larval damselflies. *Behavioral Ecology and Sociobiology*, **47**, 70–75.

Treherne, J. E. & Foster, W. A. (1981). Group transmission of predator avoidance behaviour in a marine insect: The Trafalgar effect. *Animal Behaviour*, **29**, 911–917.

Uetz, G. W., Boyle, J., Hieber, C. S. & Wilcox, R. S. (2002). Antipredator benefits of group living in colonial web-building spiders: the "early warning" effect. *Animal Behaviour*, **63**, 445–452.

Weyel, W. & Wegener, G. (1996). Adenine nucleotide metabolism during anoxia and postanoxic recovery in insects. *Experientia*, **52**, 474–480.

Wong, B. B. M., Bibeau, C., Bishop, K. A. & Rosenthal, G. G. (2005). Response to perceived predation threat in fiddler crabs: trust thy neighbor as thyself?*Behavioral Ecology and Sociobiology*, **58**, 345–350.

Zuk, M. & Kolluru, G. R. (1998). Exploitation of sexual signals by predators and parasitoids. *Quarterly Review of Biology*, **73**, 415–443.

IIc Escape trajectories and strategies during pursuit

8 Prey behaviors during fleeing: escape trajectories, signaling, and sensory defenses

Paolo Domenici and Graeme D. Ruxton

8.1 Introduction

After a prey individual has made the decision to flee from an approaching predator, a range of important behavioral options remain open to it, which can strongly influence the likelihood of flight being successful. We will explore some of these and consider signaling to the chasing predator (and to others) during flight and other ways prey may exploit the predator's sensory systems. The most obvious way in which prey behavior during flight can influence escape ability is through control of the trajectory of its escape path. We will therefore focus the bulk of the chapter on this issue, not only because it is important, but also because there are many factors that may influence escape trajectory. However, flight logically begins with the initial directional decision. At first sight it seems obvious that prey should turn and flee away from the oncoming predator, but even this is not as simple as it first seems. To discuss this decision most effectively, we first introduce the reader to the concept of directionality in the early phase of an escape response (i.e., the first detectable reaction to a threat).

We focus only on certain aspects of behavior during predation attempts in some depth rather than covering all aspects briefly. We have not necessarily chosen the behaviors that might have the strongest influence on the outcome of flight. Rather we have chosen topics where we feel we can offer a fresh perspective on how extensive research in the field could further develop. We will begin by noting a number of topics that we do not explore in detail in this chapter.

An important aspect of fleeing behavior is the decision to stop (or at least pause) fleeing. This may occur if the prey perceives that the predator has given up the chase. The factors influencing the decision of when to stop fleeing have been understudied for practical reasons. It is difficult for experimenters to keep track of a fleeing animal, and so we have much more data on flight initiation than flight termination. This imbalance is

Escaping From Predators: An Integrative View of Escape Decisions, ed. W. E. Cooper and D. T. Blumstein. Published by Cambridge University Press. © Cambridge University Press 2015.

likely to be corrected in the near future thanks to technological breakthroughs that allow the mounting of telemetric equipment on free-living animals.

One might assume that prey should flee at the highest possible speed, but this might not be the case. Slower speeds during flight may generate compensatory benefits of increased ability to monitor the chasing predator, and/or increased ability to sustain flight; it may also be related to a lower perceived risk of predation (Domenici 2010). The role of locomotor performance on the escape ability of the prey is the subject of Chapter 11 of this book, but we will briefly discuss the relative importance of speed and maneuverability, and the possibility that prey speed may be a cue that could be used by predators to assess prey palatability. Obtaining accurate speed measurements in the field from animals fleeing on trajectories that are often unpredictable and complex has been challenging; and again we expect that innovations in on-animal telemetry, GPS tracking, and accelerometry will revolutionize our understanding of this issue in the near future (Wilson *et al.* 2013).

We have not attempted to link the behavior of fleeing to life history and physiology. It is likely that flight decisions will be affected by long-term factors (e.g., ontogeny), medium-term factors (e.g., whether the animal is carrying young or not, the health status of the individual) and short-term factors (e.g., how recently the individual has previously fled, the local topography, the animal's familiarity with the local topography). We will mention these topics briefly.

Finally, we have not sought to be encyclopedic in our taxonomic coverage. Rather we focus on small invertebrates, where experimental control and replication are more practical and ethical, and lower vertebrates, which have been studied extensively. Hence this chapter does not attempt to discuss taxonomic distributions of different behaviors; data to attempt this usefully are not yet available.

8.2   Directionality of initial escape responses

8.2.1   The meaning of directionality

When startled, animals tend to change their direction, most often in a way that takes them further away from the threat. The proportion of replicates in which a prey rotates or bends (for flexible animals) its body in a direction away from the threatening stimulus during the initial phase of an escape response is called *directionality* (Blaxter & Batty 1987; Comer & Dowd 1987; Domenici & Blake 1993a; Domenici *et al.* 2011a).

Thus, *away* and *toward* responses correspond to escapes accomplished via an initial turn directed away from and toward the stimulus, respectively. It is important to note that *toward* and *away* responses do not necessarily imply that the final heading of the prey will be toward or away from the threat, respectively. If the escape turn in a *toward* response is relatively small (e.g., 10°), the prey may continue to move along a path that is in a semicircle away from the threat (Figure 8.1).

Independent of the final heading, scoring escapes in terms of initial responses *away* or *toward* provides us with a tool to investigate some of the underlying complexity of

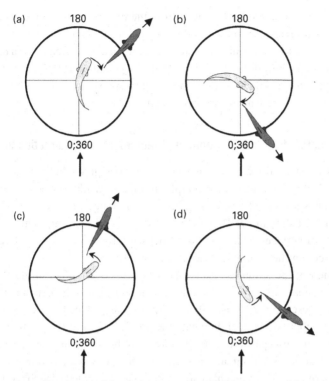

Figure 8.1   A small turn toward the threat (represented by the arrow at 0°) may result in a final heading (dark colored fish) in the semicircle away (A) or toward the stimulus (B), depending on the prey's initial orientation (light colored fish). Similarly, a small turn away from the threat may result in a final heading in the semicircle away (C) or toward (D) the threat.

escape responses. Unpredictability has been suggested as an essential element of escape responses (Humphries & Driver 1970; Godin 1997; Edut & Eilam 2004; Comer 2009). In terms of directionality, for most predator approach trajectories, a random and there-fore fully unpredictable pattern of escape would yield an equal proportion of *away* and *toward* responses. Alternatively, *away* responses may be advantageous because they allow prey to increase their distance from the threat. Most previous work (reviewed in Domenici *et al.* 2011a) shows directionality that is not completely random (i.e., 50% *away* and 50% *toward*), nor is it fully determined by the position of the threat (i.e., 100% *away*). Away responses tend to be more common than *toward* responses, and they constitute about 50 to 90% of the total escapes. From a sensory perspective, this is because the sensory system ipsilateral to the threat causes a rotation in a direction opposite to the stimulation (Domenici *et al.* 2011a). In fish, the Mauthner cells (i.e., the giant neurons that control escape responses) ipsilateral to the threatening stimulus are activated and control the contraction of the contralateral muscle, resulting in an *away* response in most cases (Eaton *et al.* 1981).

Although the presence of a small proportion of toward responses may be explained as a behavioral survival strategy, it may also be related to constraints affecting sensory performance, and these explanations need not be mutually exclusive. While *away* responses allow prey to move farther away from the threat, a small context-dependent proportion of *toward* responses may introduce a significant element of unpredictability. As we shall see, directionality is highly context dependent and is affected by a number of factors. Understanding how directionality is affected by environmental factors as well as by trade-offs with other characteristics of the escape response is fundamental to gaining some insights into the mechanisms driving directionality.

8.2.2   Individual characteristics and environmental factors affecting directionality

Accuracy is known to trade-off with the speed of a given behavioral response (Chittka *et al.* 2009). This general principle applies to work carried out on escape response, which shows that *away* responses have longer latencies than *toward* responses (in fish: Domenici & Batty 1997; Turesson *et al.* 2009). This suggests a potential trade-off between a short neural processing time (i.e., short latencies) and accuracy in directing the response away from the threat.

The orientation of the stimulus relative to the prey has an effect on directionality. In fish, when the threat comes from a direction that is approximately perpendicular to the prey's body axis, escapes are most often *away* responses. On the other hand, when the stimulation is approximately in line with the prey's body axis (i.e., within 30° from head-on or tail-on), escapes are equally likely to be *away* or *toward* responses (Domenici & Blake 1993a). From a sensory perspective, this is likely due to a decrease in left–right discrimination for mechanical stimuli that are aligned with the longitudinal axis of the fish (Domenici & Blake 1993a). However, according to a non-mutually exclusive functional explanation, when the prey is in line with the threat, executing a *toward* or an *away* response may matter very little in terms of distance gained from the predator and a similar proportion of *away* and *toward* responses may add unpredictability (Domenici 2010).

In many animal species, individuals may show task-specific lateral biases (Vallortigara & Rogers 2005). Lateralization has also been observed in escape responses, and it has been attributed to functional asymmetries in the brain (Cantalupo *et al.* 1995) or in the body/limbs (Heuts 1999, Krylov *et al.* 2008). Specialization for turning left or right may offset the disadvantages of turning toward the threat, and this may contribute to explaining why directionality is less than 100% in most species.

A predatory attack does not always trigger all sensory systems simultaneously, and different sensory channels do not necessarily yield similar levels of directionality. In a fish (herring larvae *Clupea harengus*), visual stimuli are associated with the highest directionality, compared with tactile and auditory stimuli (Blaxter & Batty 1985; Yin & Blaxter 1987; Batty 1989). Furthermore, directionality may increase across ontogenetic stages as a result of the development of sensory organs (Blaxter & Batty 1985).

Immediately prior to being startled, prey can be relatively idle or actively moving, and this can have an effect on directionality. For example, fish in the gliding phase of some swimming patterns show a higher proportion of *away* responses than actively swimming fish (Blaxter & Batty 1987). The physical environment can also affect directionality. Acute exposure to low temperature, low oxygen levels, and high CO_2 were found to decrease directionality in fish (Preuss & Faber 2003; Domenici *et al.* 2007; Allan *et al.* 2014). These acute environmental changes are likely to have a direct effect on the functioning of the sensorimotor system, suggesting that directionality can be constrained by sensory performance.

Any object or organism positioned near the prey can also affect the proportion of *away* responses. Fish show an increased proportion of *toward* response when the path directed away from the threat is obstructed by a wall (Eaton & Emberley 1991). Anurans not only avoid escaping toward a barrier, but they also avoid escaping directly away from the threat if this means moving in the direction in which a barrier had been previously positioned and then removed (Ingle & Hoff 1990).

The presence of conspecifics can affect directionality in fish. Herring startled while solitary show lower directionality (around 65%) than those in a school (around 90%; Domenici & Batty 1997). This response may reflect a need for schooling fish to stick together, and therefore to show a uniform *away* response, as opposed to solitary fish that might increase the unpredictability of their response by turning toward the threat. Another proximate explanation may be that escape latencies are longer in schooling than solitary fish, which may allow them more time for sensory processing and therefore for directional accuracy, which agrees with the speed–accuracy trade-off.

8.2.3   Should responses with a turn toward a predator be considered mistakes?

Work described above suggests that the directionality of escape responses is highly flexible. Early work on escape responses in fish and insects considered *toward* responses as potentially "incorrect," "wrong," or "apparent tactical errors" (e.g., Eaton & Emberley 1991; Tauber & Camhi 1995; King & Comer 1996). To assess the functional significance of *toward* responses, we need to assess the effect of directionality on escape success. This has rarely been done, and therefore a possible way to assess the importance of directionality is through its effect on the final escape trajectory, which is known to be a major determinant of escape success (Walker *et al.* 2005).

Can prey whose initial escape is a turn toward the predator quickly steer to produce a trajectory directed away from the threat? In schooling herring, such steering is possible, because initial escaping with *away* and *toward* responses produce similar final escape trajectories at around 150° away from the threat (Domenici & Batty 1997). In contrast, in solitary herring the escape trajectories of *toward* and *away* responses differ. Schooling herring surrounded by neighbors that, in most cases, are swimming away from the threat, may conform by swimming in the same direction. The need to remain in contact with the group may be stronger than the need for generating unpredictability in the response (Domenici & Batty 1997).

In cockroaches (*Periplaneta americana*), initial *toward* responses tend to show very small turn angles (<30°) and the final escape trajectories largely overlap with those of *away* responses. When making a *toward* response, cockroaches may therefore be minimizing the time needed for the turn, which allows them to quickly reach one of the preferred escape trajectories, in turn allowing them to produce an effective anti-predator response (Domenici *et al.* 2009). Frogs (*Rana pipiens*) show a similar pattern in

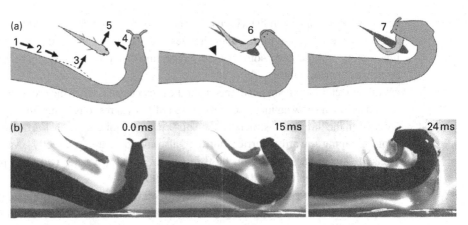

Figure 8.2   Fish escape response to tentacled snakes. The pressure wave created by the snake's body is shown in the left panels by the arrow marked as "3." The prey reacts with an "away response" (i.e., the body makes a C-shape away from the snake's body; central panels), and eventually ends up in the snake's mouth (right panels). (Reprinted from *PNAS*, Figures 3A, B in Catania, 2009 with permission from the author and publisher)

escape behavior with *toward* responses producing small turn angles and escape trajectories that overlap with those of *away* responses (Domenici *et al.* 2011b).

In addition to representing a mechanism that minimizes the time needed for reaching specific trajectories and for generating unpredictability, *toward* responses may, in some predator–prey interactions, show a higher probability of success in avoiding capture. Predator attacks may in some cases reflect relatively complex strategies, so that escaping in what may appear the most sensible direction (away from the threat) may not pay off. A good example is that of tentacle snakes (*Erpeton tentaculatum*) feeding on fish. Tentacle snakes use their body to produce a pressure wave directed toward one side of the fish's body, which triggers an *away* response in their prey in 80% of the trials (Catania 2009). In encounters with common predators, *away* responses would most likely direct the fish away from danger. However, tentacle snakes position their mouths where the fish predictably ends up when producing a response away from the snake's body wave. As a result, fish escaping with an *away* response end up moving toward the snake's open mouth (Figure 8.2). Tentacle snakes are rare predators of fish and this is most likely why they can turn the typically high proportion of *away* responses in fish to their advantage. From the prey's perspective, a small proportion of *toward* responses may be adaptive in preventing capture by rare predators. It would be interesting to investigate if the occurrence of *toward* responses varies depending on the abundance of such rare predators.

In conclusion, *toward* responses may not necessarily represent mistakes such as those derived from a misjudged assessment of the direction of the danger. At least in some cases, *toward* responses may be time-minimization strategies, may generate unpredictability, and may be adaptive responses to the attacks of rare predators. On the other hand, the low directionality caused by acute exposure to temperature, hypoxia, and elevated

CO_2, is most likely the result of malfunctioning of the sensory-motor system, which may lead to a suboptimal proportion of *away* responses. Furthermore, as we shall see in the section on escape trajectories below, escaping toward the predator in some cases (e.g., some larval fish, lizards, and small mammals attacked by birds) may represent a strategy to surprise and flee past the predator and reach safety before the predator can turn and pursue effectively (Domenici *et al.* 2011b).

8.3   Escape trajectories

8.3.1   Methodological issues

After the initial response, animals escape along a trajectory that can be evaluated using successive positions (Domenici & Blake 1993a), or by simply analyzing the heading of the body axis at a particular point in time, typically after the main initial rotational motion of the prey (Eaton & Emberley 1991). Many studies have focused on this "initial" trajectory of the escape response although some prey may undergo a series of zigzagging turns in subsequent stages of the escape (Humphries & Driver 1970). While *directionality* is based on the relative change in direction with respect to the threat (i.e., a turn may be toward or away from the threat; Figure 8.1), escape trajectories do not take into account the motion the prey has accomplished to achieve a given angle between its own heading and the position of the threat.

A number of analytical approaches have been used to study the angle of the escape trajectory in prey. Early work was based on linear statistics of turn angle (*y*-axis) as a function of stimulus angle (*x*-axis) (Camhi & Tom 1978; Eaton *et al.* 1981; Stern *et al.* 1997) (Figure 8.3A). This type of analysis allows one to test how the turn angle (i.e., the angle of turn measured relative to the prey's body axis) varies with respect to the angle at which the prey is attacked. Using this type of analysis, attack angles range from 0° (i.e., tail on) to 180° (head on). Conventionally, attacks from and responses to the right are plotted as positive values, while attacks from and responses to the left are plotted as negative values. Because prey tend to escape in a direction approximately away from the threat, this type of analysis tends to yield a general decrease from the "$-x + y$" sector to the "$+x -y$" sector, which can be tested using linear regression. However, because most points are located in two Cartesian sectors ($-x$ and y; x and $-y$) out of the four, significance may result even if, within each sector, turn angle is not related to attack angle. This problem can be overcome by testing each sector separately, or by pooling left and right stimuli in a single graph, i.e., using an axial rather than a circular scale (Eaton & Emberley 1991).

While this approach may be useful in testing how animals adjust their turn angle relative to the stimulus, it has some drawbacks: (a) the use of a linear regression is appropriate only if, for any value of x, the y values are normally distributed, which is not necessarily the case for escape responses (Domenici *et al.* 2008); and (b) the hypothesis that animals respond using one or more specific headings relative to the threat cannot be tested using linear regression of turn angle vs. attack angles.

(a)

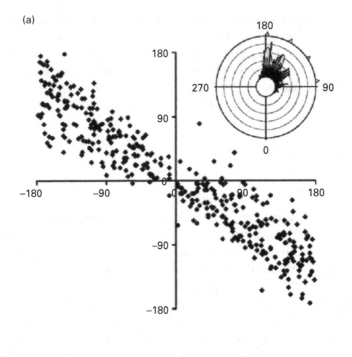

(b)

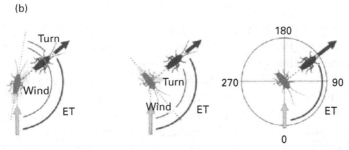

Figure 8.3   (A) Linear (cartesian) representation of turn angle (*y*-axis) and stimulus angle (*x*-axis). By convention, stimuli from and responses to the right are plotted as positive values whereas stimuli from and responses to the left are plotted as negative values (cockroach *Periplaneta americana*, data set 5i; N = 431; unpublished figure based on data from Domenici *et al.*, 2008). Inset: circular representation of the data using the convention shown in (B). In the inset, responses are plotted as if the stimulus corresponding to 0° is always coming from the right of the animal. Concentric circles represent a frequency of ten. Bin frequency is five.

(B) Definitions of escape trajectory angles in toward (left panel) and away (central panel) responses. Toward and away responses are escapes in which the turn angle achieved during the initial rotation is directed toward or away from the stimulus, respectively. In this example from the cockroach, the angle subtended by the arc labeled "wind" is the stimulus angle, that by the arc labeled "turn" is the turn angle and that by the thick arc is the final escape trajectory (ET). Away and toward responses may have the same ET (shown in the right panel). Figure 8.3A: reprinted from *Journal of Experimental Biology*, Figure 1A in Domenici *et al.* (2011b) with permission from the publisher; inset: reprinted from *Current Biology*, Figure 2A in Domenici *et al.* (2008) with permission from Elsevier; Figure 8.3B: based on Figure 5 in Booth *et al.* (1999) reproduced with permission of the *Journal of Neuroscience*.

To assess the direction of the escape trajectories (ET) relative to the predator attack direction in angelfish, Domenici and Blake (1993a) used circular statistics in which ET is defined as the angle between the threat (positioned at 0°) and the escape path of the prey once the body rotation is completed (Domenici *et al.* 2008) or at a specific kinematic stage, such as the second axial bend in the fish escape response (Domenici & Blake 1993a). This analytical approach has been used on other species (e.g., crayfish *Crangon crangon*, Arnott *et al.* 1999; cockroaches *Periplaneta americana*, Domenici *et al.* 2008; lizards *Psammodromus algirus*, Martín & López 1996). Escape trajectories can be calculated as the sum of attack angle (here ranging from 0° in head-on attacks to 180° in tail-on attacks) and turn angle, where *toward* and *away* responses bear a negative and a positive sign, respectively (Figure 8.3B).

Using this method, ET can span 360° and is treated as a circular variable (Batschelet 1981; Domenici *et al.* 2011b; Pewsey *et al.* 2013). Escape trajectories in which the position of the attack remains on the same side of the prey as at the beginning of the escape response will be placed in the 0 to 180° semicircle. Conversely, if the attack ends up on the opposite side, ETs are placed in the semicircle 180° to 360°. Unless specific asymmetries occur, by convention, right and left escapes can be pooled as if all stimuli are on the right (Domenici & Blake 1993a). This type of analysis allows the pattern of the escape heading of the prey relative to the attack direction to be assessed. Some previous work has used slightly different ways of measuring ETs (discussed in Domenici *et al.* 2011b) although in most cases these other conventions yield the same values as the ET.

8.3.2   Theory and practice: in which direction do animals flee?

Geometric arguments (see Case A, below) suggest that there is an optimal trajectory that maximizes the chances of survival. However, this approach yields a single solution in terms of ET, and therefore does not deal with unpredictability that prevents the predator taking countermeasures. Furthermore, as we shall see, many other factors can affect ET, such as the position of the sensory organs on the prey, the subsequent ET that allows prey to track the predator, as well as the presence of refugia. Given all these considerations, a number of potential theoretical distributions can be derived (Figure 8.4), most of which are used by some prey species studied in the past.

8.3.2.1   Case A: a single, optimal trajectory (Figure 8.4A)

According to geometric models (Weihs & Webb 1984; Arnott *et al.* 1999; Domenici 2002), a single trajectory allows prey to maximize the distance from the predator for any given combination of predator and prey speeds. According to these models, ETs range over 90 to 180°. While most previous work on escape responses show this range of trajectories (Domenici *et al.* 2011b), we are not aware of any study that has directly tested the relationship between the relative speeds of predator and prey and ETs, although birds, for example, are known to use different ETs depending on the approach speed of the predator (Domenici *et al.* 2011b). Furthermore, prey are able to produce a "compromise" ET when attacked by predators from two different directions

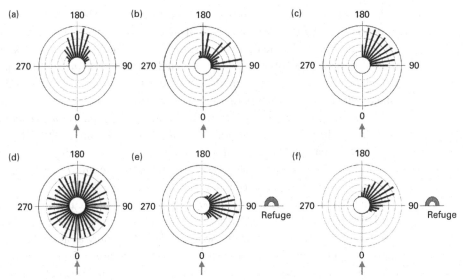

Figure 8.4   Various theoretical distributions of escape trajectories. (A) Unimodal (normal circular) distribution; (B) multimodal distribution; (C) random distribution within a limited angular range; (D) random distribution spanning 360°; (E) unimodal (normal circular) distribution directed toward the refuge; (F) unimodal (normal circular) distribution directed midway between the refuge and away from the threat. (See text for more details.) (Reprinted from *Journal of Experimental Biology*, Figure 1 in Domenici *et al.* 2011a, with permission from the publisher)

(Cooper *et al.* 2007). In addition to the idea of maximizing distance from the threat, some previous work has considered the need prey can have to track the predator while escaping. For example, whiting (*Marlangius merlangus*) escape at 135° and this was suggested to maximize distance from the threat while keeping the predator within the visual field (Hall *et al.* 1986).

Visual tracking while escaping has also been found in a number of arthropods. The haematophagous bug (*Triatoma infestans)* orients itself at an angle of about 120° relative to an approaching object (Lazzari & Varju 1990; Figure 8.5A). Because its visual field is about 140°, Lazzari and Varju (1990) suggest that keeping the threat at 120° gives the prey a safety factor of a few degrees, which prevents the predator from entering the blind zone as a result of small variations in relative motions. Nevertheless, the resulting distribution of observed ETs is quite large, spanning approximately 90°, from 70° to 160° (Lazzari & Varju 1990). In some side-walking species of crabs, escaping at approximately 180° allows tracking of the predator as a result of a combination of a translatory motion away from the threat (at 180°) and a rotation mechanism that allows the crab to keep the threat at 90° from the body axis (Layne & Land 1995; Oliva *et al.* 2007). Planktonic prey showed an escape response at 90° from the flow field of the predator, maximizing distance away from it (Jakobsen 2002). All of these examples yield a single optimal trajectory, although data show some degree of variability (Lazzari & Varju 1990). It would be interesting to test whether this variability is simply the result of noise in the system (i.e., measurement

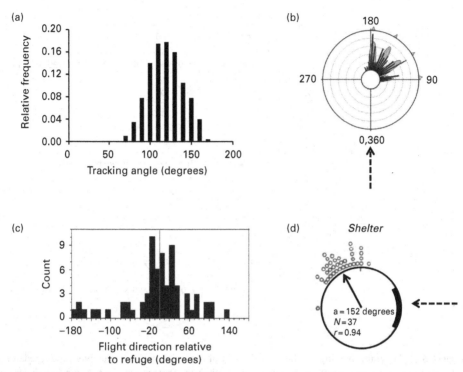

Figure 8.5 Examples of various escape strategies. (A) *Triatoma infestans* escapes using a single trajectory (about 120°) away from the stimulus, which allows tracking the threat. (B) Cockroaches (*Periplaneta americana*) escape using multimodal escape trajectories away from the threat (represented by the dashed line), thus producing unpredictability in their escape (C) Lizards (*Uta stansburiana*) escape in the direction of the refuge. (D) Blue crab *Callinestes sapidus* escape in a direction that is midway between reaching the shelter and escaping from the threat (represented by the dashed line). (Figure 8.5A modified from *Journal of Comparative Physiology A*, Figure 4B in Lazzari and Varju (1990) with permission from the publisher. Figure 8.5B reprinted from *Current Biology*, Figure 2B in Domenici *et al.* (2008) with permission from Elsevier. Figure 8.5C reprinted from *Canadian Journal of Zoology*, Figure 3A in Zani *et al.* (2009), with permission from the publisher. Figure 8.5D reprinted from *Animal Behaviour*, Figure 5D in Woodbury (1986), with permission from the publisher)

errors, limits in the animal's accuracy), or whether it has a function in increasing the unpredictability of the response.

8.3.2.2 Cases B and C: preferred trajectories (Figure 8.4B) and random ETs within a limited angular sector (Figure 8.4C)

For a single event of a predator attacking a prey, we might expect a single optimal solution. However, at least in some predator–prey systems, repeating the same strategy over and over would make the prey's response predictable, allowing learning, or even natural selection of countermeasures by predators. As alternatives to a single optimal trajectory, prey could escape using random ETs within a limited angular sector or use random selections from a finite range of preferred ETs. The

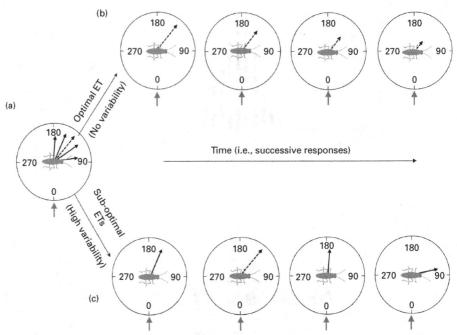

Figure 8.6 Diagram showing the theoretical effect of multiple attacks spread over time (predator positioned at 0°, grey arrow) and ETs on escape probability (represented by the length of the escape vector). (A) An ET with maximum escape probability (dotted arrow) with other ETs (full arrows) with lower probabilities of escape as a function of their angular distance from the optimal ET. (B) The ET with the highest escape probability is used in all four successive responses. Escape probability decreases as a result of predators learning to anticipate which ET will be used in successive responses. (C) Different ETs (both optimal and suboptimal) are taken in four successive responses. The escape probability does not decrease with successive responses because predators cannot learn which ET will be taken. (Reprinted from *Journal of Experimental Biology*, Figure 3 in Domenici *et al.* (2011a), with permission from the publisher)

limits in the angular sector exclude the use of trajectories toward the predator, while keeping enough variability to restrict predator countermeasures. These two strategies are discussed here together, because (a) they are likely to yield similar results in terms of prey escape success, although the neural basis of the escape behavior may differ between the two strategies, and (b) they are difficult to distinguish experimentally unless large sample sizes are used.

The different outcome, in terms of probability to escape, when using a single, optimal trajectory, vs. multiple trajectories within a given sector, is illustrated in Figure 8.6. For the "first" encounter (i.e., between a naïve predator and a naïve prey), the escape probability is higher (the length of the escape vector in Figure 8.6A) when using the optimal ET. However, when considering successive events, the probability of escape success decreases when using the "optimal ET" strategy (Figure 8.6B), because of predator countermeasures to predictable prey ETs. On the other hand, the use of variable ETs (Figure 8.6C) prevents this decrease in escape probability. As a result, although for each single predator–prey encounter, prey escape probability is lower than when using an optimal ET with a naïve predator, the mean of the escape probability calculated across all events is higher in the "high variability" than in the "optimal ET" strategy.

Escaping using variable or multiple trajectories appears to be a common strategy in many prey species from different taxa (Domenici *et al.* 2011b). In most cases, ETs tend to be within the 90 to 180° sector because prey tend to keep the threat on the side of the initial stimulation, rather than overturning (i.e., ETs in a semicircle 180 to 360° are rare) (Domenici *et al.* 2011b). A number of prey species (including fish, frogs, plankton, and deer; reviewed in Domenici *et al.* 2011b) show two main trajectories, typically at 180° and at approximately 90 to 130°. These have been observed in various species of fish, and were suggested to correspond to maximizing distance from the threat (180°) and keeping it within an angular field that allows tracking of the predator (130°) (Domenici & Blake 1993a; Domenici & Batty 1997).

Unlike side-walking crabs, soldier crabs (*Mictyris longicarpus*) walk forward, and therefore do not have the option of escaping away from a predator while maintaining visual contact. Soldier crabs show two main ETs (150° and 210°) which are symmetric with respect to 180°, and may serve to track the threat within the limits of the visual field (Domenici & Blake 1993a).

Some species of birds use different trajectories depending of the approach speed of the predator, with high and low predator speeds triggering escape response directed at 90° and 180°, respectively. This behavior is in line with the prediction of the models based on attack speeds, although only the extreme trajectories were observed. Other animals, including some larval fish, lizards, and small mammals attacked by birds, may escape using alternative directions; either away or toward the threat, where the latter may represent a strategy to surprise and flee past the predator before it can adjust its trajectory (Domenici *et al.* 2011b).

Some insect species appear to escape using more than two characteristic directions. This pattern has been fully demonstrated in cockroaches, both at the population and at the individual level (Figure 8.5B; Domenici *et al.* 2008). Each single cockroach escaped either at 90°, 120°, 150°, or 180° away from the threat. Although other insect species show highly variable ETs, whether this pattern is due to multiple peaks or random noise awaits further work using large sample sizes. Partitioning the two strategies (random noise vs. multiple peaks) will be particularly useful for elucidating the underlying mechanism generating escape variability although both tactics may allow prey to generate the unpredictability necessary to prevent predator countermeasures.

8.3.2.3 **Case D: random trajectories spanning 360° relative to the threat (Figure 8.4D)**

This strategy represents the ultimate unpredictability. Importantly, it includes situations where prey would move directly toward the predator. This creates a question: is the potential cost of occasionally going toward the predator outweighed by the extreme unpredictability? Given that responses toward the predator are rare, it appears that other strategies generating variability without including a response toward the threat are more common (e.g., Cases B and C). There are, however, a couple of specific cases that may, at least potentially, generate random trajectories when measured relative to the threat. Springtails (collembolans *Heteromurus nitidus*) and the common house mosquito (*Culex pipiens*) pupae escape in a fixed direction relative to their body axis (von Christian 1978; Brackenbury 1999), which should result in random ETs measured relative to the threat. This strategy should result in highly unpredictable directions of escape, unless the predator can forecast ETs based on the body orientation of the prey before the attack.

Another example that could, at least theoretically, yield random trajectories, is based on "nonsense orientation" exhibited by some species of birds (Thake 1981; Hart *et al.* 2013). These birds (e.g., mallards *Anas platyrhynchos*) appear to fly along a common preferred direction upon release, which does not appear to be related to the migration or homing direction. Hart *et al.* (2013) suggest that this common direction (fixed relative to cardinal points) may facilitate flock formation in an escape context. The advantage of such strategy would be that individuals of a flock will minimize decision time and will not disperse the flock. This strategy would theoretically result in random ETs when measured relative to the threat, unless the threat itself comes from a preferred geographical direction, as is the case of some predators (Červený *et al.* 2011).

8.3.2.4   Case E: ETs toward a refuge (Figure 8.4E)

Although more work is needed to test the effect of refuges in laboratory and field conditions, it is clear that the ETs of species living in a complex environment where shelters and burrows are available may be affected by such structures. This is certainly the case of many species of lizards and small mammals (see Chapters 3 and 5). A refuge may lead to ultimate protection from predators, and therefore, direction to the refuge may even override the importance of the direction of approach of a threat. The relative importance of the position of the predator and that of the refuge may depend on their distance from the prey, and in fact the effect of refuges decreases with increasing distance from the prey (e.g., in lizards *Leiocephalus carinatus*, Cooper 2007; *Uta stansburiana*, Zani *et al.* 2009; Figure 8.5C).

8.3.2.5   Case F: intermediate strategy: away from the threat and toward a refuge (Figure 8.4F)

In some cases, prey may be affected by both predator and refuge position, and the resulting ET may reflect a compromise between moving away from the threat and approaching the refuge. This is the case for blue crabs (*Callinestes sapidus*), which have an escape trajectory approximately midway between maximizing distance from the predator and reaching cover in the shortest time (Woodbury 1986; Figure 8.5D).

8.3.2.6   Overall trends

Previous work discussed above suggests that there is no single optimal ET. Rather, the ETs used by the prey will largely depend on the environmental context, the design of the prey's sensory system, and prey maneuverability. The most common escape strategies are (1) high ET variability, which may be due to multiple peaks or to wide ET distributions; (2) ETs that allow prey to continually track the threat; and (3) ETs directed toward a refuge. While high ET variability provides high unpredictability, tracking the threat and fleeing toward a refuge are relatively predictable in terms of direction.

The specific strategy used by the prey may be taxon and context specific: it may depend on the type of attack and the structural complexity of the habitat. Clearly, in some contexts, the need for unpredictability is overridden by the need to track the predator or to reach a refuge. Predator tracking may be more important in relatively slow and distant interactions, in which the prey can compensate for the motion of the predator. Similarly, reaching a refuge may be more beneficial than escaping in unpredictable directions when the refuge is nearby.

8.3.3   ### The relative importance of speed and maneuverability in predators chasing prey

Work on predator–prey interactions in fish shows that both prey speed and ET are determinants of the prey's escape success (Walker *et al.* 2005). However, in cases in which escape speed is traded off with reaching a trajectory away from the threat requiring a large turning angle, fish were shown to escape at submaximal speeds in the direction of the preferred trajectories (ranging from 130 to 180° away from the threat) (Domenici & Blake 1993a,b). Predators are usually larger than their prey, and therefore in most cases they are also faster because speed tends to increase with body size in many taxa (Peters 1983). Therefore if predator–prey gambits were to occur in a straight line, predators would generally be able to catch up with their prey. However, small animals tend to be more maneuverable than large ones, having smaller turning radii and higher turning rates (Howland 1974; Domenici 2001). From this perspective, frequent turning, such as the zigzagging, displayed by many prey when chased, may allow prey to gain ground on predators, in addition to increasing the unpredictability of their escape path.

Furthermore, it has generally been assumed that this so-called protean behavior benefits the prey. This benefit may remove the advantage the predator would have in "cutting corners" in its pursuit trajectory so as to close on its prey. Alternatively (or additionally) it may induce the predator to move more slowly so as to retain an ability to respond to changes in direction more quickly, or it may reduce the ability of the predator to quickly make good responses simply because more cognitive attention is required for tracking zigzagging prey. Any of these mechanisms might increase the time that the predator requires to capture the prey (thus making the prey less attractive) and/or increase the chance of the chase being unsuccessful from the predator's viewpoint. It is further assumed that the essence of the behavior is unpredictability (Humphries & Driver 1967; 1970), and it is this unpredictability in the future trajectory that makes capture more difficult for predators.

The term "protean behavior" was introduced by Humphries and Driver (1967), and very carefully explored in a subsequent highly influential monograph (Driver & Humphries 1988). While that book provides descriptions of a wealth of observational studies, the most explicit experimental test of the idea is much more recent (Jones *et al.* 2011). Jones *et al.* (2011) tasked human volunteers to "capture" tadpole-like representations of prey that swam around a computer screen. Capture involved moving a cursor over the prey by means of the computer's mouse. The prey's movements were varied according to a programmed algorithm. All individuals had a fixed probability per unit time of initiating a change in direction. For "control" individuals the turn angle selected was chosen randomly from within relatively narrow bounds, such that the long-term trajectory of the prey was relatively smooth; whereas "protean" individuals selected their turn angles from a much wider distribution and so had trajectories that included occasional abrupt turns. The human subjects found the "protean" prey substantially more difficult to capture. In this case, the prey moving along an unpredictable path benefitted from lower capture success. There are, however, other potential ways a prey could benefit from protean behavior. First, a given prey could benefit from a lower capture probability with a given predator that makes a second attack, since the prey response to the second attack will be different than in the first attack, avoiding costs through predator learning. Second, a given prey may benefit from its unpredictable behavior with respect to a whole population of predators. In this case, individuals in the whole prey population could benefit from protean behavior because the predator population cannot use any countermeasures for predicting the response of the prey.

Jones *et al.*'s (2011) work is a starting point for the exploration of the influence of protean behavior on predator–prey encounters. One useful extension of the work would be to allow the prey population to evolve subject to selection imposed by the human predators in order to explore what the optimal strategy is in terms of motion that hinders prey capture. This is very much like the approach that has been used to study adaptive coloration in artificial prey presented on a computer screen to birds trained to peck at discovered targets to obtain a reward (Bond & Kamil 2006). Based on analysis of the trajectory of the "predatory" cursor combined with eye-tracking equipment, it should be possible to study the gaze of human subjects to gain an improved understanding of the tactics used by humans in their prey pursuit and why protean behavior is able to exploit cognitive limitations of predators. This in turn might inform a co-evolutionary system in which the human predators are replaced by computer-generated predators whose actions are controlled by a set of rules that can be subject to selection and modification in just the same way as the prey.

However, perhaps the most exciting way to progress and expand on the work of Jones *et al.* (2011) would to be to introduce realistic physical dynamics for both the prey and the predator. In the simulations of Jones *et al.* (2011) both the prey and predators moved at a constant forward speed that is unaffected by turning. In reality there are physical constraints on individuals that determine turning rates; and trade-offs between forward speed and turning radius, and between speed and maneuverability (Domenici 2001, 2003). We see great advantage in adding realistic physical constraints to the cognitive limitations considered by Jones *et al.* (2011). Exploration of how this changes the predictions of the previous study would be very fruitful.

Methods of incorporating physical relationships and constraints have a relatively long history, stretching back at least as far as the influential modeling study of Howland (1974). This paper explored a "turning gambit" whereby prey that has a slower straight-line speed than a pursuing predator might be able to escape the predator. This is based on a number of modeling "rules." First, slower prey speed comes with a compensatory advantage of smaller turning radius. Second, the prey can gauge the correct time to initiate a turn (in terms of the proximity of the predator behind it). Third, sufficient increase in separation, as a result of this maneuver, would make the predator return to chasing it from immediately behind at greater than the critical distance at which maneuvers are triggered. Notice that these turns can be predictable and the benefit to the prey comes from physics rather than cognition. Hence, it would be a very natural extension of this work to introduce more unpredictable "protean" movements by prey and explore whether there are circumstances where the cognitive benefits of confusing the predator can overcome any dynamical costs of this behavior. Thus, the marriage of the cognitive and physical approaches to understanding maneuvering in predator–prey chases offers rewards to both theoretical traditions. Another potentially useful addition to the theory would be explicit consideration of differing rates at which energy is used in different maneuvers.

8.3.4   Modification of escape trajectories in the presence of conspecifics

For many animals that live in groups, it is not possible for the prey to detect the specific individual that has been targeted, and indeed the predator may not have selected a specific target when the point when prey start fleeing. This is especially likely when predatory attacks are launched from outside the group. Thus, a number of individuals may flee almost simultaneously. The modification of individual trajectories in the presence of conspecifics may have a number of functions: collision avoidance, placing conspecifics between a fleeing individuals and the predator (selfish herd effects), and predator confusion.

It seems clear that fleeing individuals should avoid colliding into each other, because such collisions might cause injury, attract the attention of the predator, and impair flight. It has long been postulated that avoidance of collisions might influence ETs (Hall *et al.* 1986; Domenici & Batty 1997), and that avoidance of collisions may explain the similar orientation of nearby individuals often seen in fish shoals and bird flocks. However, empirical exploration of this is exceptionally challenging and evidence of predators taking advantage of collisions is limited to a small number of anecdotal observations.

The selfish herd hypothesis was first put forward by Hamilton (1971). He proposed that when predators attack the first prey individual that comes within a certain distance of them, this behavior should select for prey aggregation by prey. By being part of an aggregation, an individual reduces the size of its "domain of danger," the region of space where, if a predator is present at any point, the focal individual would be the nearest individual to the predator. Hence, aggregations can form not necessarily as part of a collective defense mechanism, but because a number of individuals are all selfishly trying to place other individuals between themselves and possible points on the predator's expected trajectory. Increased aggregation in the face of imminent threat of predatory attack has been recorded for a number of taxa (reviewed by Krause & Ruxton 2002). Several modeling studies have explored paths that individuals might adopt, which can explain this increased aggregation through selfish-herd effects. Viscido *et al.* (2001, 2002) and Reluga and Viscido (2005), in simulations parameterized by their study of groups of fiddler crabs (*Uca*), demonstrated that even when flight away from an approaching predator occurs, selfish avoidance of danger can lead to an increase in aggregation.

The confusion effect describes the decreased likelihood that a predator will successfully catch any prey as group size of moving prey increases. The mechanism behind this is essentially "sensory overload." In predators faced with very high levels of informational input, the sensory and cognitive systems may struggle to track one particular prey item without being distracted by others. This effect has been demonstrated in simulation models that use neural networks to simulate predator sensory and cognitive systems (Krakauer 1995; Tosh *et al.* 2006). It has also been demonstrated across a wide range of predator–prey pairs (reviewed by Jeschke & Tollrian 2007; see also Ioannou *et al.* 2008) for an effective combination of modeling and empirical testing to demonstrate that reduced attack success can be linked to increased spatial targeting error. Jeschke and Tollrian (2007) made the important point that although the confusion effect is often discussed with respect to visual predators, the available empirical evidence suggests that it may be even stronger in tactile predators. The confusion effect seems particularly strong when prey individuals look and behave similarly (see Krakauer 1995 for theory and Landeau & Terborgh 1986 for empirical evidence). This may impact the behavior shown by fleeing prey, selecting for similarity in descriptors of their movement.

Recent theory and empirical evidence (Tosh *et al.* 2006; Ruxton *et al.* 2007) has demonstrated that behaviors that produce tight cohesion of a group may not be required for prey to benefit from predator confusion, and that complex coordinated behaviors between prey are not required. This issue was further explored by Jones *et al.* (2011) in experiments in which humans were challenged to capture (using a cursor controlled by a mouse) a specific target from an aggregation of targets on a computer screen. Protean prey (that showed less predictable movement trajectories) were more difficult to capture, but this effect was not influenced by the number of targets. That is, protean escape behaviors provided a direct antipredator benefit but did not enhance the confusion effect (which had previously been demonstrated to occur in a similar experimental set-up by Tosh *et al.* 2006). Recently, Ioannou *et al.* (2012) demonstrated that similarity of motion between group members could offer enhanced protection. They allowed real predators to hunt mobile virtual prey (computer-controlled images projected onto the side of the predator fish's tank). Prey whose movement rules included a tendency to be attracted toward, and to align direction of travel with, near neighbors, tended to form mobile coordinated groups that were rarely attacked compared to more isolated individuals.

The individual's ET can be influenced by the behavior of simultaneously fleeing nearby individuals. However, this can occur through a number of different and non-exclusive mechanisms, and our understanding of the relative importance of these mechanisms is still very rudimentary. A similar conclusion can be drawn at a higher level about trajectories more generally. In this section we have considered a number of factors that are likely to influence escape trajectories, but model systems have yet to emerge that would help us to probe the relative importance of these different influences.

8.4 Sensory defenses and signaling linked to fleeing

Some prey can enhance their ability to flee from predators by communicating with other individuals. Often predators may approach or chase prey that are impossible or too expensive (in time, energy, risk of injury, risk of disturbing other potential prey, and/or risk of attracting hyperpredators) to catch (see Chapters 2 and 10). If the prey can honestly inform a chasing predator of such a situation and the predator responds by breaking off the chase, then both parties benefit. However, it might appear that the prey could benefit by dishonest signaling in this regard, causing the predator to break off its attack on occasions when this would not be in the predator's best interests. In the first part of this section we explore the conditions required for more or less honest signaling of this nature to evolve and be maintained. There may also be occasions when the fleeing prey should signal to the chasing predator that although it may be possible and economic to catch the prey, subduing the caught individual will be impossible or prohibitively expensive, and we explore such signaling also. Finally, we explore signaling to other individuals that might occur because alerted individuals can be induced to break up the chase (e.g., by mobbing the predator).

8.4.1 Signaling vigor to predators

During pursuit some prey may signal to predators that the prey will be difficult to catch. The key issue for researchers is to understand under what conditions such a signal might be reliable, given that low-quality prey apparently have strong incentive to signal dishonestly. Vega-Redondo and Hasson (1993) explored this issue theoretically. Their key finding is that an evolutionarily stable signaling equilibrium exists at which the two prey types issue different signals and the predator responds differentially to those signals (attacking one type of signaler, but not the other). The equilibrium is evolutionarily stable, providing a number of conditions are satisfied. The key conditions are:

1. An attack on a higher quality individual is less likely to be successful than an attack on a poor-quality individual if both signal identically.
2. If intensity of signaling increases then the relative decrease in the probability of an attack being successful is greater for the higher quality individual than the lower quality one. Thus the cost of a more intensive signal is greater for a low-quality individual than for a high-quality individual.
3. If signal intensity becomes small enough then the predator's attack is always successful.

Tests of this theory are relatively scarce. Cresswell (1994) reported on extensive and carefully recorded naturally occurring predation events by a raptorial bird (merlin,

Falco columbarius) attacking a songbird (skylark, *Alauda arvensis*). The merlin clearly selected a skylark for pursuit before any song by the skylark was heard. If singing by the skylark was heard (by Cresswell), then it started very soon after the pursuit began. For pursuits where the merlin gave up without capture, merlins chased non-singing or poorly singing skylarks for longer periods compared to skylarks that sang well. These chases often exceeded five minutes in duration, implying that the costs of not signaling and not responding to the signal were high for the skylark and merlin, respectively. Merlins were more likely to catch non-singing than singing skylarks. Skylarks that did not sing when attacked were more likely to attempt to hide from the merlin rather than outfly it. The author noted that it has not been demonstrated that singing while being pursued is costly even though singing in the absence of pursuit is energetically demanding for skylarks (Cresswell 1994). In all other respects this study comes very close to a convincing demonstration of pursuit-deterrence signaling.

8.4.2   Cues or signals of physical or chemical defenses revealed during fleeing

For many prey, fleeing slowly on a predictable trajectory will increase their risk of predation, especially for undefended prey that can be subdued easily and consumed when caught. However, it is possible that simply fleeing slowly on a predictable trajectory (e.g., travelling slowly on a constant heading unaffected by predator position) is used as a cue (and perhaps even an evolved signal) that the fleeing organism is sufficiently defended to be difficult to subdue or unpalatable to eat if caught. Fleeing may still be advantageous to such defended individuals because attacks may be costly to the prey even if they are unsuccessful. Marden and Chai (1991) surveyed 124 Neotropical butterfly species and found that those that were sufficiently chemically defended to be unpalatable to vertebrate predators had a lower fraction of their body devoted to flight muscles than undefended species; the same was true for mimics of such species. Srygley (1994) reported similar results in a comparative study of 18 species of the butterfly tribe *Heliconiini* and 10 of their non-heliconiine co-mimics. Palatable species that were not mimics of unpalatable species had increased flight speed and maneuverability. Srygley and Dudley (1993) in experiments in cages found that relative to distasteful species, palatable butterfly species flew faster and were more able to maneuver successfully to evade attacks by insectivorous birds. Sluggish movement seems to be a cue that could be used by predators.

Hatle *et al.* (2001) demonstrated that in frog attacks on lubber grasshoppers, sluggish movement and aversive odors act together to reduce predation rates, whereas neither trait was effective alone. Hatle *et al.* (2002) explored prey selection when the Northern leopard frog (*Lithobates pipiens*) was presented aggregations of grasshoppers. The fastest moving individual in an aggregation of such aposematic individuals was most vulnerable to attack. Sluggish fleeing, then, can be used by predators as a somewhat reliable cue that the prey would be unattractive to attack. What remains unclear is if this slow flight of defended individuals is simply a cue driven by a lack of selection pressure to invest in evasion compared to the undefended, or whether this cue has evolved into a signal that has a communicative function. Sherratt *et al.* (2004) used a simulation model to show that such signals are theoretically possible, but such signaling has not been empirically demonstrated.

8.4.3   Signaling to others during fleeing

Fleeing individuals may signal to animals other than the pursuing individual. For instance, individuals might signal to request for help from individuals that might themselves benefit from the pursuit of the focal individual being unsuccessful. For example, a juvenile calling to a parent that might be able to attack the pursuer. A fleeing prey might signal to encourage conspecifics or heterospecifics to mob the pursuer because the mobbers benefit from the attack on the focal individual failing through kin selection, or because the predator is less likely to return to the same area to hunt after a failed attack. Another often-postulated idea is that calls by the fleeing individual might alert either predators or competitors of the pursuing animal. Intervention by such animals might provide increased potential for the signaler to escape.

Alarm calls (communicating information about imminent danger of predation) have been intensively studied with respect to their informational content, the ecological correlates of their use, and the responsiveness of conspecific and heterospecific receivers (see Caro 2005, for an overview). However, the linkage between calling and any other antipredatory behaviors of the caller have been almost entirely neglected. In particular, it is likely that some callers will also flee from the predator, and some calling may occur during flight. It would be interesting to explore whether such calling is different from calls emitted prior to fleeing or those emitted by non-fleeing individuals.

So called "distress calls" or "fear screams" that are produced by a range of birds, mammals, and anurans when physically contacted by a predator have also been studied widely (see Ruxton *et al.* 2004; Caro 2005, for reviews). Such screams are variously suggested to startle predators, attract competitors of the predator, encourage mobbing, or act as a warning to kin. Many of these benefits might be enhanced if such calls were initiated prior to the prey actually falling into the grip of the predator. However, such anticipatory distress calls have not been widely reported, nor has there been considera- tion of whether such anticipation might be excessively costly or ineffective. We would welcome exploration of the effects of distress calls on probability of escape and of whether distress calls are initiated prior to capture (while the prey is still in flight from the predator) and if not, why not.

8.5   Conclusions

Behavioral choices by prey during fleeing can influence the chance of being captured in multiple ways. In terms of the locomotor component of fleeing, prey have to deal with the laws of biomechanics, the performance of their sensory systems, and the need to generate unpredictability. Signaling while fleeing may increase the chances of survival because signaling then can deter a predator from chasing and it can strengthen the effect of collective antipredator behaviors. We believe that progress in this field will require integration of a number of fields of biology, such as behavioral ecology, biomechanics, and sensory biology. We thus hope to have pointed to some relatively tractable areas where current understanding of fleeing could be strengthened.

References

Allan, B. J. M., Miller, G. M., McCormick, M. I., Domenici, P. & Munday, P. L. (2014). Parental effects improve escape performance of juvenile reef fish in a high-CO_2 world. *Proceedings of the Royal Society B: Biological Sciences*, **281**, 2013–2179.

Arnott, S. A., Neil, D. M. & Ansell, A. D. (1999). Escape trajectories of the brown shrimp *Crangon crangon*, and a theoretical consideration of initial escape angles from predators. *Journal of Experimental Biology*, **202**, 193–209.

Batschelet, E. (1981). *Circular Statistics in Biology*. New York: Academic Press.

Batty, R. S. (1989). Escape responses of herring larvae to visual stimuli. *Journal of the Marine Biological Association of the United Kingdom*, **69**, 647–654.

Blaxter, J. H. S. & Batty, R. S. (1985). The development of startle responses in herring larvae. *Journal of the Marine Biological Association of the United Kingdom*, **65**, 737–750.

Blaxter, J. H. S. & Batty, R. S. (1987). Comparisons of herring behavior in the light and dark: Changes in activity and responses to sound. *Journal of the Marine Biological Association of the United Kingdom*, **67**, 849–859.

Bond, A. B. & Kamil, A. C. (2006). Spatial heterogeneity, predator cognition, and the evolution of color polymorphism in virtual prey. *Proceedings of the National Academy of Sciences of the United States of America*, **103**, 3214–3219.

Booth, D., Marie, B., Domenici, P., Blagburn, J. M. & Bacon, J. P. (1999). Transcriptional control of behavior: Engrailed knock-out changes cockroach escape trajectories. *Journal of Neuroscience*, **29**, 7181–7190.

Brackenbury, J. (1999). Regulation of swimming in the *Culex pipiens* (Diptera, Culicidae) pupa: Kinematics and locomotory trajectories. *Journal of Experimental Biology*, **202**, 2521–2529.

Camhi, J. M. & Tom, W. (1978). The escape behaviour of the cockroach *Periplaneta americana*. 1. Turning response to wind puffs. *Journal of Comparative Physiology A*, **128**, 193–201.

Cantalupo, C., Bisazza, A. & Vallortigara, G. (1995). Lateralization of predator-evasion response in a teleost fish (*Girardinus falcatus*). *Neuropsychologia*, **33**, 1637–1646.

Caro, T. M. (2005). *Antipredator Defenses in Birds and Mammals*. Chicago, IL: University of Chicago Press.

Catania, K. C. (2009). Tentacled snakes turn C-starts to their advantage and predict future prey behavior. *Proceedings of the National Academy of Sciences of the United States of America*, **106**, 11183–11187.

Červený, J., Begall, S., Koubek, P., Nováková, P. & Burda, H. (2011). Directional preference may enhance hunting accuracy in foraging foxes. *Biology Letters*, **7**, 355–357.

Chittka, L., Skorupski, P. & Raine, N. E. (2009). Speed-accuracy tradeoffs in animal decision making. *Trends in Ecology & Evolution*, **24**, 400–407.

Comer, C. M. & Dowd, J. P. (1987). Escape turning behaviour of the cockroach. Changes in directionality induced by unilateral lesions of the abdominal nervous system. *Journal of Comparative Physiology A*, **160**, 571–583.

Comer, C. (2009). Behavioral biology: Inside the mind of Proteus? *Current Biology*, **19**, R27–R28.

Cooper, W. E. (2007). Escape and its relationship to pursuit-deterrent signalling in the cuban curly-tailed lizard *Leiocephalus carinatus*. *Herpetologica*, **63**, 144–150.

Cooper, W. E., Perez-Mellado, V. & Hawlena, D. (2007). Number, speeds, and approach paths of predators affect escape behavior by the Balearic Lizard, *Podarcis lilfordi*. *Journal of Herpetology*, **41**, 197–204.

Cresswell, W. E. (1994). Song as a pursuit-deterrent signal, and its occurrence relative to other anti-predator behaviours of skylark (*Alauda arvensis*) on attack by merlins (*Falco columbarius*). *Behavioral Ecology & Sociobiology*, **23**, 217–223.

Domenici, P. (2001). The scaling of locomotor performance in predator prey encounters: From fish to killer whales. *Comparative Biochemistry and Physiology A*, **131**, 169–182.

Domenici, P. (2002). The visually mediated escape response in fish: Predicting prey responsiveness and the locomotor behaviour of predators and prey. *Marine and Freshwater Behaviour and Physiology*, **35**, 87–110.

Domenici, P. (2003). Habitat, body design and the swimming performance of fish. In *Vertebrate Biomechanics and Evolution*. Oxford: Bios Scientific Publishers, pp. 137–160.

Domenici, P. (2010). Context-dependent variability in the components of fish escape response: Integrating locomotor performance and behavior. *Journal of Experimental Zoology*, **313A**, 59–79.

Domenici, P. & Batty, R. S. (1997). Escape behaviour of solitary herring (*Clupea harengus*) and comparisons with schooling individuals. *Marine Biology*, **128**, 29–38.

Domenici, P. & Blake, R. W. (1993a). Escape trajectories in angelfish (*Pterophyllum eimekei*). *Journal of Experimental Biology*, **177**, 253–272.

Domenici, P. & Blake, R. W. (1993b). The effect of size on the kinematics and performance of angelfish (*Pterophyllum eimekei*). *Canadian Journal of Zoology*, **71**, 2319–2326.

Domenici, P., Lefrançois, C. & Shingles, A. (2007). Hypoxia and the anti-predator behaviour of fishes. *Philosophical Transactions of the Royal Society, B*, **362**, 2105–2121.

Domenici, P., Booth, D., Blagburn, J. M. & Bacon, J. P. (2008). Cockroaches keep predators guessing by using preferred escape trajectories. *Current Biology*, **18**, 1792–1796.

Domenici, P., Booth, D., Blagburn, J. M. & Bacon, J. P. (2009). Escaping away from and towards a threat: The cockroach's strategy for staying alive. *Communicative and Integrative Biology*, **2**, 497–500.

Domenici, P., Blagburn, J.M. & Bacon, J.P. (2011a). Animal escapology I: Theoretical issues and emerging trends in escape trajectories. *Journal of Experimental Biology*, **214**, 2463–2473.

Domenici, P., Blagburn, J.M. & Bacon, J.P. (2011b). Animal escapology II: Escape trajectorycase studies. *Journal of Experimental Biology*, **214**, 2474–2494.

Driver, P. M. & Humphries, D. A. (1988). *Protean Behavior*. Oxford: Clarendon Press.

Eaton, R. C. & Emberley, D. S. (1991). How stimulus direction determines the trajectory of the Mauthner-initiated escape response in a teleost fish. *Journal of Experimental Biology*, **161**, 469–487.

Eaton, R. C., Lavender, W. A. & Wieland, C. M. (1981). Identification of Mauthner-initiated response patterns in goldfish: Evidence from simultaneous cinematography and electrophysiology. *Journal of Comparative Physiology A*, **144**, 521–531.

Edut, S. & Eilam, D. (2004). Protean behavior under barn-owl attack: Voles alternate between freezing and fleeing and spiny mice flee in alternating patterns. *Behavioural Brain Research*, **155**, 207–216.

Godin, J.-G. J. (1997). Evading predators. In *Behavioural Ecology of Teleost Fishes*. Oxford: Oxford University Press, pp. 191–236.

Hall, S. J., Wardle, C. S. & Maclennan, D. N. (1986). Predator evasion in a fish school: Test of a model for the fountain effect. *Marine Biology*, **91**, 143–148.

Hamilton, W. D. (1971). Geometry of the selfish herd. *Journal of Theoretical Biology*, **31**, 295–311

Hart, V., Malkemper, E. P., Kusta, T. *et al.* (2013). Directional compass preference for landing in water birds. *Frontiers in Zoology*, **10**, 38.

Hatle, J. D., Salazar, B. A. & Whitman. D. W. (2001). Sluggish movement and repugnant odor are positively interacting insect defensive traits in encounters with frogs. *Journal of Insect Behaviour*, **14**, 479–496.

Hatle, J. D., Salazar, B. A. & Whitman, D. W. (2002). Survival advantage of sluggish individuals in aggregations of aposematic prey, during encounters with ambush predators. *Evolutionary Ecology*, **16**, 415–431

Heuts, B. A. (1999). Lateralization of trunk muscle volume, and lateralization of swimming turns of fish responding to external stimuli. *Behavioural Processes*, **47**, 113–124.

Howland, H. C. (1974). Optimal strategies for predator avoidance: The relative importance of speed and manoeuvrability. *Journal of Theoretical Biology*, **134**, 56–76.

Humphries, D. A. & Driver, P. M. (1967). Erratic display as a device against predators. *Science*, **156**, 1767.

Humphries, D. A. & Driver, P. M. (1970). Protean defence by prey animals. *Oecologia*, **5**, 285–302.

Ingle, D. J. & Hoff, K. V. (1990). Visually elicited evasive behavior in frogs. *Bioscience*, **40**, 284–291.

Ioannou, C. C., Tosh, C. R., Neville, L. & Krause, J. (2008). The confusion effect: From neural networks to reduced predation risk. *Behavioral Ecology*, **19**, 126–130.

Ioannou, C. C., Guttal, V. & Couzin, I. D. (2012). Predatory fish select for coordinated collective motion in virtual prey. *Science*, **337**, 1212–1215

Jakobsen, H. H. (2002). Escape of protists in predator-generated feeding currents. *Aquatic Microbial Ecology*, **26**, 271–281.

Jeschke, J. M. & Tollrian, R. (2007). Prey swarming: Which predators become confused and why? *Animal Behaviour*, **74**, 387–393.

Jones, K. A., Jackson, A. L. & Ruxton, G. D. (2011). Prey jitters: Protean behavior in grouped prey. *Behavioral Ecology*, **22**, 831–836.

King, J. R. & Comer, C. M. (1996). Visually elicited turning behavior in *Rana pipiens*: Comparative organization and neural control of escape and prey capture. *Journal of Comparative Physiology A*, **178**, 293–305.

Krakauer, D. C. (1995). Groups confuse predators by exploiting perceptual bottlenecks: A connectionist model of the confusion effect. *Behavioural Ecology & Sociobiology*, **36**, 421–429.

Krause, J. & Ruxton, G. D. (2002). *Living in Groups*. Oxford: Oxford University Press.

Krylov, V. V., Nepomnyashchikh, V. A., Izvekov, E. I., Izyumov, Y. G. & Chebotareva, Y. V. (2008). Asymmetry of escape behavior of the roach (*Rutilus rutilus*, Cyprinidae): Correlation with morphological asymmetry. *Zoologichesky Zhurnal*, **87**, 573–577.

Land, M. & Layne, J. (1995). The visual control of behavior in fiddler-crabs.2. Tracking control-systems in courtship and defense. *Journal of Comparative Physiology A*, **177**, 91–103.

Landeau, L. & Terborgh, J. (1986). Oddity and the confusion effect in predation. *Animal Behaviour*, **34**, 1372–1380.

Lazzari, C. & Varju, D. (1990). Visual lateral fixation and tracking in the hematophagous bug *Triatoma infestans*. *Journal of Comparative Physiology A*, **167**, 527–531.

Marden, J. H. & Chai, P. (1991). Aerial predation and butterfly design: How palatability, mimicry, and the need for evasive flight constrain mass allocation. *American Naturalist*, **138**, 15–36.

Martin, J. & Lopez, P. (1996). The escape response of juvenile *Psammodromus algirus* lizards. *Journal of Comparative Psychology*, **110**, 187–192.

Oliva, D., Medan, V. & Tomsic, D. (2007). Escape behavior and neuronal responses to looming stimuli in the crab *Chasmagnathus granulatus* (Decapoda : Grapsidae). *Journal of Experimental Biology*, **210**, 865–880.

Peters, R. H. (1983). *The Ecological Implications of Body Size*. Cambridge: Cambridge University Press.

Pewsey, A., Neuhauser, M. & Ruxton, G. D. (2013). *Circular Statistics, in R*. Oxford: Oxford University Press.

Preuss, T. & Faber, D. S. (2003). Central cellular mechanisms underlying temperature-dependent changes in the goldfish startle-escape behavior. *Journal of Neuroscience*, **23**, 5617–5626.

Reluga, T. C. & Viscido, S. (2005). Simulated evolution of selfish herd behavior. *Journal of Theoretical Biology*, **234**, 213–235.

Ruxton, G. D., Sherratt, T. N. & Speed, M. P. (2004). *Avoiding Attack: The Evolutionary Ecology of Crypsis, Warning Signals & Mimicry*. Oxford: Oxford University Press.

Ruxton, G. D., Jackson, A. L. & Tosh, C. R. (2007). Confusion of predators does not rely on specialist coordinated behavior. *Behavioral Ecology*, **18**, 590–596.

Sherratt, T. N., Rashed, A. & Beatty, C. D. (2004). The evolution of locomotory behavior in profitable and unprofitable simulated prey. *Oecologia*, **138**, 143–150.

Srygley, R. B. (1994). Locomotory mimicry in butterflies: The associations of positions of centers of mass among groups of mimetic unprofitable prey. *Philosophical Transactions of the Royal Society of London B*, **343**, 145–155.

Srygley, R. B. & Dudley, R. (1993). Correlations of the position of centre of body-mass with butterfly escape tactics. *Journal of Experimental Biology*, **174**, 155–166.

Stern, M., Ediger, V. L., Gibbon, C. R., Blagburn, J. M. & Bacon, J. P. (1997). Regeneration of cercal filiform hair sensory neurons in the first-instar cockroach restores escape behavior. *Journal of Neurobiology*, **33**, 439–458.

Thake, M.A. (1981). Nonsense orientation: An adaptation for flocking during predation? *Ibis*, **123**, 47–248.

Tauber, E. & Camhi, J. M. (1995). The wind-evoked escape behavior of the cricket *Gryllus bimaculatus*: Integration of behavioral elements. *Journal of Experimental Biology*, **198**, 1895–1907.

Tosh. C. R., Jackson, A. L. & Ruxton, G. D. (2006). The confusion effect in predatory neural networks. *American Naturalist*, **167**, E52–E65.

Turesson, H., Satta, A. & Domenici, P. (2009). Preparing for escape: anti-predator posture and fast-start performance in gobies. *Journal of Experimental Biology*, **212**, 2925–2933.

Vallortigara, G. & Rogers, L. J. (2005). Survival with an asymmetrical brain: Advantages and disadvantages of cerebral lateralization. *Behavioral Brain Science*, **28**, 575–633.

Vega-Redondo, F. & Hasson, O. (1993). A game-theoretic model of predator–prey signaling. *Journal of Theoretical Biology*, **162**, 309–319.

Viscido, S. V., Miller, M. & Wethey, D. S. (2001). The response of a selfish herd under attack from outside the group perimeter. *Journal of Theoretical Biology*, **208**, 315–328.

Viscido, S. V., Miller, M. & Wethey, D. S. (2002). The dilemma of the selfish herd: the search for a realistic movement rule. *Journal of Theoretical Biology*, **217**, 183–194.

Walker, J. A., Ghalambor, C. K., Griset, O. L., McKenney, D. & Reznick, D. N. (2005). Do faster starts increase the probability of evading predators? *Functional Ecology*, **19**, 808–815.

Von Christian, E. (1978). The jump of springtails. *Naturwissenschaft*, **65**, 495–496.

Weihs, D. & Webb, P. W. (1984). Optimal avoidance and evasion tactics in predator–prey interactions. *Journal of Theoretical Biology*, **106**, 189–206.

Wilson, A. M, Lowe, J. C., Roskilly, K. *et al.* (1013). Locomotion dynamics of hunting in wild cheetahs. *Nature*, **498**, 185–189.

Woodbury, P. B. (1986). The geometry of predator avoidance by the blue-crab, *Callinectes sapidus* Rathbun. *Animal Behaviour*, **34**, 28–37.

Yin, M. C. & Blaxter, J. H. S. (1987). Escape speeds of marine fish larvae during early development and starvation. *Marine Biology*, **96**, 459–468.

Zani, P. A., Jones, T. D., Neuhaus, R. A. & Milgrom, J. E. (2009). Effect of refuge distance on escape behavior of side-blotched lizards (*Uta stansburiana*). *Canadian Journal of Zoology-Revue Canadienne De Zoologie*, **87**, 407–414.

IId Refuge use

9 Hiding time in refuge

José Martín and Pilar López

9.1 Introduction

In most cases, prey animals do not escape randomly, but toward a refuge such as a rock crevice, burrow, tree, or a patch of thick vegetation. Safer habitats where animals restrict most of their activity to avoid exposure to potential predators found in other places are often called refuges or refugia (e.g., Werner *et al.* 1983). That is not our meaning of refuge in this chapter. Here, a refuge refers to small portions of the habitat where a prey hides temporarily after escaping from a predator that has been detected or that has attacked the prey. By definition, a refuge is a physical structure or some part of a habitat where the predator cannot enter to follow and capture the prey, or is at least impeded from doing so. Therefore predation risk immediately decreases, sometimes to zero, when the prey enters a refuge and hides inside it.

Numerous studies have shown that prey often respond to predator presence by increasing their use of refuges or safe microhabitats (Lima & Dill 1990; Sih *et al.* 1992). However, most prey animals do not spend their lives in the safety of a refuge (Sih 1997) because by staying in refuges prey often incur some fitness costs that should be minimized (e.g., the loss of time available for foraging; Godin & Sproul 1988; Koivula *et al.* 1995; Dill & Fraser 1997; Martín *et al.* 2003a; Blumstein & Pelletier 2005; or mate searching; Sih *et al.* 1990; Martín *et al.* 2003b; Reaney 2007). Unfavorable conditions in refuges (e.g., suboptimal temperatures or oxygen levels) might also entail physiological costs, such as hypothermia or hypoxia (Wolf & Kramer 1987; Martín & López 1999b; Polo *et al.* 2005). And, finally, refuges are often useful against some types of predators, but can expose of prey to other type of predators, which can cause a conflict in refuge use (Soluk 1993; Sih *et al.* 1998; Amo *et al.* 2005).

9.2 The optimal hiding time

Because refuge use is often costly, prey should optimize the time spent hiding inside a refuge and elect to use alternative escape strategies if refuge costs are too high. Some theoretical models have analyzed when prey should decide to leave the refuge and

Escaping From Predators: An Integrative View of Escape Decisions, ed. W. E. Cooper and D. T. Blumstein. Published by Cambridge University Press. © Cambridge University Press 2015.

resume their behavior after a predator's unsuccessful attack (see Chapter 2 for details). The hiding decision should be made based on the balance between the cost of being outside the refuge (i.e., predation risk) and the costs of refuge use. This decision is very important, as suggested by a state-dependent dynamic model that explored potential fitness consequences of hiding decisions in yellow-bellied marmots (*Marmota flaviventris*; Rhoades & Blumstein 2007). This model suggested that the overall survival of a population is substantially reduced when individuals make suboptimal hiding decisions (e.g., hiding 50% less or 200% more than the optimal hiding time substantially decreases the likelihood of survival). Because individuals need simultaneously to acquire energy and avoid predation, individuals making incorrect decisions could either starve or be killed.

Economic models of refuge use predict that prey should choose to leave a refuge when the cost of refuge use is higher than the risk to fitness of predation outside (Martín & López 1999a; Cooper & Frederick 2007; see Chapter 2 for details and graphs). The optimal hiding time will be modified in two ways. First, when the rate of reduction of predation risk decreases, the time spent in the refuge should increase. Second, when the costs of refuge use increase, the time spent in the refuge should decrease.

Economic models make three predictions. (1) Time spent in the refuge should be longer when the threat of the initial attack has been higher, and therefore the subsequent diminution of risk is slower (i.e., the probability of a new attack after emergence is higher). (2) Time spent in the refuge should be longer when costs of refuge use are lower. (3) The effects of costs of refuge use should be more important in the high-risk situation. In the low-risk situation, prey should emerge after a short period of time (when predation risk level drops), regardless of levels of costs of refuge use.

Optimality models consider the costs and benefits of all the possible strategies an animal could adopt, and predict which should be the optimal decision that maximizes fitness. These models predict that the optimal hiding time should increase with initial fitness and decrease as the maximum benefit that can be obtained by not hiding increases (Cooper & Frederick 2007; see Chapter 2 for details and graphs). Initial fitness is important because prey having high residual reproductive value should be more cautious to protect this "reproductive asset" (Clark 1994) by remaining hidden for longer. However, when the benefits obtainable by emerging are greater, prey should accept greater risk, and have shorter hiding times. If large benefits are retainable after death, prey may emerge and allow themselves to be killed. These predictions are similar to those from the previous economic models. However, optimality models make the new predictions. One is that emergence time increases with initial fitness and varies with the exponent in the benefit function. The second prediction, that prey may risk being killed by emerging for large benefits retainable after death, is unique to the optimal hiding time model.

9.3   Experimental tests of the predictions of hiding time models

Models of refuge use make many ordinal level and quantitative predictions about hiding or emergence time based on the balance between the benefits of staying hidden (i.e., risk

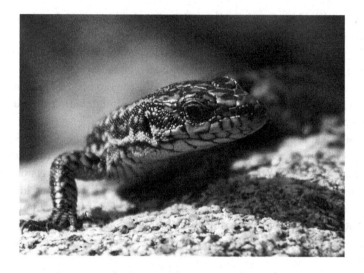

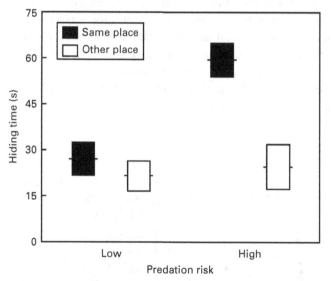

Figure 9.1   (a) Predation risk level affects refuge use by the Iberian rock lizard, *Iberolacerta cyreni*. (b) Hiding times (mean ± SE) in a refuge after a predatory attack are shown under two levels of risk. Responses change depending on whether lizards emerge from the site of refuge entry or at a different site. (Figure 9.1a: photograph by J. Martín; Figure 9.1b: redrawn from Martín & López 1999a)

of emerging) and the costs incurred while hiding in the refuge (i.e., cost of not emerging) (Sih 1992; Martín & López 1999a; Cooper & Frederick 2007).

One example of an experimental test of the predictions from optimal hiding models (see Chapter 2) is a field study that analyzed the variation in hiding time in a refuge (rock crevices) in the Iberian rock-lizard, *Iberolacerta cyreni,* under two different simulated predation risk levels and under different thermal costs of refuge use (Martín & López

1999a). As predicted by the economic models, lizards hid longer when the risk level of the initial attack was high, and therefore the subsequent reduction of risk with time is slower (Figure 9.1b). However, lizards may reduce hiding time in the refuge while also minimizing predation risk by walking while hidden under rock screes to reappear at a different place, leaving the predator waiting for the prey to appear at the wrong place (Figure 9.1). Interestingly, only individuals with initial high body temperatures seem able to adopt this alternative strategy.

On the other hand, effects of thermal costs are more important in high-risk situations. Under high-risk situations, time spent in the refuge increases when thermal conditions of the refuge are more similar to thermal conditions outside (i.e., when physiological costs of refuge use are lower) (Figure 9.2). Under these high-risk situations, hiding time is correlated with the temperature differential if lizards emerge from the point of refuge entry, but not when lizards emerge from different places. In low-risk situations, the place of emergence has no effect on the relationship between temperature differential and hiding time.

In addition to this first test of the economic model by Martín and López (1999a) that examined effects of both predation risk and cost of hiding, predictions of models of optimal hiding time have been verified consistently for various specific costs and benefits in several observational and experimental studies (Table 9.1). These are discussed in the remaining sections of this chapter. Of the studies carried out on hiding behavior, there has been a strong bias toward a few species of lizards, with only a minor fraction of studies made with other animals, such as fish, crabs, insects, marmots, etc.

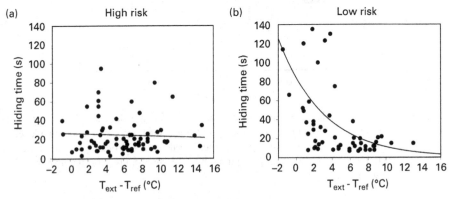

Figure 9.2   Thermal costs affect refuge use by Iberian rock lizards, *Iberolacerta cyreni*. Relationships observed between hiding time in a refuge after a predatory attack and the difference between the external temperature (T_{ext}) and the refuge temperature (T_{ref}) under two levels of risk. Thermal cost of refuge use is higher when this difference is greater because body temperature decreases faster in refuge as refuge temperature decreases relative to the outside temperature. (Redrawn from Martín & López 1999a)

Table 9.1 Studies examining variation in hiding time (or related variables) depending on several factors in different taxa. Results of these studies are useful to test the predictions of models of optimal refuge use.

Species	Factors examined	Reference
PLANTS:		
Mimosa pudica	"Foraging" costs	Jensen *et al.* 2011
INVERTEBRATES:		
Polychaetes:		
Balanus glandula	Foraging costs. Nutritional state. Body size	Dill & Gillet 1991
Serpula vermicularis	Foraging costs	Dill & Fraser 1997
Mollusks:		
Corbicula fluminea	Physiological costs (oxygen availability)	Saloom & Duncan 2005
Margaritifera margaritifera	Group size (risk dilution)	Wilson *et al.* 2003
Crustaceans:		
Uca lactea perplexa	Predators' risk level. Handling	Jennions *et al.* 2003
Uca mjoebergi	Foraging and reproductive costs	Reaney 2007
Pagurus filholi	Predators' risk level. Alternative tactics	Mima *et al.* 2003
Pagurus acadianus	Foraging costs	Scarratt & Godin 1992)
Heteroptera:		
Notonecta maculata	Predators' risk level. Foraging costs. Nutritional state. Competition with conspecifics	Martín & López 2004b
Notonecta hoffmani	Predator density. Body size. Nutritional state	Sih 1992
Gerris remigis	Reproductive costs	Sih *et al.* 1990
Lepidoptera:		
Achroia grisella	Costs of intrasexual competition between males	Brunel-Pons *et al.* 2011
Orthoptera:		
Gryllus integer	Prey's conspicuous calling	Hedrick 2000
	Long-term differences in predation pressure	Hedrick & Kortet 2006
Gryllus bimaculatus	Limb autotomy on calling behavior	Bateman & Fleming 2006
Teleogryllus oceanicus	Prey's conspicuous calling. Differences in parasitism pressure	Lewkiewicz & Zuk 2004

Table 9.1 (cont.)

Species	Factors examined	Reference
Trichoptera:		
Halesus radiatus (larvae)	"Waiting games" between predator and prey	Johansson & Englund 1995
Ephemeroptera:		
Baetis tricaudatus (larvae)	Multiple types of predators	Soluk 1993
Ephemerella subvaria (larvae)	Multiple types of predators	Soluk 1993
Diptera:		
Culex pipiens (larvae)	Predators' risk level. Physiological costs (oxygen availability)	Rodríguez-Prieto *et al.* 2006
VERTEBRATES:		
Fish:		
Colisa lalia	Physiological costs (oxygen availability)	Wolf & Kramer 1987
Fundulus diaphanus	Predators' risk level. Body size. Nutritional state	Dowling & Godin 2002
	Foraging costs. Nutritional state	Metcalfe & Steele 2001
Gasterosteus aculeatus	Foraging costs	Godin & Sproul 1988
	Body size. Foraging costs. Body condition	Krause *et al.* 1998
	Predators' risk level. Body size. Foraging costs. Nutritional state	Krause *et al.* 2000a,b
Phoxinus phoxinus	Predators' risk level. Body size. Foraging costs. Nutritional state	Krause *et al.* 2000a
Poecilia reticulata	Long-term differences in predation pressure	Harris *et al.* 2010
Semotilus atromaculatus	Foraging costs	Gilliam & Fraser 1987
Frogs:		
Lithobates catesbeianus	Predators' risk level	Cooper 2011b
Lizards:		
Plesiodon laticeps	Predators' risk level. Multiple attacks	Cooper 1998
Eulamprus heatwolei	Costs of intrasexual competition between males	Stapley & Keogh 2004
Pseudemoia entrecasteauxii	Multiple types of predators	Stapley 2004

Table 9.1   (cont.)

Species	Factors examined	Reference
Sceloporus jarrovii	Predators' risk level. Multiple attacks	Cooper & Avalos 2010
Sceloporus virgatus	Thermal costs	Cooper & Wilson 2008
	Predators' risk level. Thermal and foraging costs	Cooper 2009a
	inter-individual differences (personalities)	Cooper 2009c
	Predator's risk level and starting distance. Thermal costs	Cooper 2011a
	Tail autotomy and handling	Cooper & Wilson 2010
Tropidurus hispidus	Costs of intrasexual competition between males	Díaz-Uriarte 1999
Acanthodactylus erythrurus	Multiple attacks	Martín & López 2003a
Lacerta schreiberi	Thermal costs. Body size	Martín & López 2010
Podarcis lilfordi	Long-term differences in predation pressure	Cooper et al.2009
	Predator's risk level. Multiple attacks	Cooper et al.2010
Podarcis muralis	Predation pressure and thermal and foraging costs	Martín & López 1999b
	Predator's risk level. Thermal costs	Amo et al. 2003
	Predator's risk level. Multiple attacks	Martín & López 2005
	Multiple types of predators	Amo et al. 2004, 2005
Iberolacerta cyreni	Predator's risk level. Thermal costs. Economic model of refuge use	Martín & López 1999a
	Predator's risk level. Thermal costs. Multiple attacks	Martín & López 2001
	Predator's risk level. Thermal costs. Multiple attacks	Polo et al. 2005
	Body size related thermal costs	Martín & López 2003b
	Thermal and foraging costs. Body condition	Amo et al. 2007a,b
	Predator's risk level. Different individual predators	Cooper et al. 2003
	Foraging costs. Nutritional state	Martín et al. 2003a

Table 9.1 (cont.)

Species	Factors examined	Reference
	Predator's risk level. Reproductive costs	Martín *et al.* 2003b
	Prey's conspicuous coloration	Cabido *et al.* 2009
	inter-individual differences (personalities)	López *et al.* 2005
	Predator's risk level. Multiple attacks	Martín & López 2004a
	Temporal patterns of risk	Martín *et al.* 2009
	Predator's risk level. Monitoring from refuge	Polo *et al.* 2011
Iberolacerta monticola	Prey's conspicuous coloration	Cabido *et al.* 2009
Turtles:		
Mauremys leprosa	Predator's risk level. Handling. Alternative tactics	Martín *et al.* 2005
	Predator's risk level	Polo-Cavia *et al.* 2008
Trachemys scripta	Predator's risk level	Polo-Cavia *et al.* 2008
Birds:		
Poecile montanus	Foraging costs. Nutritional state	Koivula *et al.* 1995
Mammals:		
Marmota flaviventris	Foraging costs. Body size. inter-individual differences (personalities)	Blumstein & Pelletier 2005
	Predator's risk level. Foraging costs. Body size. Fitness consequences of hiding decisions	Rhoades & Blumstein 2007

9.3.1   Factors affecting risk of emergence on hiding time

Immediately after a prey hides in a refuge after escaping from a predator, risk of predation (i.e., costs of emergence) outside the refuge is highest; thereafter, risk level decreases gradually as time spent hidden in the refuge increases. This occurs because after some waiting time most predators will leave the area (Hugie 2003). Thus the probability that the predator is waiting for the prey outside the refuge (i.e., probability of a new attack) decreases as hiding time increases. All theoretical models of refuge use predict that hiding time should increase as the initial risk increases or the rate of diminution of predation risk with time decreases (Martín & López 1999a; Cooper & Frederick 2007; see Chapter 2). This has been confirmed for several types of risks in many studies cited below.

9.3.1.1   Risk due to the predator's behavior

After entering a refuge, prey may assess predation risk level in the exterior from the characteristics of the predator's behavior during approach, or the predator's attack behavior before the prey hides. Predation risk may vary in relation to the threat and characteristics of the immediately previous encounter with the predator (Stankowich & Blumstein 2005). The reduction of predation risk might be very fast when the prey has retreated into the refuge as a preventive strategy to elude a detected predator that has not yet attacked. In contrast, in a high predation risk situation (e.g., a direct attack by the predator), the initial level of predation risk is higher, and risk will diminish more slowly with time because the predator is known to pose a greater threat to the prey.

When a simulated predator approaches the prey faster, which indicates higher risk, subsequent hiding times are longer in several species of lizards (broad-headed skinks, *Plestiodon laticeps*:Cooper 1998; Iberian rock lizards, *Iberolacerta cyreni*: Cooper *et al.* 2003; Martín & López 1999a, 2001; wall lizards, *Podarcis muralis*: Martín & López 2005; striped plateau lizards, *Sceloporus virgatus*: Cooper 2009a; and Balearic lizards, *Podarcis lilfordi*: Cooper *et al.* 2010; Figure 9.3). In contrast, yellow-bellied marmots hide longer in response to a slower approach of the predator (Rhoades & Blumstein 2007), probably because marmots may consider a slow approach more dangerous as many of their predators slowly stalk their prey.

The directness of a predator's approach is another cue that prey use to assess risk. Predators approaching tangentially might not be attacking, whereas directly approaching predators are more likely to have detected the prey and be preparing to attack. Therefore hiding time is predicted to be longer for direct than indirect approaches. As predicted, when a predator has approached directly, fiddler crabs (*Uca lactea perplexa*; Jennions *et al.* 2003) and several lizards (Martín & López 1999a, 2004a, 2005; Cooper *et al.* 2003, 2010; Cooper 2009a) have longer hiding times than when a predator has approached indirectly (Figure 9.3).

A predator that is closer when first detected or that remains closer to the refuge after the attack may be considered a higher risk leading to longer hiding times in fiddler crabs (Jennions *et al.* 2003), skinks and other lizards (Cooper 1998, 2009a; Cooper *et al.* 2010; Figure 9.3). However, in American bullfrogs, *Lithobates catesbeianus*, time spent submerged after escaping by jumping into water was uncorrelated with proximity of the predator upon escape (Cooper 2011b). This contradiction may be explained because frogs may need to surface to determine whether the predator remains nearby, and can submerge themselves again if so.

Prey responses may also depend on the subtle characteristics of each individual predator, which may be considered to pose different risk levels (Cooper *et al.* 2003). Also, a prey that was able to escape from a predator that has captured it temporarily may, in a subsequent encounter, assess that this predator, or a similar one, poses a greater risk, and therefore increase hiding time (Cooper & Wilson 2010; Figure 9.4). Duration of handling by the predator before escaping also affected hiding times in fiddler crabs (Jennions *et al.* 2003) and turtles (Martín *et al.* 2005).

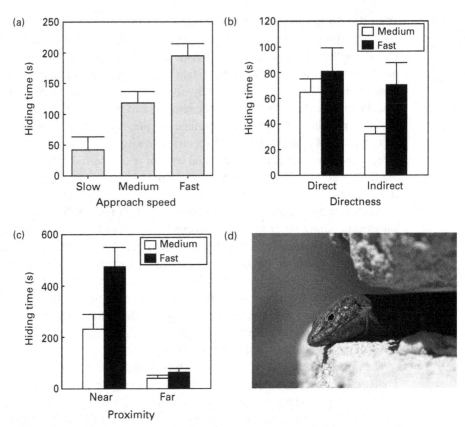

Figure 9.3   Effects of several risk factors on refuge use by Balearic lizards, *Podarcis lilfordi* (d). Time spent hiding in refuges (mean + SE) by lizards (a) increases linearly with predator approach speed; (b) is greater following direct than indirect approaches that bypass the prey without contact at medium approach speed, but not at the fast approach speed; and (c) is longer when the predator stays near the refuge than farther from it, and the difference between proximity levels of the predator is greater after approaches at the fast than the medium speed. (Graphs redrawn from Cooper *et al.* 2010; photograph by J. Martín)

Multiple repeated approaches also may represent a higher risk, which results in longer hiding times for the second of two consecutive attacks in several lizard species (Cooper 1998, 2011a; Martín & López 2001, 2004a, 2005; Cooper & Avalos 2010; Cooper *et al.* 2010). Similarly, after the first attack, most individuals of the lizard *Acanthodactylus erythrurus* do not hide, but stop after running in the open and remain vigilant; whereas in subsequent attacks within a brief interval, lizards use increasingly safer, structurally more complex bush refuges (i.e., larger and with more obstructive cover; Martín & López 2003a). These data suggest that persistent predatory attacks increase predation risk and prey adjust hiding time to correspond with the risk level. However, the outcome of several multiple attacks may be harder to predict than for only two successive attacks because there are usually interactions with other predation risk factors or changes in risk

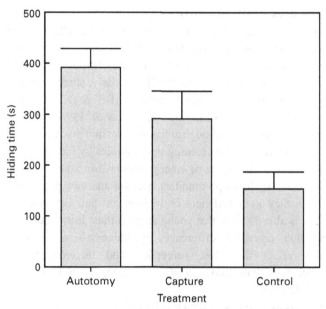

Figure 9.4   Effects of a previous capture by the predator and tail autotomy on refuge use by striped plateau lizards, *Sceloporus virgatus*. Hiding time (mean + SE) is longer following both tail autotomy and capture than in the uncaptured, unhandled control treatment, and longer following autotomy than just capture and handling. (Redrawn from Cooper & Wilson 2010)

level between attacks (Martín & López 2001, 2004a, 2005; Polo *et al.* 2005). These combined multiple effects will be examined below in more detail (see section 9.6).

Prey may perceive a higher risk when a given individual predator is persistent. Individual recognition of the predator may not be needed if the assessment is based solely on attack rate. Similarly, prey might respond to an increase in the density of different individual predators (Cooper 1998). Thus aquatic bugs *Notonecta hoffmani*, increase hiding time in response to increased predator density (Sih 1992). Nevertheless, some prey may be able to use the time interval between successive attacks to estimate whether repeated attacks are originated by the same individual predator, which would indicate persistence of the same individual predator (i.e., high risk), or as independent single attacks by different predators or by the same predator but with low motivation (i.e., low risk) (Martín & López 2004a).

Finally, in contrast to flight initiation distance (see Chapter 2), hiding time seems unaffected by the predator's starting distance (predator to prey distance when approach begins) in the lizard *Sceloporus virgatus* (Cooper 2011a), which suggests that once a prey enters refuge, the SD is irrelevant to predation risk upon emergence. However, it is likely that prey dynamically increase their assessed risk such that when there are longer approach times (which should be correlated with SD), there is greater perceived risk (Cooper & Blumstein 2014). Under such conditions, hiding time should also increase as SD increases, just as it increases with increases in other risk factors during the approach.

9.3.1.2   Risk due to the prey's characteristics

The prey's own characteristics, such as body size and age, may affect risk perception and refuge use. Small juvenile aquatic bugs *Notonecta hoffmani* (instar 1) are more susceptible to predation by adults than are large juveniles (instar 3); accordingly, small juveniles show longer hiding times (Sih 1992). Similarly, smaller barnacles, *Balanus glandula*, have longer hiding times than larger ones (Dill & Gillett 1991). In contrast, large fish often hide longer than small ones (Krause *et al.* 1998, 2000a,b; Dowling & Godin 2002), possibly because, although at higher risk from predators upon emergence, small fish have higher costs of lost feeding opportunities by hiding than do large fish. Similarly, yellow-bellied marmot pups emerge sooner than adults, which is also consistent with the costs of lost opportunities because marmot pups will not survive hibernation unless they gain sufficient body mass in their first year (Blumstein & Pelletier 2005). It is also possible that young animals must learn about how to respond to risks. In addition, consistent differences in boldness between otherwise similar individuals may affect their risk perception and therefore their refuge use (Blumstein & Pelletier 2005; López *et al.* 2005; Cooper 2009c; see Chapter 14 for more studies and details).

More conspicuous individuals suffer a greater risk of being detected by predators and therefore should increase hiding time. Male rock lizards, *Iberolacerta monticola*, have bright-blue UV lateral ocelli that serve as sexual signals, but also make males conspicuous to predators. They seem to compensate for greater conspicuousness by increasing hiding time in proportion to the number of these conspicuous ocelli (Cabido *et al.* 2009). By contrast, males of a sister lizard species, *I. cyreni*, that have fewer and less conspicuous ocelli, do not vary hiding time (Cabido *et al.* 2009). Similar behavioral compensation for increasing conspicuousness of displaying males to predators or parasites has been reported in other animals. For example, male field crickets, *Gryllus integer*, with longer, more conspicuous, songs behave more cautiously than males with shorter songs; they take longer to emerge from a shelter within a novel, potentially dangerous environment, and they cease calling for a longer time when their calls are interrupted by a predator cue (Hedrick 2000). Similarly, in the field cricket, *Teleogryllus oceanicus*, latency to resume calling after disturbance corresponds to population-level differences in risk of being parasitized (Lewkiewicz & Zuk 2004). And vividly colored birds are more responsive to the sounds of their aerial predators (Journey *et al.* 2013).

The ability of the prey to escape again from a predator after emerging from a refuge also influences predation risk and may affect hiding times. For example, lizards that escape by autotomizing their tails subsequently have decreased escape speed and lose the ability to use autotomy again. Thus the risk of being captured upon emergence is greater after an experimentally induced autotomy, which leads to longer hiding times in the lizard *Sceloporus virgatus* (Cooper & Wilson 2010) (Figure 9.4). Also, field crickets, *Gryllus bimaculatus*, that have lost legs by autotomy have longer hiding times than intact individuals (Bateman & Fleming 2006).

Finally, the risk dilution effect of being in a group remains almost unexplored in relation to hiding time after a predator attack. However, freshwater pearl mussels,

Margaritifera margaritifera, that were in a group closed their valves for shorter times than solitary mussels after experiencing potentially dangerous novel stimuli (Wilson *et al.* 2012).

9.3.1.3 "Waiting games" between predator and prey

Hiding in a refuge increases safety, but may restrict further information from being obtained about the risk associated with the waiting predator. When this occurs, the individual predator and prey involved become opponents in a "waiting game" (Hugie 2003). The prey must decide how long to wait for the predator to depart before emerging and potentially exposing itself to attack. The predator must decide how long to wait for the prey to emerge before departing in search of other foraging opportunities. Waiting is assumed to be costly to both players. Hugie (2003) used a game-theoretical model to determine the evolutionarily stable waiting strategy of both players. The model predicts that each player's waiting distribution (i.e., the distribution of waiting times expected for individuals in each role) will have a characteristic shape: the predator's distribution should resemble a negative exponential function, whereas the waiting time of the prey is predicted to be more variable and follow a positively skewed distribution. The model also predicts that the predator will rarely outwait the prey.

Illustrating this relationship, Johansson and Englund (1995) studied a waiting game between bullheads, *Cottus gobio,* which are predatory fish, and casemaking caddis fly larvae, *Halesus radiatus.* After an unsuccessful attack by a bullhead, a larva remains motionless with its head and legs hidden in a case of organic debris. The bullhead usually responds by orienting toward the larva and remaining motionless. Measures of waiting times of prey and predator reveal a good fit with the predictions of Hugie's (2003) waiting-game model. Furthermore, as predicted, the predator rarely outwaited the prey: only 1.5% of larvae re-emerged before the bullhead had departed.

9.3.2 Costs of refuge use determining hiding time

When deciding hiding times, prey should consider several costs of refuge use, which are mainly the loss of opportunities for obtaining food or reproductive benefits outside the refuge, and the physiological costs associated with unfavorable conditions inside refuges. The potential for encountering other types of predators inside the refuge is another cost in some situations. Theoretical models predict that the optimal hiding time should decrease as the costs of refuge use increase (Sih 1992; Martín & López 1999a; Cooper & Frederick 2007, see Chapter 2). Several empirical studies have examined how specific costs affect hiding decisions.

9.3.2.1 Loss of foraging opportunities

The cost of remaining hidden in a refuge often varies with food availability outside the refuge, especially when food becomes available in a food-limited environment. Therefore many animals take more risks when food levels are high. For example, the tubeworm, *Serpula vermicularis,* alters hiding time inside its tube with fluctuating food

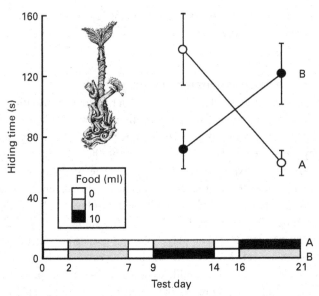

Figure 9.5   Effects of loss of opportunities for foraging by polychaete worms, *Serpula vermicularis*, on time spent retreated inside their calcareous tubes. Hiding times (mean ± SE) of two groups of serpulids before and after a change in food availability (A) from 1 ml of food suspension to 10 ml or (B) from 10 ml to 1 ml. Values plotted are the means of the average hiding times in several test days for individual tubeworms in the two treatment groups. The low horizontal bars represent the amount of a standard algal suspension provided daily to each tank. (Redrawn from Dill & Fraser 1997)

levels in the environment. It emerges from its tube sooner when food is abundant, thereby avoiding greater opportunity cost of remaining in the tube than when food is scarce (Dill & Fraser 1997; Figure 9.5). Moreover, tubeworms adjust their hiding times in response to short-term experimental changes in food availability. Similarly, juveniles of a small freshwater minnow, *Semotilus atromaculatus*, spent less time in a safe area that protected them from predators as food level increased outside in the riskier environment (Gilliam & Fraser 1987).

Iberian rock lizards, *Iberolacerta cyreni*, have shorter hiding times when they have detected food before entering refuge than when they have not (Martín *et al.* 2003a). This was demonstrated by experimentally introducing a mealworm or control stimulus outside the refuge immediately before a simulated attack ("R" and "RNW" treatments vs. "NF" treatment in Figure 9.6). Avoiding the approaching predator is probably the main priority in the absence of food. However, when a lizard hidden in refuge can observe that the prey that it was trying to capture before the predator attacked ("R" treatment), or a new food item provided after the attack ("RNW" treatment) is available outside the refuge, the benefit expected to be gained by emerging from the refuge is presumably higher than the expected cost due to predation risk. Based on this assessment, lizards rapidly emerge. Furthermore, the success of the encounter with food before the attack, and the added possibility of capturing either a new food item, or one that had been available, but not captured when the

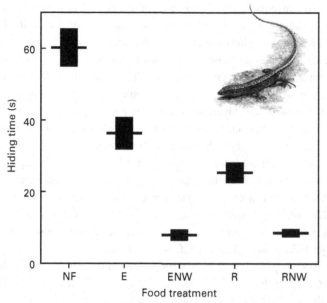

Figure 9.6 Effects of the loss of opportunities for foraging on refuge use by rock lizards, *Iberolacerta cyreni*. Hiding times (mean ± SE) of lizards after a predatory attack under different experimental treatments of food availability and satiation (NF: no food; E: lizards eat a prey before the attack; ENW: lizards eat a prey before the attack and new food offered after the attack; R: food presented but removed before eating and before the attack; RNW: food removed before eating but new food offered after the attack. (Redrawn from Martín *et al.* 2003a)

lizard hid after the predator appeared, differentially affects the magnitude of the costs of refuge use and, consequently, hiding duration. Lizards that have just eaten a prey before the attack ("E" treatment) have longer hiding times than lizards that have not eaten it ("R" treatment) (Figure 9.6). Lizards with a better nutritional state may delay resuming foraging to decrease predation risk. However, when a new prey is offered after the attack ("ENW" and "RNW" treatments), hiding times decrease greatly in both groups independently of the nutritional state (Martín *et al.* 2003a; Figure 9.6).

Similarly, hiding times of striped plateau lizards, *Sceloporus virgatus*, in rock crevices are shorter when a cricket is placed in front of the crevice opening where it can be seen by the lizard (Cooper 2009a). Food addition also reduces hiding times in fiddler crabs, *Uca mjoebergi*, but only during periods when food is naturally abundant and foraging is optimal (Reaney 2007). Food additions, however, have no noticeable effect on hiding times of crabs when food levels are naturally low and foraging efficiency is low, probably because the food added only has a weak effect on the benefits of quick emergence after being attacked by a predator. Size of food items near the shell refuge of hermit crabs, *Pagurus acadianus*, does not affect hiding time (Scarratt & Godin 1992). However, this is consistent with predictions because all food items were larger than could be eaten entirely.

Yellow-bellied marmots emerged sooner from refuges when supplemental food was experimentally placed next to their burrows than when food was absent (Blumstein & Pelletier 2005; Rhoades & Blumstein 2007). However, there is an intriguing interaction; bold individuals that tolerate close approaches before hiding (i.e., with short FIDs) emerge sooner when food is present, while those that are shy and intolerant of approaching humans (i.e., with longer FIDs) take longer to emerge and, in contrast, emerge sooner when food is not present. The latter observation does not apparently fit the expectations of refuge use models. However, it has been suggested (Cooper 2009a) that this finding would be consistent with theory if the placement of food by researchers before the trials in the experimental treatment increased perceived risk more for shy than bold marmots. Another possibility is that individuals that escaped later were hungrier, which would explain why they delayed fleeing and had shorter hiding times. By contrast, those that had longer FIDs might not need the food as much at the moment of attack, but might consider it as a harvestable asset that would reduce foraging costs upon emergence, allowing longer hiding times than when food was absent.

Optimality models predict that prey with greater initial fitness should have longer hiding times (Cooper & Frederick 2007). This is based on the asset protection principle (Clark 1994) that predicts that individuals with greater assets should protect them more carefully. Empirical evidence supports this expectation that prey state (i.e., initial fitness) affects hiding decisions. For example, hungry prey have shorter hiding times. This has been observed in barnacles, *Balanus glandula* (Dill & Gillett 1991), insects (water striders, *Notonecta hoffmani*: Sih 1992; *N. maculata*: Martín & López 2004b), lizards (*Iberolacerta cyreni*: Martín et al. 2003a), birds (willow tits, *Parus montanus*: Koivula et al. 1995), and in several species of fish (minnows, *Phoxinus phoxinus*, and three-spined sticklebacks, *Gasterosteus aculeatus*: Krause et al. 2000a; Metcalfe & Steele 2001), but not in others (Dowling & Godin 2002). Another observation that supports this prediction is that prey animals with a lower body condition or that have experienced greater weight loss (i.e., that have lower fitness) have shorter hiding times (fish: Krause et al. 1998; lizards: Amo et al. 2007a, b).

Finally, even some plants might adjust for "foraging" cost of being hidden. The plant *Mimosa pudica* displays a defensive behavior of rapidly folding its leaves when stimulated by touch, thereby decreasing visibility to herbivores, but at the cost of reducing light acquisition and photosynthesis. The time that these plants take to reopen leaves following a disturbance is longer under high light conditions than under more light-limited conditions (Jensen et al. 2011). This suggests that this plant can balance the risk and benefits of antiherbivore behavior in relation to current environmental light conditions.

9.3.2.2   Loss of reproductive opportunities

The loss of reproductive opportunities may also influence hiding times. Many animals are less responsive to predators during the reproductive seasons (Brown & Shine 2004), and this response may differ between sexes. For example, during the mating season, male Iberian rock lizards have shorter hiding times than females at any time and than males outside of the breeding season (Martín et al. 2003b). Furthermore, during the

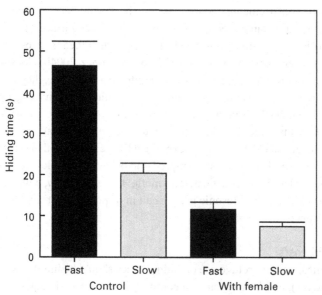

Figure 9.7   Effects of the loss of opportunities for reproduction on refuge use by rock lizards, *Iberolacerta cyreni*. Hiding times (mean + SE) in a refuge by male lizards in presence or absence (control) of a tethered female after being approached directly by an experimenter at one of two different approach speeds (slow vs. fast) in the mating season. (Redrawn from Martín *et al.* 2003b)

mating season, males have shorter hiding times when a tethered unfamiliar female (i.e., a potential mate) is experimentally placed nearby on their territories territory (Martín *et al.* 2003b; Figure 9.7). Moreover, in the absence of a female (control situation), males delay emergence when the approach speed of the simulated predator is fast (i.e., high risk) than when it is slow (low risk), but hiding times do not differ between approach speeds or risk levels when a female is present (Figure 9.7). Therefore variation in hiding times seem to reflect different balances between the costs of losing mating opportunities and the benefit of a reduction of predation risk over time.

Similarly, when mating opportunities for male fiddler crabs, *Uca mjoebergi*, are experimentally increased by introducing a tethered female, actively courting males engage in highly risky behavior and re-emerge a few seconds after an attack, considerably sooner than males not presented with a female; some males even abandon refuge use completely if a female is present (Reaney 2007). This latter observation confirms the prediction from optimality models (Cooper & Frederick 2007) that prey may risk being killed by leaving the refuge if it may obtain reproductive benefits that are retainable after death.

Hiding time may also be reduced by recent interactions with conspecific competitors due to an increased perceived need to defend feeding or reproductive opportunities, given that a hiding territorial resident is unable to monitor its territory or defend it from conspecific intrusions. The presence of an intruder in the near past can indicate an increased probability of future intrusions. Therefore following a conspecific intrusion, territorial residents should minimize costs from future intrusions at the cost of higher predation risks (Díaz-Uriarte 2001). Thus when a predator attack occurs immediately after an agonistic conspecific interaction, foraging backswimmers, *Notonecta maculata*, hide underwater, but resume feeding positions at the water surface more quickly and closer to the original position from which they were disturbed, suggesting short-term defense of particular foraging positions (Martín & López 2004b). When male lava lizards, *Tropidurus hispidus*, have recently encountered a rival male, they emerge sooner after a simulated predator attack, presumably to avoid losing mating opportunities (Díaz-Uriarte 1999, 2001). Similarly, territorial male water skinks, *Eulamprus heatwolei*, are less likely than non-territorial floaters to hide in refuges and return faster to a basking site after an attack. This may be explained by the trade-off that territorial lizards face between territorial defense and antipredator behavior (Stapley & Keogh 2004). Also, "singing" males of the acoustic pyralid moth, *Achroia grisella*, within leks respond with shorter pauses in their ultrasonic mating call in response to bat sounds than solitary individuals (Brunel-Pons *et al.* 2011).

9.3.2.3   Physiological costs

The physiological costs of refuge use on hiding times should be influenced by temperature (in ecotherms), and by oxygen concentration in the water (in aquatic animals). In ectotherms, such as reptiles, the attainment and regulation of an optimal body temperature is essential to maximize physiological and ecological processes, which may conflict with costs expected due to predation risk (Christian & Tracy 1981; Huey 1982). When a lizard or other ectothermic animal hides in a cold refuge (e.g., a rock crevice), its body temperature will quickly fall below optimal values (Polo *et al.* 2005). This may affect general physiological performance, such as somatic growth (Martín & López 1999b; Amo *et al.* 2007a,b), and may increase susceptibility to predators after emergence due to a reduced escape speed at low body temperatures (Christian & Tracy 1981). Therefore hiding decisions of ectotherms should reflect the thermal costs of refuge use.

Theoretical models predict, and empirical studies have shown, that as the difference between temperatures inside cold refuges and outside environmental temperatures increases (i.e., when the physiological cost of refuge use increases), hiding times decrease in rock lizards, *Iberolacerta cyreni* (Martín & López 1999a; Polo *et al.* 2005; see Figures 9.1 and 9.2), wall lizards, *Podarcis muralis* (Amo *et al.* 2003), and striped plateau lizards, *Sceloporus virgatus* (Cooper & Wilson 2008; Cooper 2009a, 2011a). A lizard's body temperature that before entering the refuge was correlated with the outside environmental temperature, will decrease more quickly and to a greater extent inside the refuge when the difference in ambient temperatures between the exterior and the refuge is greater. The empirical results suggest that optimization of refuge-use strategies may help lizards to cope with changes in predation risk without incurring excessive physiological costs associated with a lowered body temperature.

Predictions for the effect of difference between body and refuge temperatures in ectotherms are similar in all models, and optimality models predict that hiding times should be strongly affected by the cooling rate inside the refuge (Cooper and Frederick 2007). In lizards, ontogenetic changes in body size affect thermal exchange rates, with smaller individuals having a lower thermal inertia (i.e., they heat and cool faster). This simple physical property may have consequences for thermoregulation, and also for antipredator behavior. Therefore ontogenetic differences in thermal properties might affect costs of refuge use. In comparison with large adults, smaller juvenile rock lizards, *Iberolacerta cyreni*, delay fleeing to a refuge and have shorter hiding times in cold refuges, probably because their costs of hiding are higher, because they experience faster cooling rates than adults (Martín & López 2003b).

The effect of temperature on hiding decisions may be more complicated in ectothermic animals because they may partially emergence to assess risk prior to complete emergence. In such cases, hiding time has two components. First, *appearance time* is the time between refuge entry and appearance of a prey without fully emerging. Second, *waiting time* is the time between appearance and full emergence.

In Schreiber's green lizards, *Lacerta schreiberi*, appearance time increases as temperature outside the refuge increases, body mass increases, and temperature inside the refuge decreases (Martín & López 2010). Waiting time is longer when temperature in the refuge is lower, but is not affected by exterior temperature or body mass. Consequently, the total hiding time before complete emergence is longer when the exterior temperature is higher and the interior temperature is lower. The results show that interior and exterior temperatures have opposite effects on appearance time, and that waiting time increases as interior temperature decreases. The increase in appearance time as exterior temperature and body mass increase are consistent with the hypothesis that lizards can spend longer in refuge without suffering great loss of performance capacity when their body temperatures are higher and cooling rates are lower when they enter refuges. Warmer lizards with slower cooling rates take longer to reach a critically low body temperature requiring partial emergence. The increase in appearance time as interior temperature decreases is opposite to previous findings that hiding time increases as interior temperature increases.

Because waiting time also increases as interior temperature decreases, hiding time is longer when refuge temperature is lower and exterior temperature is higher (Martín & López 2010). If lizards allow body temperature to fall lower before appearing at the refuge's entrance when refuge temperature is lower, cooler lizards may require more time to assess risk prior to full emergence. Furthermore, body temperature might increase during the waiting interval while lizards are partially emerged. This is more likely if the lizards can bask, but also happens because the environmental temperature at the entrance may be higher than the temperature deeper in the refuge. The longer waiting times of lizards that enter cooler refuges may account for the absence of any effect of body mass on hiding time despite the increase in appearance time as body mass increases. Alternatively, lizards having greater thermal inertia take longer to cool, but also take longer to warm, which may lead to countervailing effects on appearance time and waiting time. Although only interior temperature is significantly related to waiting time, possible differences in body temperature upon emerging between smaller and larger lizards could obscure a relationship between body mass and waiting time.

Further research is needed to develop a comprehensive understanding of these findings. However, it is clear that when making decisions regarding refuge use, *Lacerta schreiberi* lizards seem to consider the physiological costs of being at low temperatures and also the risk of emerging with low escape performance that results from low body temperature.

In some cases, hiding in refuges may preclude breathing or make it difficult to breathe. This too can increase the physiological costs of refuge use. For example, air-breathing dwarf gouramis fish, *Colisa lalia,* increase their air-breathing frequency at low dissolved oxygen concentrations in water. These gouramis increase their use of refuges (submerged vegetation) and thus decrease their frequency of surfacing events to breathe air in the presence of predatory fish (Wolf & Kramer 1987). The freshwater clam, *Corbicula fluminea,* protects its soft tissues from small predators by closing its protective valves. This reduces predation risk, but ventilation and oxygen uptake are suspended. Clams reopen their valves sooner when under lower than higher oxygen concentrations; a finding that suggests that hypoxia increases costs of refuge use and increases vulnerability to predation (Saloom & Duncan 2005). Mosquito pupae, *Culex pipiens,* get aerial oxygen by sticking their air siphons above water. When undisturbed, pupae rest at the surface, but react to physical and visual disturbance by swimming down. The time interval between two consecutive surfacing events (hiding time) is longer under high risk, suggesting, but not demonstrating, a possible trade-off between risk and tolerance of oxygen deficit (Rodríguez-Prieto *et al.* 2006). Nevertheless, time spent on the surface does not vary with risk levels.

9.3.2.4   Multiple types of predators and conflicting refuge use

A prey's defenses against one predator may put it at greater risk of being killed by other predators. Some types of refuges may be useful only against particular types of predators or may expose prey to different predators (Sih *et al.* 1998). For example, mortality of mayfly larvae in the presence of both predaceous fish and stonefly larvae is greater than expected because stoneflies in refuges cause mayflies to come out of hiding, thus increase their exposure to fish (Soluk 1993).

Prey exposed to multiple types of predators can experience conflicts. Enhanced survival from one predator may simultaneously increase vulnerability to another predator, especially if prey can deploy defense against only one type of predator at a time (Sih *et al.* 1998). In such cases, prey should use tactics to defend against the most dangerous predator and ignore the less dangerous predators (McIntosh & Peckarsky 1999; Bouwma & Hazlett 2001). In many cases prey should decide to use a refuge against an exterior predator if the risk of being captured by this predator is higher than the risk of being captured by another type of predator inside the refuge.

Wall lizards, *Podarcis muralis,* respond to simulated predatory attacks of birds and mammals by hiding inside the nearest rock crevice, but this may expose them to increased risk of predation by the saurophagous smooth snake, *Coronella austriaca,* which ambushes lizards inside rock crevices. Thus wall lizards employ different alternative escape strategies in relation to their reliance on refuge safety (Amo *et al.* 2005). Lizards basking close to refuges that they have used recently, hide in them again when attacked. By contrast, lizards that are moving do not always enter the closest refuge, but often run away without hiding. This behavior may be a strategy to avoid entering refuges in which the absence of predators has not been recently ascertained.

Similarly, the gecko *Oedura lesueurii* uses the same types of refuges as one of its main snake predators, *Holocephalus bungaroides.* These geckos use their chemosensory ability to avoid entering rock crevices covered with the scent of *H. bungaroides* (Downes & Shine 1998). Log skinks, *Pseudemoia entrecasteauxii*, use snake-scented refuges less than predator-free refuges (Stapley 2004). However, when skinks are exposed to risk of predation by a snake inside the refuge and by a bird in the open, skinks do not decrease their use of snake-scented refuges (Stapley 2004), suggesting that predation by birds is more dangerous than the risk of encountering a snake inside a refuge.

Hiding time in refuges should depend on the probability that another type of potential predator is in the refuge. When a refuge is potentially unsafe (e.g., because the prey detects predator cues inside), the probability of being detected by a second type of predator hidden in that refuge increased with time spent in the refuge. Hence, a prey hidden in an unsafe refuge will have increased costs of refuge use and should emerge sooner than from a predator-free refuge. However, the presence of different predator cues may modify a prey's reliance on refuge safety by altering its assessment of the risk associated with entering a refuge as well as the cost of remaining in one in relation to the risk outside the refuge. For example, after a simulated attack outside a laboratory refuge, wall lizards hid longer when there were no snake cues inside than when chemical or visual snake cues were added to the refuge. Moreover, when visual and chemical snake cues were combined, hiding times were even shorter, supporting an additive effect of several cues to risk assessment (Amo *et al.* 2004).

9.4   Hiding behavior when in morphological and constructed refuges

Many animals flee to refuges, but are also able to escape by fleeing without hiding, to choose the refuge type, and to change refuges after persistent attacks (Cooper 1998; Martín & López 1999a, 2003a). Other species that are relatively sessile, such as polychaete tubeworms, caddis-fly larvae, mollusks, and barnacles, can only take refuge in a protective structure surrounding their bodies (Dill & Gillett 1991; Johansson & Englund 1995; Dill & Fraser 1997). An intermediate situation occurs when animals have morphological or protective structures that provide partial protection, but are also able to escape actively to safer refuges in their habitat. Examples are hermit crabs, hedgehogs, pangolins, porcupines, armadillos, some fishes, skin-armoured lizards (e.g., the armadillo girdled lizard, *Cordylus cataphractus*; horned lizards, *Phrynosoma* spp.) and turtles (McLean & Godin 1989; Doncaster 1993; Losos *et al.* 2002; Mima *et al.* 2003; Martín *et al.* 2005). However, factors that modulate refuge use in these animals remain largely unknown, and characteristics of such prey could complicate escape and hiding decisions predicted by optimal refuge use theory (Martín & López 1999a; Hugie 2003; Cooper & Frederick 2007).

Hermit crabs, *Pagurus filholi*, have two antipredator tactics: taking refuge in their shells and fleeing. When hermit crabs are dropped into seawater containing chemical stimuli from a predatory crab, they prefer hiding in shells of species that provide more effective protection against crab predators, and hiding times are shorter in the shells of mollusks where they are more vulnerable. However, hermit crabs have shorter hiding

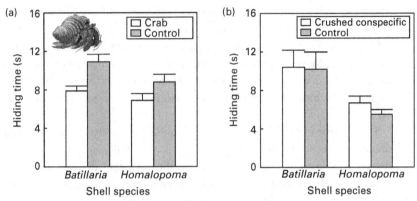

Figure 9.8   Hiding time before active fleeing by hermit crabs, *Pagurus filholi*, in the shells of *Batillaria cumingi* (heavy and highly protective) or *Homalopo masangarense* (light and vulnerable) after being dropped into seawater control or seawater containing (a) stimulus of a predatory crab or (b) stimulus of crushed conspecific. (Redrawn from Mima *et al.* 2003)

times in shells and switch to active fleeing earlier when predator stimuli are present than absent (Mima *et al.* 2003; Figure 9.8).

Spanish terrapins, *Mauremys leprosa*, adjust their hiding behavior by assessing the risk of emerging before the predator has left the area. Turtles hide longer in their shells when risk level is higher, as indicated by the predator's behavior (i.e., longer handling duration during the attack, proximity as the turtle hides, and persistence after the attack; Martín *et al.* 2005). However, because the shell offers only partial protection, increasing hiding time may also increase the risk that the predator is able to injure or kill the turtle. Therefore the possibility of switching from hiding to active escape to a safer refuge (e.g., into water) also shortens hiding times.

In turtles, interspecific differences in hiding behavior appear to be related to the presence of different types of predators in different habitats (Martín *et al.* 2005; Polo-Cavia *et al.* 2008). After an attack by a terrestrial predator, basking sliders, *Trachemys scripta*, remain hidden inside the shell for long periods delaying or avoiding active escape toward the water (Polo-Cavia *et al.* 2008). In contrast, basking Spanish terrapins, *Mauremys leprosa*, typically flee toward the safety of deep water immediately, remaining hidden in the shell only when they are far from water (Martín *et al.* 2005). Sliders hide in the shell before entering water because diving may expose them to dangerous aquatic predators, but for *M. leprosa* fleeing to water immediately is favored because aquatic predators are relatively uncommon in their habitat (Martín *et al.* 2005; Polo-Cavia *et al.* 2008).

9.5   Hiding under simultaneous risks and costs

During an interaction with a predator, prey must simultaneously assess risks and costs for multiple risk factors and several types of costs, and adjust hiding time accordingly. For example, a prey might accurately assess risk level based on predator behavior during the attack, increasing hiding time with increasing directness and approach speeds, but the prey has to simultaneously assess the risk posed by a predator waiting close to the refuge to avoid being captured immediately upon emergence. Conversely, if the prey assesses risk associated with the predator's distance to the refuge, but fails to consider the predator's approach speed, it might be captured due to misjudging the predator's speed.

The "threat-sensitivity hypothesis" (Helfman 1989) predicts that multiple risk factors have additive effects on the intensity of antipredatory responses. This implies that all predator traits contribute to risk in an additive fashion and simultaneous risks must therefore have additive effects (Smith & Belk 2001). However, optimal refuge use theory suggests that interaction between factors should be more common (Cooper & Frederick 2007; Chapter 2): additive effects are predicted to occur only if the differences in curves of risk diminution with time for different risk levels of one risk factor are identical to those for the second risk factor. Effects should be interactive when risk decreases faster with time for one factor than the other, which is a more likely situation given the different characteristics and effects of each risk factor.

A review of empirical studies examining effects of multiple risks and costs on FID and hiding time (Cooper 2009b) revealed far more frequent interactive than additive effects between two risk factors, as predicted by optimality theory. For example, approach speed during the attack and predator proximity after the attack have additive effects on hiding times of rock lizards, but approach speed and directness interact with predator persistence (Martín & López 2004a), with place of emergence (Martín & López 1999a), and with the peculiar characteristics of each individual predator (Cooper et al. 2003). Similarly, in wall lizards, directness interacts with proximity and with persistence of the predator (Martín & López 2005), and in Balearic lizards approach speed interacts with both directness of approach and predator proximity (Cooper et al. 2010) (see Figure 9.3). In Spanish terrapins, risk level (handling duration) and proximity of the predator interacts with the microhabitat where the attack occurs because hiding time inside the shell increases with risk on land, but not in water where emergence could facilitate an alternative active escape (Martín et al. 2005).

However, additive and interactive effects seem to be equally common when a risk and a cost factor are considered simultaneously (Cooper 2009b). In this case, if there are unequal slopes of the risk curves for different risk levels, the cost curves for different magnitudes of costs, or both, we could expect an interaction between risks and costs. If curves for different levels of risks or costs have equal slopes, or differences are too small to be noted, we could expect additive effects. For example, risk due to lower escape ability after tail loss and thermal costs of refuge use have additive effects on hiding time in striped plateau lizards (Cooper & Wilson 2010). Thermal costs interact with directness and speed of the approach in lizards (Martín & López 1999a, 2005), but when there are persistent repeated attacks of a predator, the effects are additive with thermal costs (Polo et al. 2005). More studies of diverse taxa are required to determine the shapes of risk and cost curves. These are needed by optimality models of refuge use to predict joint effects of multiple risks and costs.

9.6   Repeated attacks and multiple hiding decisions

9.6.1   Optimal multiple hiding decisions

In some circumstances, if predators remain waiting outside the refuge and try new attacks or if predator density increases, a particular prey may suffer successive attacks in a short time. Successive attacks may be assessed as indicating increase in the risk of predation, but the costs of refuge use also increase with time spent in the refuge. Thus prey should make new, but related, decisions on when to emerge after each attack. In a field experiment, rock lizards, *Iberolacerta cyreni*, were approached ten times in a short interval. Hiding times increased progressively with successive attacks, but only when the thermal cost of refuge use was low, as lizards tended to maintain or even to decrease hiding times between approaches when cost of refuge use increased (Martín & López 2001).

Polo *et al.* (2005) modified previous economic models of hiding time to include the case of a high, sustained level of predation risk during repeated attacks. The model assumes that prey perceive that the probability of a new attack decreases more slowly with time after each successive attack, that costs of refuge use increase with time at the same rate after each attack, and that hiding cost does not start from zero except after the first attack, but accumulates across approaches and begins each time at the maximum level reached in the previous episode of hiding (Figure 9.9). The model predicts that the optimal hiding time should increase following successive attacks and that this increase should not be linear but accelerating (i.e., the rate of increase in hiding time increases over successive emergences).

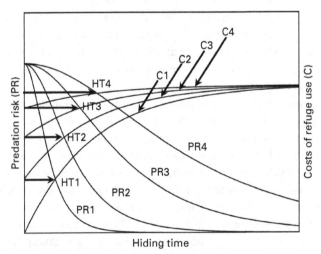

Figure 9.9   An economic model to predict the hiding times of lizards in a refuge after successive continuous attacks as a function of the expected fitness effects of the diminution of the risk of predation in the exterior with time (PR) after each attack (successive PR curves), and variations with time in costs (C) of refuge use after each attack (successive C curves). The optimal hiding times (HT) after each successive attack are shown. (Redrawn from Polo *et al.* 2005)

In a laboratory experiment using male Iberian rock lizards, predation risk was identical in two treatments in which temperature inside the refuge was high or low. As predicted, successive hiding times increased in an accelerating rather than linear manner and were shorter when thermal cost of refuge use was higher (Polo *et al.* 2005). This is similar to previous field observations (Cooper 1998; Martín & López 1999a, 2001). However, in the laboratory, potential confounding variables were held constant and changes from low to high thermal cost were observed consistently in the same individuals.

Assessed risk presumably was higher in the laboratory study (Polo *et al.* 2005) than in the field (Martín & López 2001) because only one refuge was available in a terrarium and persistent attacks were made from close range in the laboratory, whereas multiple refuges were present and attacks were launched from longer distance in the field. Greater risk explains the increase in laboratory hiding times even when thermal cost was high. Alternatively stated, when predation risk is very high, prey may adopt a conservative strategy and remain inactive in the refuge for very long periods and conserve energy (Polo *et al.* 2005). But this strategy is dependent on temperature inside the refuge. When refuge temperature is low, lizards should initially emerge as soon as possible to avoid heat loss. However, after repeated attacks, it might be more favorable to remain inactive until risk decreases because emerging with a low body temperature, and thus having poor locomotor performance, may be more dangerous than risking starvation by remaining in the burrow. In contrast, in a refuge with a high temperature, where body temperature does not decrease, prey can resume normal activity immediately after emerging (Polo *et al.* 2005).

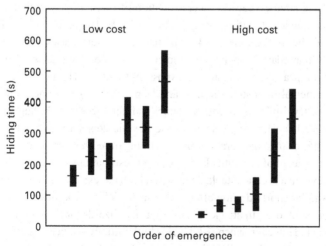

Figure 9.10   Multiple hiding decisions by rock lizards *Iberolacerta cyreni*. Successive hiding times in a refuge (mean ± SE) after multiple predatory attacks and under low or high thermal costs of refuge use. (Redrawn from Polo *et al.* 2005)

9.6.2   Risk assessment affecting multiple hiding decisions

Although not responding to predator cues appropriately can be lethal, an excessive or unnecessary hiding response also can have detrimental effects for prey (Rhoades & Blumstein 2007). Thus when there are multiple persistent predatory attacks it is important to determine whether prey use fixed behaviors or respond flexibly to short-term changes in perceived predation risk by changing their hiding times.

Prey might assess predation risk during successive attacks in several ways. (1) Fixed independent estimation: prey might estimate that each successive attack is independent of the previous one and adjust hiding time to the current risk level in each attack without considering previous risk estimates. (2) Accumulative dependent estimation: prey might consider that each successive attack represents an increase in risk level with respect to the previous estimation regardless of the actual risk level of each single attack. Thus successive hiding times would increase. (3) Flexible dependent estimations: dynamic models have suggested that animals will show tolerance to imperfect information (Bouskila & Blumstein 1992), but that the extent of this tolerance may change from one situation to the next, and that the rules of thumb used to assess risk should be flexible enough to correspond to current conditions (Koops & Abrahams 1998). After a second successive attack indicating predator persistence, it may be necessary to assess risk more accurately. An individual might remember its estimate of the risk level in one attack, compare it with the estimated risk in the current attack, and modify hiding time accordingly. If the second risk level is estimated to be higher than the previous one, prey might consider that it has underestimated the previous risk level and increase hiding time more than expected. If the second risk level is estimated to be lower, then prey might consider that it has overestimated the first risk level and show shorter hiding times than expected. A more conservative option might be to maintain at least the response to the risk level estimated in the first attack, even if the second attack was estimated to be of lower intensity. This could be a viable strategy because overestimation of risk may have milder fitness consequences than underestimating danger (Bouskila & Blumstein 1992; Rhoades & Blumstein 2007; but see Abrams 1994). Alternatively, in some cases, prey may habituate and reduce its antipredator responses to a potential predator that ceases to be regarded as dangerous after repeated non-threatening exposures to it (e.g., Hemmi & Merkle 2009).

In an experimental field study, Martín and López (2004a) examined how short-term changes in risk level of two successive attacks affect successive hiding times of rock lizards (Figure 9.11). The lizards seem to use flexible dependent estimations of risk in each attack. They change the duration of their hiding times through successive attacks as a function of risk level of each attack, but previous estimations of risk are used to assess the new risk level in a second attack. Thus when both attacks are of low intensity, hiding times are of similar short duration after both attacks. When risk increases from the first attack to the second, or both attacks are of high risk, lizards increase hiding times after the second attack. However, when risk level is high initially but decreases for the second attack, lizards maintain the hiding time required for the risk level assessed in the first attack. This might seem to imply overestimation of risk, but the cost of ignoring persistent attack may be higher (Bouskila & Blumstein 1992).

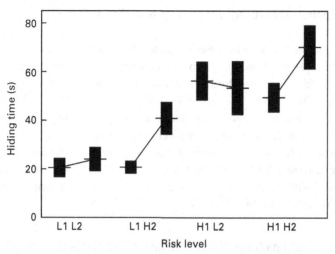

Figure 9.11 Multiple hiding decisions by rock lizards, *Iberolacerta cyreni*. Successive hiding times in a refuge (mean ± SE) in four treatments in which two successive predatory attacks were both of low risk level (L1L2), increasing in risk level (L1H2), decreasing in risk level (H1L2), or both of high risk level (H1H2). (Redrawn from Martín & López 2004a)

In contrast, wall lizards, *Podarcis muralis*, seem to consider each of three successive attacks to be independent. They adjust hiding time to current risk in each attack without considering the risk levels in previous attacks (Martín & López 2005). This indicates that lizards may track short-term changes in risk level through time and modify their initial responses when required. This might occur if lizards considered that a predator should usually not outwait the prey after an unsuccessful attack (Hugie 2003), but depart to look for other potential prey, which is plausible because lizard density is very high in this population. For this species, two successive attacks are likely to come from different individual predators, in which case risk may be assessed again in each attack independently of previous estimates.

9.6.3 Monitoring from the refuge to determine hiding time

Most studies of refuge use have analyzed situations in which information on predator behavior is unavailable to hiding prey. In this case current risk of being killed upon emergence can only be estimated by prey based on time elapsed since the attack and characteristics of the attack (Sih 1992; Martín & López 1999a; Hugie 2003). In other cases, prey can monitor predators from the refuge safely and use information gained to decide hiding times (Cooper 2008; Polo *et al.* 2011). Nevertheless, monitoring predators from the refuge entails costs, such as revealing the refuge's position to the predator while scanning for the predator presence.

When monitoring behavior is possible for lizards at, or partially outside, the refuge's entry, hiding time, as noted previously, can be divided into appearance time and waiting or monitoring time. These different times may be differentially affected by risk and costs of refugia.

For example, in response to series of simulated attacks (low vs. high risks), rock lizards, *Iberoalcerta cyreni*, have appearance times that do not differ between risk levels, but have longer monitoring times after a single low-risk approach of the predator than after a direct unsuccessful attack (Polo *et al.* 2011). This may occur because, if there has not been a clear attack, uncertainty about future risk would be greater, and prey may need more time before leaving the refuge to ensure that a predator has not detected the lizard and that it is not lying in wait nearby. These results suggest that different levels of uncertainty about future risks, rather than just the previous risk level during the attack, seem to modulate monitoring time from the refuge and, thereby, total hiding times.

9.6.4   Long-term temporal patterns of risk affecting hiding decisions

Prey in nature experience a broad range of temporal patterns of predation risk, and it is not entirely clear how prey respond to these variations (Lima & Bednekoff 1999; Sih *et al.* 2000). This is important because it has been predicted that antipredator behavior in situations with different levels of predation risk should vary with not just the immediate level of risk but also with the preceding temporal pattern of perceived risk (i.e., risk allocation hypothesis; *sensu* Lima & Bednekoff 1999).

Rock lizards, *Iberolacerta cyreni*, were subjected to a series of simulated repeated predatory attacks in the laboratory (24 attacks in a four-hour period) of different risk level (i.e., low vs. high), with similar overall numbers of low-risk and high-risk attacks across a trial, but with three different temporal patterns of presentation (i.e., a series of low-risk approaches and then a series of high-risk attacks, or the opposite pattern, or successive attacks where risk level changed randomly; Martín *et al.* 2009). Under predictable temporal patterns of risk (i.e., multiple attacks with the same risk level in the recent past) lizards show accurate antipredator responses to each of the successive attacks. However, when risk is random, individuals are not able to predict the level of the next predatory attack and adopt a conservative strategy with longer hiding times than required by the actual current risk level.

On the other hand, hiding times may be shaped by natural selection or maternal effects. These may act through long-term differences in exposure to predation between populations. For example, the first-generation of male crickets, *Gryllus integer*, reared in the laboratory from field-caught mothers from a high-predation habitat hide longer when placed in a novel environment in the laboratory than male crickets born from mothers from a low-predation habitat (Hedrick & Kortet 2006). Therefore differences in behavior are due to either non-genetic environmental–maternal effects or genetic effects. Similarly, Balearic lizards, *Podarcis lilfordi*, from two islet populations with different predation pressure differ in hiding time (almost nine times longer under high predation pressure) (Cooper *et al.* 2009). And wild-caught guppies, *Poecilia reticulata*, from high-predation localities emerge sooner from shelter compared to those from low-predation localities (Harris *et al.* 2010).

9.7 Conclusions and future directions

Many predictions from theoretical models of hiding time have been successfully tested using simply designed studies that measured hiding behavior, but many topics require research in the future. First, the emphasis of available studies is heavily on lizards. Studies of a wide range of different taxa, in different environments and with different physiological and morphological constrains may impart more useful knowledge and help to assess the range of applicability of the predictions of theoretical models. Second, new, probably more elaborated and complex, models and experiments are needed to understand hiding behavior in situations when several risk and costs factors act simultaneously and when mutliple responses depend of previous decisions. In addition, variation in decisions about refuge use may interact with other antipredatory behaviors, such as FID and DF, and may also depend on differences in personality that are not considered in current models. Encounters with predators often involve multiple, complex successive chases and escape sequences. In such cases, prey should continuously assess and track changes in risk level, consider potential accumulative costs of refuge use, and estimate the relative success of its previous antipredatory decisions to modify them accordingly. The ability to monitor predators and quality of the information about predator behavior and "intentions" have been considered little. Although the waiting-game model (Hugie 2003) predicts that hiding time is longer than a predator's giving-up time, very little empirical attention has been paid to understanding why predators should not be able to predict hiding times of their prey better (as human researchers seem to do) and counteract their antipredatory strategies. This points out the need for models and studies that consider the actions of both prey and predator behavior simultaneously. New models and experiments using hiding time and related variables will lead to a greater understanding of many aspects of risk-taking decisions.

References

Abrams, P. A. (1994). Should prey overestimate the risk of predation? *American Naturalist*, **144**, 317–328.

Amo, L., López, P. & Martín, J. (2003). Risk level and thermal costs affect the choice of escape strategy and refuge use in the wall lizard, *Podarcis muralis. Copeia*, **2003**, 899–905.

Amo, L., López, P. & Martín, J. (2004). Wall lizards combine chemical and visual cues of ambush snake predators to avoid overestimating risk inside refuges. *Animal Behaviour*, **67**, 647–653.

Amo, L., López, P. & Martín, J. (2005). Flexibility in antipredatory behavior allows wall lizards to cope with multiple types of predators. *Annales Zoologici Fennici*, **42**, 109–121.

Amo, L., López, P. and Martín, J.(2007a). Refuge use: a conflict between avoiding predation and losing mass in lizards. *Physiology and Behavior*, **90**, 334–343.

Amo, L., López, P. & Martín, J. (2007b). Pregnant female lizards *Iberolacerta cyreni* adjust refuge use to decrease thermal costs for their body condition and cell mediated immune response. *Journal of Experimental Zoology A*, **307**, 106–112.

Bateman, P. W. & Fleming, P. A. (2006). Sex, intimidation and severed limbs: The effect of simulated predator attack and limb autotomy on calling and emergence behaviour in the field cricket *Gryllus bimaculatus*. *Behavioral Ecology and Sociobiology*, **59**, 674–681.

Blumstein, D. T. & Pelletier, D. (2005). Yellow-bellied marmot hiding time is sensitive to variation in costs. *Canadian Journal of Zoology*, **83**, 363–367.

Bouskila, A. & Blumstein, D. T. (1992). Rules of thumb for predation hazard assessment: Predictions from a dynamic model. *American Naturalist*, **139**, 161–176.

Bouwma, P. & Hazlett, B. A. (2001). Integration of multiple predator cues by the crayfish *Orconectes propinquus*. *Animal Behaviour*, **61**, 771–776.

Brown, G. P. & Shine, R. (2004). Effects of reproduction on the antipredator tactics of snakes (*Tropidonophis mairii*, Colubridae). *Behavioral Ecology and Sociobiology*, **56**, 257–262.

Brunel-Pons, O., Alem, S. & Greenfield, M. D. (2011). The complex auditory scene at leks: Balancing antipredator behaviour and competitive signalling in an acoustic moth. *Animal Behaviour*, **81**, 231–239.

Cabido, C., Galán, P., López, P. & Martín, J. (2009). Conspicuousness-dependent antipredatory behavior may counteract coloration differences in Iberian rock lizards. *Behavioral Ecology*, **20**, 362–370.

Christian, K. A. & Tracy, C. R. (1981). The effect of the thermal environment on the ability of Galapagos land iguanas to avoid predation during dispersal. *Oecologia*, **49**, 218–223.

Clark, C. W. (1994). Antipredator behavior and the asset protection principle. *Behavioral Ecology*, **5**, 159–170.

Cooper, W. E., Jr. (1998). Risk factors and emergence from refuge in the lizard *Eumeces laticeps*. *Behaviour*, **135**, 1065–1076.

Cooper, W. E., Jr. (2008). Visual monitoring of predators: occurrence, cost and benefit for escape. *Animal Behaviour*, **76**, 1365–1372.

Cooper, W. E., Jr. (2009a). Theory successfully predicts hiding time: new data for the lizard *Sceloporus virgatus* and a review. *Behavioral Ecology*, **20**, 585–592.

Cooper, W. E., Jr. (2009b). Fleeing and hiding under simultaneous risks and costs. *Behavioral Ecology*, **20**, 665–671.

Cooper, W. E., Jr. (2009c). Variation in escape behavior among individuals of the striped plateau lizard *Sceloporus virgatus* may reflect differences in boldness. *Journal of Herpetology*, **43**, 495–502.

Cooper, W. E., Jr. (2011a). Risk, escape from ambush, and hiding time in the lizard *Sceloporus virgatus*. *Herpetologica*, **68**, 505–513.

Cooper, W. E., Jr. (2011b). Escape strategy and vocalization during escape by American Bullfrogs (*Lithobates catesbeianus*). *Amphibia-Reptilia*, **32**, 213–221.

Cooper, W. E., Jr. & Avalos, A. (2010). Predation risk, escape and refuge use by mountain spiny lizards (*Sceloporus jarrovii*). *Amphibia-Reptilia*, **31**, 363–373.

Cooper, W. E., Jr. & Blumstein, D. T. (2014). Novel effects of monitoring predators on costs of fleeing and not fleeing explain flushing early in economic escape theory. *Behavioral Ecology*, **25**, 44–52.

Cooper, W. E., Jr. & Frederick, W. G. (2007). Optimal time to emerge from refuge. *Biological Journal of The Linnean Society*, **91**, 375–382.

Cooper, W. E., Jr. & Wilson, D. S. (2008). Thermal cost of refuge use affects refuge entry and hiding time by striped plateau lizards *Sceloporus virgatus*. *Herpetologica*, **64**, 406–412.

Cooper, W. E., Jr. & Wilson, D. S. (2010). Longer hiding time in refuge implies greater assessed risk after capture and autotomy in striped plateau lizards (*Sceloporus virgatus*). *Herpetologica*, **66**, 425–431.

Cooper, W. E., Jr., Martín, J. & López, P. (2003). Simultaneous risks and differences among individual predators affect refuge use by a lizard, *Lacerta monticola*. *Behaviour*, **140**, 27–41.

Cooper, W. E., Jr., Hawlena, D. & Pérez-Mellado, V. (2009). Islet tameness: Escape behavior and refuge use in populations of the Balearic lizard (*Podarcis lilfordi*) exposed to differing predation pressure. *Canadian Journal of Zoology*, **87**, 912–919.

Cooper, W. E., Jr., Hawlena, D. & Pérez-Mellado, V. (2010). Influence of risk on hiding time by Balearic lizards (*Podarcis lilfordi*): Predator approach speed, directness, persistence, and proximity. *Herpetologica*, **66**, 131–141.

Díaz-Uriarte, R. (1999). Anti-predator behaviour changes following an aggressive encounter in the lizard *Tropidurus hispidus*. *Proceedings of the Royal Society of London Series B, Biological Sciences*, **266**, 2457–2464.

Díaz-Uriarte, R. (2001). Territorial intrusion risk and antipredator behaviour: A mathematical model. *Proceedings of the Royal Society of London Series B, Biological Sciences*, **268**, 1165–1173.

Dill, L. M. & Fraser, A. H. G. (1997). The worm re-turns: hiding behavior of a tube-dwelling marine polychaete, *Serpula vermicularis*. *Behavioral Ecology*, **8**, 186–193.

Dill, L. M. & Gillet, J. F. (1991). The economic logic of the barnacle *Balanus glandula* (Darwin) hiding behaviour. *Journal of Experimental Marine Biology and Ecology*, **153**, 115–127.

Doncaster, C. P. (1993). Influence of predation threat on foraging pattern: The hedgehog's gambit. *Revue d Ecologie-la Terre et la Vie*, **48**, 207–213.

Dowling, L. M. & Godin, J.-G. J. (2002). Refuge use in a killifish: influence of body size and nutritional state. *Canadian Journal of Zoology*, **80**, 782–788

Downes, S. & Shine, R. (1998). Sedentary snakes and gullible geckos: Predator–prey coevolution in nocturnal rock dwelling reptiles. *Animal Behaviour*, **55**, 1373–1385.

Godin, J. G. L. & Sproul, C. D. (1988). Risk taking in parasitized sticklebacks under threat of predation: Effects of energetic need and food availability. *Canadian Journal of Zoology*, **66**, 2360–2367.

Guliam, J. F. & Fraser, D. F. (1987). Habitat selection under predation hazard: Test of a model with foraging minnows. *Ecology*, **68**, 1856–1862.

Harris, S., Ramnarine, I. W., Smith, H. G. & Pettersson, L. B. (2010). Picking personalities apart: estimating the influence of predation, sex and body size on boldness in the guppy *Poecilia reticulata*. *Oikos*, **119**, 1711–1718.

Hedrick, A. V. (2000). Crickets with extravagant mating songs compensate for predation risk with extra caution. *Proceedings of the Royal Society of London. Series B: Biological Sciences*, **267**, 671–675.

Hedrick, A. V. & Kortet, R. (2006). Hiding behaviour in two cricket populations that differ in predation pressure. *Animal Behaviour*, **72**, 1111–1118.

Helfman, G. S. (1989). Threat-sensitive predator avoidance in damselfish–trumpetfish interactions. *Behavioral Ecology and Sociobiology*, **24**, 47–58.

Hemmi, J. & Merkle, T. (2009). High stimulus specificity characterizes anti-predator habituation under natural conditions. *Proceedings of the Royal Society of London Series B, Biological Sciences*, **276**, 4381–4388.

Huey, R. B. (1982). Temperature, physiology and the ecology of reptiles. In Gans, C. & Pough, F. H. (ed.), *Biology of the Reptilia, Vol. 12*, pp. 25–91. New York: Academic Press.

Hugie, D. M. (2003). The waiting game: A "battle of waits" between predator and prey. *Behavioral Ecology*, **14**, 807–817.

Jennions, M. D., Backwell, P. R. Y., Mourai, M. & Christy, J. H. (2003). Hiding behaviour in fiddler crabs: How long should prey hide in response to a potential predator? *Animal Behaviour*, **66**, 251–257.

Jensen, E. L., Dill, L. M. & Cahill, J. F., Jr. (2011). Applying behavioral–ecological theory to plant defense: Light-dependent movement in *Mimosa pudica* suggest a trade-off between predation risk and energetic reward. *American Naturalist*, **177**, 377–381.

Johansson, A. & Englund, G. (1995). A predator–prey game between bullheads and case-making caddis larvae. *Animal Behaviour*, **50**, 785–792.

Journey, L., Drury, J. P., Haymer, M., Rose, K. & Blumstein, D. T. (2013). Vivid birds respond more to acoustic signals of predators. *Behavioral Ecology and Sociobiology*, **67**, 1285–1293.

Koivula, K., Rytkönen, S. & Orell, M. (1995). Hunger dependency of hiding behaviour after a predator attack in dominant and subordinate willow tits. *Ardea*, **83**, 397–404.

Koops, M. A. & Abrahams, M. V. (1998). Life history and the fitness consequences of imperfect information. *Evolutionary Ecology*, **12**, 601–613.

Krause, J., Loader, S. P., McDermott, J. & Ruxton, G. D. (1998). Refuge use by fish as a function of body length-related metabolic expenditure and predation risks. *Proceedings of the Royal Society of London. Series B: Biological Sciences*, **265**, 2373–2379.

Krause, J., Cheng, D. J.-S., Kirkman, E. & Ruxton, G. D. (2000a). Species-specific patterns of refuge use in fish: The role of metabolic expenditure and body length. *Behaviour*, **137**, 1113–1127.

Krause, J., Longworth, P. & Ruxton, G. D. (2000b). Refuge use in sticklebacks as a function of body length and group size. *Journal of Fish Biology*, **56**, 1023–1027.

Lewkiewicz, D. A. & Zuk, M. (2004). Latency to resume calling after disturbance in the field cricket, *Teleogryllus ocanicus*, corresponds to population-level differences in parasitism risk. *Behavioral Ecology and Sociobiology*, **55**, 569–573.

Lima, S. L. & Bednekoff, P. A. (1999). Temporal variation in danger drives antipredator behavior: The predation risk allocation hypothesis. *American Naturalist*, **153**, 649–659.

Lima, S. L. & Dill, L. M. (1990). Behavioral decisions made under the risk of predation: A review and prospectus. *Canadian Journal of Zoology*, **68**, 619–640.

López, P., Hawlena, D., Polo, V., Amo, L. & Martín, J. (2005). Sources of interindividual shy–bold variations in antipredatory behaviour of male Iberian rock-lizards. *Animal Behaviour*, **69**, 1–9.

Losos, J. B., Mouton, P. le F. N., Bickel, R., Cornelius, I. & Ruddock, L. (2002). The effect of body armature on escape behaviour in cordylid lizards. *Animal Behaviour*, **64**, 313–321.

Martín, J. & López, P. (1999a). When to come out from a refuge: risk-sensitive and state-dependent decisions in an alpine lizard. *Behavioral Ecology*, **10**, 487–492.

Martín, J. & López, P. (1999b). An experimental test of the costs of antipredatory refuge use in the wall lizard, *Podarcis muralis*. *Oikos*, **84**, 499–505.

Martín, J. & López, P. (2001). Repeated predatory attacks and multiple decisions to come out from a refuge in an alpine lizard. *Behavioral Ecology*, **12**, 386–389.

Martín, J. & López, P. (2003a). Changes in the escape responses of the lizard *Acanthodactylus erythrurus* under persistent predatory attacks. *Copeia*, **2003**, 408–413.

Martín, J. & López, P. (2003b). Ontogenetic variation in antipredatory behavior of Iberian-rock lizards (*Lacerta monticola*): Effects of body-size-dependent thermal-exchange rates and costs of refuge use. *Canadian Journal of Zoology*, **81**, 1131–1137.

Martín, J. & López, P. (2004a). Iberian rock lizards (*Lacerta monticola*) assess short-term changes in predation risk level when deciding refuge use. *Journal of Comparative Psychology*, **118**, 280–286.

Martín, J. & López, P. (2004b). Balancing predation risk, social interference and foraging opportunities in backswimmers, *Notonecta maculata*. *Acta Ethologica*, **6**, 59–63.

Martín, J. & López, P. (2005). Wall lizards modulate refuge use through continuous assessment of predation risk level. *Ethology*, **111**, 207–219.

Martín, J. & López, P. (2010). Thermal constraints of refuge use by Schreiber's green lizards, *Lacerta schreiberi*. *Behaviour*, **147**, 275–284.

Martín, J., López, P. & Cooper, W. E., Jr. (2003a). When to come out from a refuge: Balancing predation risk and foraging opportunities in an alpine lizard. *Ethology*, **109**, 77–87.

Martín, J., López, P. & Cooper, W. E., Jr. (2003b). Loss of mating opportunities influences refuge use in the Iberian rock lizard, *Lacerta monticola*. *Behavioral Ecology and Sociobiology*, **54**, 505–510.

Martín, J., Marcos, I. & López, P. (2005). When to come out from your own shell: Risk sensitive hiding decisions in terrapins. *Behavioral Ecology and Sociobiology*, **57**, 405–411.

Martín, J., López, P. & Polo, V. (2009). Temporal patterns of predation risk affect antipredatory behaviour allocation by Iberian rock-lizards. *Animal Behaviour*, **77**, 1261–1266.

McIntosh, A. R. & Peckarsky, B. L. (1999). Criteria determining behavioural responses to multiple predators by a stream mayfly. *Oikos*, **85**, 554–564.

McLean, E. B. & Godin, J. G. J. (1989). Distance to cover and fleeing from predators in fish with different amounts of defensive armour. *Oikos*, **55**, 281–290.

Metcalfe, N. B. & Steele, G. I. (2001). Changing nutritional status causes a shift in the balance of nocturnal to diurnal activity in European minnows. *Functional Ecology*, **15**, 304–309.

Mima, A., Wada, S. & Goshima, S. (2003). Antipredador defence of the hermit crab *Pagurus filholi* introduced by predator crabs. *Oikos*, **102**, 104–110.

Polo, V., López, P. & Martín, J. (2005). Balancing the thermal costs and benefits of refuge use to cope with persistent attacks from predators: A model and an experiment with an alpine lizard. *Evolutionary Ecology Research*, **7**, 23–35.

Polo, V., López, P. & Martín, J. (2011). Uncertainty about future predation risk modulates monitoring behaviour from refuges in lizards. *Behavioral Ecology*, **22**, 218–223.

Polo-Cavia, N., López, P. & Martín, J. (2008). Interspecific differences in responses to predation risk may confer competitive advantages to invasive freshwater turtle species. *Ethology*, **114**, 115–123.

Reaney, L. T. (2007). Foraging and mating opportunities influence refuge use in the fiddler crab, *Uca mjoebergi*. *Animal Behaviour*, **73**, 711–716.

Rhoades, E. & Blumstein, D. T. (2007). Predicted fitness consequences of threat-sensitive hiding behavior. *Behavioral Ecology*, **18**, 937–943.

Rodríguez-Prieto, I., Fernández-Juricic, E. & Martín, J. (2006). Anti-predator behavioral responses of mosquito pupae to aerial predation risk. *Journal of Insect Behavior*, **19**, 373–381.

Saloom, M. E. & Duncan, R. S. (2005). Low dissolved oxygen levels reduce antipredation behaviours of the freshwater clam *Corbicula fluminea*. *Freshwater Biology*, **50**, 1233–1238.

Scarratt, A. M. & Godin, J.-G. J. (1992). Foraging and antipredator decisions in the hermit crab *Pagurus acadianus* (Benedict). *Journal of Experimental Marine Biology and Ecology*, **156**, 225–238.

Sih, A. (1992). Prey uncertainty and the balancing of antipredator and feeding needs. *American Naturalist*, **139**, 1052–1069.

Sih, A. (1997). To hide or not to hide? Refuge use in a fluctuating environment. *Trends in Ecology and Evolution*, **12**, 375–376.

Sih, A., Krupa, J. & Travers, S. (1990). An experimental study on the effects of predation risk and feeding regime on the mating behavior of the water strider, Gerris remigis. *American Naturalist*, **135**, 84–290.

Sih, A., Kats, L. B. & Moore, R. D. (1992). Effects of predatory sunfish on the density, drift and refuge use of stream salamander larvae. *Ecology*, **73**, 1418–1430.

Sih, A., Englund, G. & Wooster, D. (1998). Emergent impacts of multiple predators on prey. *Trends in Ecology and Evolution*, **13**, 350–355.

Sih, A., Ziemba, R. & Harding, K. C. (2000). New insights on how temporal variation in predation risk shapes prey behavior. *Trends in Ecology and Evolution*, **15**, 3–4.

Smith, M. E. & Belk, M. C. (2001). Risk assessment in western mosquito fish (*Gambusia affinis*): Do multiple cues have additive effects. *Behavioral Ecology and Sociobiology*, **51**, 101–107.

Soluk, D. A. (1993). Multiple predator effects: Predicting combined functional response of stream fish and invertebrate predators. *Ecology*, **74**, 219–225.

Stankowich, T. & Blumstein, D. T (2005). Fear in animals: A review and metaanalysis of risk assessment. *Proceedings of the Royal Society of London. Series B: Biological Sciences*, **272**, 2627–2634.

Stapley, J. (2004). Do log skinks (*Pseudemoia entrecasteauxii*) modify their behaviour in the presence of two predators? *Behavioral Ecology and Sociobiology*, **56**, 185–189.

Stapley, J. & Keogh, J. S. (2004). Exploratory and antipredator behaviours differ between territorial and nonterritorial male lizards. *Animal Behaviour*, **68**, 841–846.

Werner, E. E., Gilliam, J. F., Hall, D. J. & Mittelbach, G. G. (1983). An experimental test of the effects of predation risk on habitat use. *Ecology*, **64**, 1540–1548.

Wilson, C. D., Arnott, G. & Elwood, R. W. (2012). Freshwater pearl mussels show plasticity of responses to different predation risks but also show consistent individual differences in responsiveness. *Behavioural Processes*, **89**, 299–303.

Wolf, N. G. & Kramer, D. L. (1987). Use of cover and the need to breathe: The effects of hypoxia on vulnerability of dwarf gouramis to predatory snakeheads. *Oecologia*, **73**:127–132.

Part III

Related behaviors and other factors influencing escape

10 Vigilance, alarm calling, pursuit deterrence, and predation inspection

Guy Beauchamp

10.1 Introduction

Prey species that detect predators late in the predation sequence have little option but to flee as soon as possible. However, prey species may exercise some control over the timing of predator detection, which can free up time to evaluate the threat that the predator poses and even alter the outcome of the encounter with the predator (Caro 2005). The purpose of this chapter is to examine factors that influence predator detection and the options available to a prey animal between the detection of a predator and escape.

The ability to detect predators early in the predation sequence depends on the amount of time allocated to antipredator vigilance. Maintaining a vigilant state allows prey animals to detect predators earlier but at a cost. Indeed, vigilance often conflicts with other fitness-enhancing activities, such as foraging and sleeping, and, generally, prey species must make a trade-off between their various time demands (Caraco 1979). Any factor that influences how much time individuals can allocate to antipredator vigilance will have an impact on the distance at which a predator can be detected on average. I shall review some of the major factors that affect vigilance, such as group size, and highlight some recent developments in vigilance research with a direct bearing on escape behavior. In particular, vigilance may be expected to fluctuate through time within the same group, implying that the ability to detect predators may also vary on a short time scale.

Prey species can manipulate the outcome of an encounter with a predator after detection. Many prey species produce alarm calls upon detection of a predator (Bradbury & Vehrencamp 2011). Such signals may be aimed at the predator to indicate detection, but they often transfer information to nearby conspecifics. Recent work has shown that alarm calls can convey information about predator size and distance and even behavior, which may be crucial to receivers in determining the best course of action as the predator approaches (Zuberbühler 2009). Upon hearing an alarm call, individuals may flee immediately or assess the situation before initiating flight. The second part of this chapter focuses on the properties of alarm calls and their effects on conspecifics.

Escaping From Predators: An Integrative View of Escape Decisions, ed. W. E. Cooper and D. T. Blumstein.
Published by Cambridge University Press. © Cambridge University Press 2015.

Signals produced after predator detection can also convey information to the predator (Shelley & Blumstein 2005). Prey animals that are likely to escape following detection may signal to the predator that it has been detected. In addition, they can signal their quality to the predator. Predators may use information from these signals to abandon chases that would most likely be futile. The third part of this chapter examines the effects of signals produced by prey on their predators.

Many prey species approach detected predators rather than flee (Pitcher *et al.* 1986; FitzGibbon 1994). This counterintuitive tactic, which brings the prey closer to a potentially harmful predator, illustrates the notion that prey are willing to take risk to gather information about the motivation of a predator. Predator inspection behavior is common in fish and some mammals, and I close this chapter by evaluating the costs and benefits of this behavior.

10.2   Antipredator vigilance

If prey animals were in predator detection mode at all times, the distance at which a predator would be detected would simply reflect the ability of the prey to extract threat signals from other non-predator related environmental stimuli, or noise. Basic predator detectability would vary among individuals, and from species to species, reflecting sensory processing ability. In birds, for instance, greater visual acuity associated with larger eyes allows earlier detection (Fernández-Juricic *et al.* 2004). Sensory processing ability would interact with the degree of noise that characterizes the habitat to determine when an approaching predator first becomes detectable to the prey. For example, visual detection may be less effective in cluttered habitats (Devereux *et al.* 2006) and aural detection may deteriorate in noisier settings (Quinn *et al.* 2006).

This ideal scenario is unlikely to apply under most circumstances for at least two reasons. First, rival sources of attention are almost always present in the lives of prey animals. Their attention may be diverted to monitor the activity of neighbors (Favreau *et al.* 2010) or to fulfill other fitness-enhancing needs such as grooming, sleeping or foraging (Caraco 1979). In fact, the ability to detect predators may be severely compromised when performing these activities. For instance, the senses of a sleeping prey animal are at best intermittently available, which may allow predators to approach undetected more easily (Lima *et al.* 2005). Animals also need to forage, and again the effectiveness of predator detection may be limited when resource exploitation interferes with detection (Lima & Bednekoff 1999; Kaby & Lind 2003). Second, the ability to detect stimuli may, paradoxically, decrease when vigilance for predation threats is maintained for too long a period of time due to habituation or fatigue (Dimond & Lazarus 1974). This physiological response may entice prey animals to reduce to some extent the total amount of time allocated to predator detection so as to maintain a high level of detectability. This discussion emphasizes that the time available to detect predators is most likely limited.

Overall, the distance at which a predator can be first detected will reflect the interplay between sensory processing ability, the amount of environmental noise, and the time that can be devoted to predator detection. All else being equal, animals that invest less time in predator detection may be expected to detect predators later on average. Any factor that influences the time devoted to predator detection, which is typically referred to as vigilance, is thus likely to impact the ability to detect predators early. In the following, I explore some attributes of vigilance and the role of several ecological and physiological variables known to influence its expression in the context of escape behavior.

10.2.1   What is vigilance?

Vigilance is a state of alertness that allows the detection of relevant stimuli. It is practically measured using external expressions of alertness, such as when an animal raises its head to scan the surroundings. Indeed, a posture with the head up was used to define vigilance in the very first model of vigilance (Pulliam 1973). The focus on head position assumes that vigilance is mostly performed visually, but acoustic vigilance may be a common feature in animals and need not be performed head up (Ridgway *et al.* 2006). In this case, it may be difficult to assess when an animal is vigilant.

Two types of vigilance are generally distinguished: routine or induced vigilance (Blanchard & Fritz 2007). Routine vigilance occurs during spare time while induced vigilance is viewed as a direct reaction to an imminent predation threat. It is the investment in routine vigilance that matters in the context of predator detection. Induced vigilance would occur after a threat is detected and allow animals to weigh their options before escaping.

10.2.2   Can detection of predators occur when non-vigilant?

Vigilance was initially viewed as being entirely incompatible with other activities such as foraging. This simple dichotomy made it very easy to determine the amount of time spent vigilant by an individual. The incompatibility assumption probably reflects the fact that early models of vigilance focused on species of birds feeding with the head down, a posture thought to impair their ability to detect threats. However, recent research with birds, and other species as well, implies that some level of vigilance may be maintained during other activities. Some species of animals can be alert for predators even when asleep (Rattenborg *et al.* 1999). When foraging, animals with laterally facing eyes can monitor areas directly above them to some extent (Lima & Bednekoff 1999; Fernández-Juricic *et al.* 2008; Wallace *et al.* 2013). Many species can also monitor their surroundings while searching or handling food in a head-up posture (Kaby & Lind 2003; Fortin *et al.* 2004).

The fact that some level of vigilance may be maintained by non-overtly vigilant animals suggests that predator detection is possible regardless of head position. However, it appears that the ability to detect predators is weaker when the head is down. In an influential series of experiments, Lima and Bednekoff aimed to determine the extent to which non-overtly vigilant animals can detect a predator. When head up, dark-eyed juncos (*Junco hyemalis*) can detect a fast approaching mounted hawk very

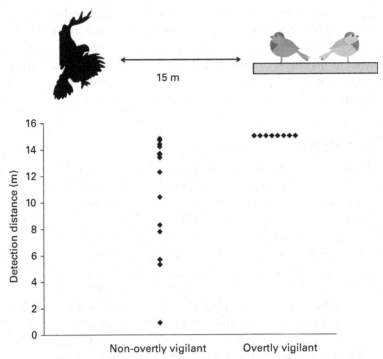

Figure 10.1 Dark-eyed juncos detect a mounted hawk more quickly when overtly vigilant with their head up rather than with their head down. The attack started 15 m away from a feeding platform upon which targeted birds fed. (After Lima & Bednekoff 1999)

rapidly. By contrast, birds with their head down detected the hawk less rapidly, suggesting a less than optimal detection response (Lima & Bednekoff 1999; Figure 10.1). In a further experiment with the same species, individuals increased the duration of their scans to compensate for the addition of visual barriers that prevented head-down vigilance (Bednekoff & Lima 2005), implying that these birds value the information they can acquire when non-overtly vigilant. At least in this species, detection of predators is possible when non-overtly vigilant, but appears less than optimal. Whether this is the case in other species remains to be established. Generally, it may not be obvious to determine when a predator has been detected.

10.2.3   The effect of group size on vigilance

As long as the probability of predator detection is higher during overt vigilance, any factor that reduces time spent vigilant will reduce the ability to detect threats. Vigilance can be influenced by many variables, but the effect of group size has attracted the most attention in the literature (Beauchamp 2008). Models of vigilance predict that individual investment in vigilance should decrease as group size increases for two main reasons (McNamara & Houston 1992). First, as group size increases, more eyes and ears become available to monitor the surroundings so that threats are less likely to go undetected.

Once a threat is detected, the fright responses of detectors can warn the non-detectors rapidly, allowing all group members to flee rapidly. Second, the presence of several potential targets in a group effectively dilutes predation risk for each prey as long as the rate of encounter with predators does not increase with group size and predators capture at most one individual per attack. In view of the decreased risk of capture in a group, individuals can reduce their investment in vigilance. As long as the vigilance at the group level is high enough, individuals in larger groups should enjoy greater safety than when foraging alone or in small groups.

Predator detection should thus typically occur sooner in larger groups, which benefit from the presence of many potential detectors. In a classic experiment, Kenward used a trained goshawk (*Accipiter gentilis*) to attack wood pigeons (*Columba palumbus*) in groups of varying sizes from a standard distance. As the number of pigeons increased in the group, individuals detected the predator at a greater distance, as predicted from the pooling of individual detection effort (Kenward 1978). While this study only relied on one trained predator, results along these lines have been obtained in other species (Caro 2005).

Detection of threats will not necessarily always occur earlier in larger groups. What matters for detection is the level of vigilance maintained at the group level, which is known as collective vigilance. Detection will occur sooner in larger groups as long as collective vigilance increases with group size. However, as I explained earlier, individuals are expected to be less vigilant in larger groups, implying that collective vigilance is unlikely to increase linearly with group size. Moreover, the time freed by a reduction in vigilance becomes available to increase fitness through other activities, such as foraging. Under some circumstances, the fitness gains that accrue from an increase in foraging may allow individuals to sacrifice safety, leading to a lower level of collective vigilance in large groups. Sacrifices in safety may make sense in various situations, including when foragers have low energy reserves or exploit resources in rich food patches (McNamara & Houston 1992). In such cases, detection ability could, theoretically, be lower in larger groups. Further research should allow us to determine whether the advantages in having more eyes and ears in a larger group always translate into faster detection.

10.2.4   Temporal changes in vigilance

Two recent developments in vigilance research are especially relevant to escape behavior. Collective vigilance is a key factor in determining the ability to detect predators early. These recent developments suggest that collective vigilance may in fact fluctuate through time, which implies that the ability to detect predators may not be constant within the same group. Such fluctuations have been related to two factors: vigilance copying and predation risk assessment.

Temporal fluctuation in collective vigilance is predicted to occur when individuals copy the vigilance of one another (Beauchamp *et al.* 2012; Sirot & Touzalin 2009). To put matters into perspective, models of vigilance typically assume that vigilance should be independent among group members. Sirot and Touzalin (2009) suggested that

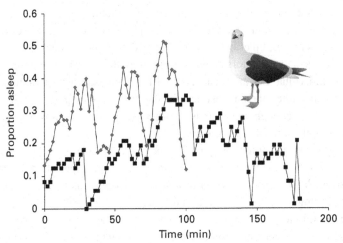

Figure 10.2   Collective temporal waves of sleeping, a low vigilant state, in two roosting flocks of gulls (*Larus* spp.). Time series analysis revealed a statistically significant periodicity of 46 min in one flock of 72 gulls (dark squares) and of 34 min in a flock of 150 gulls (gray squares). (After Beauchamp 2011)

individuals in a group should, instead, copy the vigilance of their neighbors under some circumstances detailed below. When copying occurs, collective vigilance will be less than predicted under independent vigilance because there will be more bouts than expected with few or no group members vigilant at the same time.

Why would individuals copy the vigilance of their neighbors if it compromises the detection of predators? As I pointed out earlier, direct detection of threats allows a quicker escape. If predators preferentially target those that escape more slowly, an individual should be more vigilant when its neighbors are vigilant to avoid being left behind when the group is attacked. Copying vigilance is expected to produce rises and falls in the proportion of vigilant group members through time, temporal waves as it were. Copying vigilance has been documented recently in many species of birds and mammals (Beauchamp 2009b; Ge *et al.* 2011; Michelena & Deneubourg 2011; Öst & Tierala 2011; Pays *et al.* 2012), where it has been possible to eliminate the possibility that outside stimuli triggered synchronized vigilance. One study also provided evidence for temporal waves of vigilance in sleeping gulls (Beauchamp 2011; Figure 10.2). The implication for escape behavior research is that the ability to detect predators may fluctuate on a short time scale within the same group.

Copying vigilance should produce rises and falls in collective vigilance but about the same mean. Recent models suggest that collective vigilance may also be expected to decrease systematically with time since a group started to forage. A decrease in individual vigilance with time may reflect the outcome of an arms race between predators and prey (Beauchamp & Ruxton 2012). Prey species often have little information about current predation risk in the food patches they visit. In particular, a group that arrives at a new patch must determine whether a predator lurks nearby – like a lion (*Panthera leo*) hiding in the bushes (Périquet *et al.* 2010). The predator must decide when to break cover, and the prey animals must choose the level of vigilance to adopt as a function of time. If the hiding predator always broke cover at the same time, individuals in the group will be selected to be extra-vigilant until that very time. Predators should thus keep the group guessing about attack time. However, waiting too long may not be desirable as group members may be more likely to detect the predator. Group members should also keep the predator guessing about when vigilance will decrease to avoid the situation in which the predator simply waits for vigilance to come down before launching an attack. The predicted solution to this war of attrition between predator and prey takes the following form: predators attack at unpredictable times but typically early and group members adopt a high vigilance early and then switch unpredictably later to lower vigilance (Beauchamp & Ruxton 2012).

Prey animals in groups do not always face observant predators, but still need to assess predation risk. As time goes by without an attack, individuals may feel safer and progressively and adaptively lower their vigilance (Sirot & Pays 2011). The implication of these directional changes in vigilance is that the ability to detect predators may decrease as foraging progresses in the same group. Lack of control over time since a feeding bout started will thus generally increase the amount of noise in detection distance. In addition, predator detection distance is expected to decrease gradually during a feeding bout. Empirical studies with simulated attacks would be useful to establish whether detection ability and escape behavior change at times where the group is expected to be less vigilant, say, during a trough in collective vigilance or later in a feeding bout.

10.2.5   Other factors that affect vigilance

Many factors other than group size are known to influence the allocation of time to vigilance. All these factors will have an impact on the ability to detect threats by reducing the time devoted to predator detection. Lack of control over these factors can introduce additional variation among samples of detection distance.

Habitat characteristics that influence the ability of escape, time of day, and food availability are three examples of environmental factors that influence vigilance. The ability to escape may vary in certain habitats, due to the presence of obstacles or because protective cover is further away (Lima 1992), for instance, which should influence the level of vigilance that prey animals adopt. Detection ability may thus increase in habitats where the probability of escaping is slighter. Time of day can influence vigilance through many means. Predation risk may vary throughout the day as some predators are more active at particular times of the day or more difficult to detect due to poor light condition (Lima 1988). When predation risk is perceived to be higher, prey animals are expected to increase vigilance, which may allow them to detect predators sooner. Vigilance may also vary on a daily basis in response to changing energy requirements (Pravosudov & Grubb 1998). For instance, vigilance may increase from early morning to the afternoon as animals become more satiated.

Samples of detection distances may often be taken from areas that differ markedly in resource availability and quality. Food patch characteristics can also influence vigilance levels, and thus indirectly detection distances (Beauchamp 2009a). Models indicate that when animals face time constraints or, in other words, when there is a tangible risk of starvation, the level of vigilance should decrease as the rate of food intake increases (McNamara & Houston 1992). As patches of higher quality typically allow foragers to obtain food more rapidly, vigilance is thus expected to decrease with food density. In conclusion, several environmental factors are known to influence vigilance and must be properly controlled, either statistically or experimentally, to reduce the amount of noise in detection distance.

10.3   Alarm calling

Vigilance is an investment in time prior to predator detection. It increases the chances of detecting the predator before it is too late. The following sections focus on what happens after predator detection but prior to the actual escape. After detection, prey animals often emit alarm calls or produce other signals. Here, I am concerned with signals aimed at conspecifics. In the following section, I shall deal with signals aimed at the predator.

In view of the limited amount of time allocated to vigilance by each group member, few prey animals are expected to detect an approaching predator at the same time. Nevertheless, the detection of a threat by a few spreads rapidly throughout the group. Detectors provide indirect cues of detection to non-detectors through their behavior (Lima 1995). For instance, eastern gray kangaroos (*Macropus giganteus*) that have detected a snake stare intently at the predator and this cue soon alerts the others in the group (Pays *et al.* 2013). A more active system to alert neighbors is the use of alarm calls, which can reach other group members rapidly even when they are not in direct visual contact. In the context of escape behavior, the occurrence of alarm calls can change the costs and benefits of the options available to group members prior to fleeing, and thus affect the course of action selected.

10.3.1   Alarm calls can convey information about the type of threat

Alarm calls can provide crucial information about the type of threat the group faces and eventually which reaction is the most appropriate. In a classic paper, Seyfarth *et al.* (1980) showed that different types of predators elicited different alarm calls in free-living vervet monkeys (*Chlorocebus pygerythrus*). With the use of playbacks, the authors subsequently demonstrated that vervet monkeys adapted their escape tactics to the type of alarm calls broadcasted: climbing in a tree when they heard the playback of an alarm call associated with a leopard (*Panthera pardus*), looking down when they heard the alarm call elicited by a snake, and running to cover and looking up when they heard the alarm call produced after spotting an eagle (Seyfarth *et al.* 1980; Figure 10.3). In other species, acoustic features of alarm calls have been shown to convey information about predator size (Templeton *et al.* 2005), distance to the predator (Wilson & Evans 2012), urgency to respond (Manser *et al.*

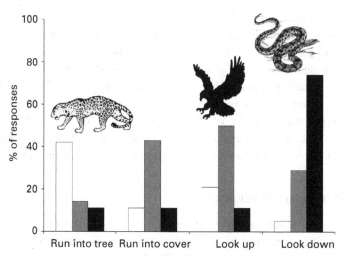

Figure 10.3   Vervet monkeys respond differently to playbacks of alarm calls elicited by a leopard, an eagle, or a snake. The percentage of trials where at least one individual showed a given response for longer after than before the playback is shown for each type of predator ($n = 19$ for the leopard (white bars), 14 for the eagle (gray bars), and 19 for the snake (black bars)). (After Seyfarth *et al.* 1980)

2002), and even predator behavior (Griesser 2008), all of which could allow signal receivers to better choose their escape tactics.

This degree of sophistication in alarm calling probably matches the variety of escape tactics available to a species. A single kind of alarm call may be sufficient to all types of predators when there is only one way to escape (Blumstein & Armitage 1997), but different alarm calls matched to a predator or a specific situation may be beneficial when prey animals can respond to a threat in many different ways, as the vervet example clearly illustrates.

10.3.2   False alarm calls

Alarm calls are notoriously unreliable. Indeed, a high percentage of all alarm calls in many species are actually false alarms attributable to non-threatening stimuli (Cresswell *et al.* 2000; Blumstein *et al.* 2004). Upon hearing an alarm call, it would make sense for non-detectors to evaluate the potential threat by themselves rather than flee immediately.

One way to reduce superfluous escapes is to adjust the strength of responses to the number of alarm callers. When many individuals sound the alarm at the same time, it is probably more likely that the threat is real. Supporting this hypothesis, yellow-bellied marmots (*Marmota flaviventris*) were found to be more vigilant after hearing two alarm callers at the same time rather than one (Blumstein *et al.* 2004). In birds, flushes to safety by several individuals at the same time are also more effective in triggering responses by nearby companions than single flushes (Lima 1995; Cresswell *et al.* 2000).

In many species, alarm calls have been reported to be individually distinctive, which raises the possibility that signal receivers may respond differently according to the reliably of alarm callers. Indeed, some individuals may have a higher ratio of false to real alarms due to their lack of experience or a lower threshold for responding to potentially threatening stimuli. This idea was tested by associating the individually distinct calls of some yellow-bellied marmots to a real threat and others to harmless stimuli, varying the reliability of alarm callers (Blumstein *et al.* 2004). Marmots discriminated among reliable and less reliable callers and spent more time investigating the source of disturbance following broadcasts of calls from the unreliable callers.

10.3.3   Alarm calls and antipredator ploys

Alarm calls may signal an imminent threat to which immediate action is required. However, the threat may not always be urgent, and in this case alarm calling may be useful to deploy antipredator tactics that will reduce the chances of a successful attack. Alarm calls in many species cause signal receivers to adopt cryptic behavior such as crouching, whose purpose appears to be to reduce the likelihood of detection by the predator (Evans *et al.* 1993). Long-distance alarm calls in one species of monkey, indicative of a distant threat, causes individuals to bunch together, increasing the effectiveness of factors such as collective detection and risk dilution (Shultz *et al.* 2003). Alarm calls often trigger an increase in vigilance in signal receivers thus increasing the number of individuals actually monitoring the threat (Loughry & McDonough 1988). Increased vigilance may be useful to better assess a threat (perhaps reducing the rate of false alarms) or to ready all group members for mass flight (see below).

10.3.4   Alarm calls and mass flight

By warning other group members rapidly, alarm calls may play yet another function prior to escape. Rather than fleeing alone, an alarm caller can effectively recruit all group members for mass flight (Owens & Goss-Custard 1976; Sherman 1985), potentially reducing the chances of capture through the confusion or selfish-herd effects.

Confusion acts when the predator closes in on a group of prey and attempts to capture a particular individual from a fleeing group. Reduced capture rate after initiating a chase is thought to reflect distraction of attention from the targeted prey by the presence of several non-target companions (Neill & Cullen 1974; Landeau & Terborgh 1986). Recent research suggests that confusion is a line of defense that works by exploiting the cognitive limitations of the predator (Tosh *et al.* 2006). The empirical evidence that confusion plays a role during escape behavior following an alarm call is rather anecdotal (Leger *et al.* 1980; Sherman 1985). To be more convincing, we would need data on the effect of prey density on predator success rate with the prediction that capture rate should decrease when prey are closer to one another.

The alarm caller could also benefit by seeking protection inside the group, effectively using other group members as a shield (Hamilton 1971). To invoke the selfish-herd effect, we need direct evidence that alarm callers select particular trajectories in space that would reduce their domain of danger when fleeing. It is interesting to note that if an alarm caller chooses to flee, the range of options for signal receivers becomes very limited. As Sherman (1985) pointed out, a signal receiver that fails to flee cannot benefit from the confusion or selfish-herd effects and may also provide a more inviting target to the predator.

10.4   Pursuit-deterrence signals

I explore signals made by prey animals upon detection of a predator focusing this time on their potential effects on predators. As with alarm calling, these signals can change the value of the choices available to prey after detection. If the predator, say, abandons the chase after receiving the signal, the prey animals may choose to maintain vigilance rather than flee.

The logic of signaling to an approaching predator is simple: when an individual is quite likely to avoid capture, it makes sense for the individual to produce a signal to dissuade the predator from attacking. Capture may be unlikely if, for example, the predator has been detected early and lost the element of surprise or if the prey animal possesses attributes, such as speed, that make capture more challenging. With such a signal, prey can avoid the energy and time costs of an actual escape while the predator avoids the costs of a most likely futile pursuit (Ruxton *et al.* 2004). Such signals have been referred to as pursuit-deterrent signals. Pursuit-deterrence signals come in two types: signals that advertise detection to the predator and those that signal the condition of the signaler to the predator.

10.4.1   Perception advertisement

This type of signal may be produced in two contexts. The most obvious one is when the predator is detected outside the typical range of attack distances. Beyond this range, the risk of capture is low and producing the signal does not reduce the ability to escape should the predator choose to attack. Other means of dissuading the predator from attacking after detection include mobbing by the prey (Tan *et al.* 2012) or hiding in a refuge, both of which significantly reduce the chances of capture. Examples of detection signals involve visual signals such as tail flagging in deer (Caro *et al.* 1995) and ground squirrels (Barbour & Clark 2012), tail wagging in lizards (Cooper 2010), or auditory signals such as long-distance calling in primates (Zuberbühler *et al.* 1997).

Perception advertisement signals may also be produced when the prey animals strongly suspect that a predator is present (Bergstrom & Lachmann 2001). This mechanism involves parsing information from the environment and producing the signal when a threshold of perceived risk has been crossed. These perception advertisement signals may thus be made in the absence of a predator.

The costs of a perception advertisement signal for the prey involve the production of the signal and the risk of inadvertently attracting the attention of other predators.

Producing the signal itself is probably inexpensive, certainly in comparison to avoiding the costs of a chase altogether. Signaling, especially by mistake, can be costly if it attracts the attention of undetected predators. This potential cost may not apply when predator density is low and when the risk of mistaking harmless stimuli as real is also low. From the predator point of view, the benefits include the probability of capture during a chase and the costs include the time and energy involved in the chase. Mathematical modeling reveals that a perception advertisement signal can be evolutionarily stable if the benefits of producing the signals exceed the costs for the signaler and if the costs of chasing are high and the probability of capture is low for the predator (Bergstrom & Lachmann 2001).

While it is clear that both predator and prey can benefit from perception advertisement signals, it is less clear what prevents prey from cheating. Indeed, prey animals could produce signals of detection more frequently than needed in the odd chance that a predator has approached undetected. However, this is not a stable solution in view of the time costs involved in the production of needless signals and the chances that the signal may attract the attention of other predators, thus increasing predation risk inadvertently. Nevertheless, pre-emptive perception signals may work if signals have a short range, which makes them unlikely to attract other predators, and if the signal is typically associated with honest detection (Murphy 2007).

10.4.2   Quality advertisement

If the odds of capture after detecting the predator are high, it would seem at first ill-advised for the prey to take the time to produce a pursuit-deterrent signal when it could flee instead and gain more ground on the predator. Individuals that have the ability to escape at closer distances may still benefit from producing such signals, effectively advertising their quality to the predator. To evolve, such signals must be costly otherwise all individuals, those able to escape or not, will produce the signal making it useless (Grafen 1990). Honest signals may include those that are condition dependent. For example, the length or frequency or intensity of a signal may be indicative of the condition of the signaler, which would allow the predator to judge the quality of the prey. Mathematical modeling reveals that such signals can evolve as long as there is a close relationship between features of the signal and condition of the prey, and that the risk of capture for signaling prey decreases as the condition of the signaler increases (Vega-Redondo & Hasson 1993). These signals are considered quality advertisement signals, and tend to be more costly than the perception advertisement signals discussed above (Caro 2005).

What prevents cheating in this signaling system is the relationship between specific features of the signal and individual quality. A low-quality individual is simply unable to produce signals that would deceive the predator (Zahavi & Zahavi 1997). Intriguingly, cheating may be preventable even if the relationship between signal features and individual quality is rather weak. Consider a situation in which low- and high-quality individuals produce the same signal. If a low-quality individual finds itself in a group with $n - 1$ high-quality companions, the low-quality individual will still have a $1/n$ chance of being targeted by a predator that attacks any group member with the same probability. The risk of capture for the low-quality individual is higher now because the predator has been allowed much closer during the display. In addition, the poor quality of the prey animal will hamper its escape. Cheating of this type may only be possible in very large groups in which the risk of being targeted is much lower.

While predators should give up quite readily after a perception advertisement signal, there should be a close relationship between abandoning a hunt and some definable features of a quality advertisement signal. The difficulty is to distinguish between the two types of signals. It is not always obvious to determine the costs of a signal, and, moreover, the quality of the prey may not be easy to assess in the field. Stotting is a good case in point. When stotting, an animal jumps up in the air with all four legs held stiffly. The success rate of attacks by cheetahs (*Acynonyx jubatus*) on Thomson's gazelles (*Gazella thomsoni*) decreases from 21 to 0% when the quarry stots (Caro 1986). Stotting may signal to the predator that it has been detected, but may also signal the quality of the signaler. The crucial data on the relationship between stotting performance and condition of the prey species come from a study involving African wild dogs (*Lacyon pictus*), another predator of Thomson's gazelles (FitzGibbon & Fanshawe 1988). Indeed, African wild dogs were more likely to chase gazelles that stotted at a lower rate (Figure 10.4). After being targeted, gazelles that eventually escaped stotted longer during the chase than those that were captured (Figure 10.4). Supporting the hypothesis that stotting reveals the condition of the prey, stotting was more common during the wet season when body condition generally improves. In other species, stotting rate correlates positively with body condition (Caro 1994).

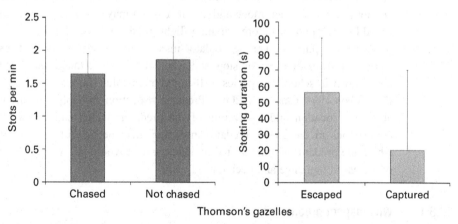

Figure 10.4   African wild dogs prefer to chase Thomson's gazelles that stotted at a lower rate on average (left panel). Error bars show one standard deviation. Gazelles that stotted longer during the chase were less likely to be captured (right panel). The median and the 75th percentile are illustrated. (After FitzGibbon & Fanshawe 1988)

10.4.3   Evolution of pursuit-deterrent signals

Signals produced by a solitary animal after the detection of a predator, such as an alarm call, can only be aimed at the predator. By contrast, signals produced by animals living in groups may be aimed at companions as well as the predator. To distinguish between the two potential targets of such signals, it is necessary to understand the context of signaling. If group-living animals produce such signals when they are alone, the predator is certainly a potential target (Murphy 2006) although this does not rule out that the signal may also be useful to warn companions.

As signals that evolved in one context may be co-opted by another, the current target of a signal may not reflect very well the selection pressures that led to its evolution in the first place. A good example of this comes from the evolution of white tails in rails, a clade of reclusive semi-aquatic birds (Stang & McRae 2009). Rails flick their tails when disturbed and this behavior is more common in species with white tails, which contrast sharply with their overall dark plumage. This display may be used to signal to the predator that it has been detected and/or to alert companions in social species. A phylogenetic reconstruction showed that rails living in open habitats are more likely to have white tails. In addition, the transition to open habitats tended to precede the evolution of white tails while gregariousness evolved later in some lineages. This ordering of events indicates that white tails probably evolved as an antipredator signal needed in the more risky open habitats, and any current use by conspecifics reflects a co-option of the signal for other purposes.

10.5   Predator inspection

After detecting a predator, several options are available to prey animals in groups. When an attack is imminent, the only option is to flee as soon as possible. However, predators are not always in attack mode and, in this case, it may pay foragers to assess the risk posed by the predator before initiating flight. Predator inspection behavior appears to play just this purpose. During predator inspection, a subset of individuals leave the group, approach the predator, stop, and eventually return to the group. This behavior is best known in schooling species of fish and mammalian herbivores (Magurran 1986; FitzGibbon 1994; Caro *et al.* 2004). Predator inspection probably provides information about the location and motivation of the predator, which can be passed along to companions in the group. Predator inspection may be helpful to identify situations where the predator is uninterested in attack, which would allow prey to save the cost of increased vigilance and fleeing needlessly.

10.5.1   Why inspect predators?

At first sight, predator inspection appears ill-advised. Why risk death by approaching a potentially dangerous predator rather than simply hide in the safety of the group? Early research showed that inspectors do assess the risk associated with approaching a

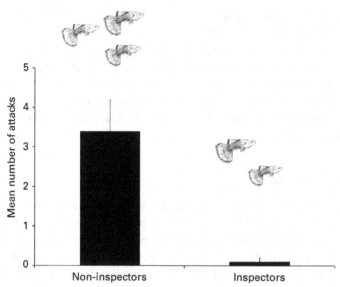

Figure 10.5   Guppies that inspect a fish predator are attacked less often than those that remain behind. Error bars show one standard deviation. (After Godin & Davis 1995)

predator. In one fish species, predator inspection was indeed more likely in less threatening situations (e.g., immobile predator) and when many individuals joined the inspection party (Pitcher *et al.* 1986). Fish also tend to avoid the cone of attack of a predator during inspection by biasing their approach toward the tail rather than the head (Brown & Dreier 2002). Similarly, Thomson's gazelles are more likely to approach a predator when in large groups and in a terrain that reduces the probability of ambush. Nevertheless, predator inspection is riskier than remaining behind in the group (FitzGibbon 1994; Milinski *et al.* 1997), suggesting that predator inspection must provide compensating benefits.

One possibility is that predator inspection can actually reduce predation risk for the inspectors. Indeed, guppies (*Poecilia reticulata*) that inspected a predator were less likely to be attacked and killed than those that remained behind (Godin & Davis 1995; Figure 10.5). Similar findings have been reported in European minnows (*Phoxinus phoxinus*; Magurran 1990) and Thomson's gazelles (FitzGibbon 1994).

Predator inspection can reduce predation risk through many means. The approach of several inspectors may confuse the predator, which may then prefer to attack those that remain behind (Curio 1978). Inspection may signal to the predator that it has been detected and that an attack on them rather than on those left behind is most likely futile.

Supporting the idea that inspection reduces the probability of attack, cheetahs tended to move to a different area after having been approached by inspecting Thomson's gazelles. Finally, inspection may also be a signal of quality to discourage the predator from attacking those that comes closest. Support for the quality advertisement hypothesis comes from the observation that larger three-spined sticklebacks

(*Gasterosteus aculeatus*) and those in better condition are more likely to approach predators (Külling & Milinski 1992).

Predator inspection is often performed in groups and appears relatively contagious. In Thomson's gazelles, for example, all members of a group typically approach the predator and other groups nearby are also likely to join (FitzGibbon 1994). Approaching in groups certainly reduces the probability of attack for any individual group member through a simple dilution of risk. Risk dilution reduces the costs of predator inspection.

10.5.2   Preferences for partners

In the preceding section, I showed that individuals can discriminate among alarm callers on the basis of their reliability. Research on predator inspection behavior has also examined whether the choices of partners during approaches to a predator are similarly biased. As predator inspection involves risks, an individual that remains slightly behind during predator inspection would gain all the benefits from the inspection without incurring the risks. To avoid such cheating, it was proposed that individuals should seek partners that have proven reliable during previous predator inspection bouts, a tit-for-tat like behavior (Milinski 1987). Evidence from the laboratory and the field suggests that fish can form strong ties with one another while foraging and during predator inspection, which suggests that reciprocity may be involved in choosing partners for inspection (Croft *et al.* 2006). However, crucial evidence that individuals are less likely to carry out predator inspection with partners that have defected in the past is generally lacking (Thomas *et al.* 2008). These issues suggest at the very least that group composition may influence the occurrence of predator inspection.

10.6   Future directions

The amount of time between predator detection and escape is under the control of the prey animals to some extent and can be increased by allocating more time to antipredator vigilance. This period allows individuals to assess the threat posed by a predator and to communicate through signals with nearby conspecifics and the predator. The risks of being attacked and of escaping can be manipulated by using signals after predator detection. In the following, I highlight some specific challenges for future work on the topics covered in this chapter.

Antipredator vigilance represents an option to increase the distance at which predators are detected on average. It is not an easy task to determine detection distance since vigilance serves many purposes and varies as a function of several environmental variables. A greater understanding of the factors that influence collective vigilance will be needed to make more precise predictions. Recent work also suggests that different individuals may vary consistently in their vigilance (Carter *et al.* 2009; Mathot *et al.* 2011). This finding fits with the observation that animals can vary in the level of risk they are prepared to accept (Reale *et al.* 2007). This raises the fascinating possibility that detection at the group level may vary as a function of the phenotypic composition of the group, and that different individuals may be able to detect predators more quickly than others. Future work along these lines will probably challenge the assumption that all individuals adopt the same vigilance in a group.

The type of information conveyed by alarm calls has been studied intensely, but we still know little about the costs and benefits of uttering alarm calls. It is usually thought that such signals reduce the personal safety of the callers, but the evidence is limited at the moment (Caro 2005). Many of the mechanisms that may allow prey animals to escape following an alarm, such as the confusion and selfish-herd effects, remain to be demonstrated convincingly. Complicating matters, alarm calls may not only warn conspecifics but also act concomitantly as a signal to the predator, making it difficult to disentangle the respective selection pressures. The information from alarm calls can also be used by nearby individuals from different species to mount effective antipredator responses (Goodale *et al.* 2010), effectively increasing the audience network for such calls. It will be interesting to determine in the future what information members of different species can extract from alarm calls developed for members of one species, and whether such calls can influence the detection ability and escape behavior of other species.

By contrast to other means of dissuading predators from attacking, such as crypsis or aposematic signals, pursuit-deterrent signals are displayed on a facultative basis, which highlights the costs of using such signals at all times and also makes it possible to show graded signals that are condition dependent. It would be interesting to investigate why a facultative tactic serves the purposes of predator deterrence to a greater extent in some species.

Predator inspection behavior can also be viewed as a pursuit-deterrent signal. If it serves as a detection signal, it is not clear why detection cannot be signaled from the confine of the group at a safe distance from the predator. Coming closer to the predator is risky, but in fish at least inspection behavior deflects the costs to those behind. This situation would make sense if inspection behavior is a quality advertisement signal. However, the costs and benefits of predator inspection behavior are known to some extent in a relatively small number of species and general conclusions are difficult to draw.

References

Barbour, M. A. & Clark, R. W. (2012). Ground squirrel tail-flag displays alter both predatory strike and ambush site selection behaviours of rattlesnakes. *Proceedings of the Royal Society B: Biological Sciences*, **279**, 3827–3833.

Beauchamp, G. (2008). What is the magnitude of the group-size effect on vigilance? *Behavioral Ecology*, **19**, 1361–1368.

Beauchamp, G. (2009a). How does food density influence vigilance in birds and mammals? *Animal Behaviour*, **78**, 223–231.

Beauchamp, G. (2009b). Sleeping gulls monitor the vigilance behaviour of their neighbours. *Biology Letters*, **5**, 9–11.

Beauchamp, G. (2011). Collective waves of sleep in gulls (*Larus* spp.). *Ethology*, **117**, 326–331.

Beauchamp, G., Alexander, P. & Jovani, R. (2012). Consistent waves of collective vigilance in groups using public information about predation risk. *Behavioral Ecology*, **23**, 368–374.

Beauchamp, G. & Ruxton, G. D. (2012). Changes in anti-predator vigilance over time caused by a war of attrition between predator and prey. *Behavioral Ecology*, **23**, 368–374.

Bednekoff, P. A. & Lima, S. L. (2005). Testing for peripheral vigilance: do birds value what they see when not overtly vigilant? *Animal Behaviour*, **69**, 1165–1171.

Bergstrom, C. T. & Lachmann, M. (2001). Alarm calls as costly signals of antipredator vigilance: The watchful babbler game. *Animal Behaviour*, **61**, 535–543.

Blanchard, P. & Fritz, H. (2007). Induced or routine vigilance while foraging. *Oikos*, **116**, 1603–1608.

Blumstein, D. T. & Armitage, K. B. (1997). Does sociality drive the evolution of communicative complexity: A comparative test with ground-dwelling sciurid alarm calls. *American Naturalist*, **150**, 179–200.

Blumstein, D. T., Verneyre, L. & Daniel, J. C. (2004). Reliability and the adaptive utility of discrimination among alarm callers. *Proceedings of the Royal Society of London – Series B: Biological Sciences*, **271**, 1851–1857.

Bradbury, J. W. & Vehrencamp, S. L. (2011). *Principles of Animal Communication*, 2nd edn. Sunderland: Sinauer.

Brown, G. E. & Dreier, V. M. (2002). Predator inspection behaviour and attack cone avoidance in a characin fish: The effects of predator diet and prey experience. *Animal Behaviour*, **63**, 1175–1181.

Caraco, T. (1979). Time budgeting and group size: A theory. *Ecology*, **60**, 611–617.

Caro, T. M. (1986). The functions of stotting in Thomson's gazelles: Some tests of the predictions. *Animal Behaviour*, **34**, 663–684.

Caro, T. M. (1994). Ungulate antipredator behaviour: Preliminary and comparative data from African bovids. *Behaviour*, **128**, 189–228.

Caro, T. M. (2005). *Antipredator Defenses in Birds and Mammals*. Chicago, IL: University of Chicago Press.

Caro, T. M., Lombardo, L., Goldizen, A. W. & Kelly, M. (1995). Tail-flagging and other antipredator signals in white-tailed deer: New data and synthesis. *Behavioral Ecology*, **6**, 442–450.

Caro, T. M., Graham, C. M., Stoner, C. J. & Vargas, J. K. (2004). Adaptive significance of antipredator behaviour in artiodactyls. *Animal Behaviour*, **67**, 205–228.

Carter, A. J., Pays, O. & Goldizen, A. W. (2009). Individual variation in the relationship between vigilance and group size in eastern grey kangaroos. *Behavioral Ecology & Sociobiology*, **64**, 237–245.

Cooper, W. E. (2010). Timing during predatorprey encounters, duration and directedness of a putative pursuit-deterrent signal by the zebra-tailed lizard, *Callisaurus draconoides*. *Behaviour*, **147**, 1675–1691.

Cresswell, W., Hilton, G. M. & Ruxton, G. D. (2000). Evidence for a rule governing the avoidance of superfluous escape flights. *Proceedings of the Royal Society B: Biological Sciences*, **267**, 733–737.

Croft, D., James, R., Thomas, P. *et al.* (2006). Social structure and co-operative inter-actions in a wild population of guppies (*Poecilia reticulata*). *Behavioral Ecology and Sociobiology*, **59**, 644–650.

Curio, E. (1978). The adaptive significance of avian mobbing: I. Teleonomic hypothesess and predictions. *Zeitscrift fur Tierpsychologie*, **48**, 175–183.

Devereux, C. L., Whittingham, M. J., Fernández-Juricic, E., Vickery, J. A. & Krebs, J. R. (2006). Predator detection and avoidance by starlings under differing scenarios of predation risk. *Behavioral Ecology*, **17**, 303–309.

Dimond, S. & Lazarus, J. (1974). The problem of vigilance in animal life. *Brain, Behavior and Evolution*, **9**, 60–79.

Evans, C. S., Evans, L. & Marler, P. (1993). On the meaning of alarm calls: Functional reference in an avian vocal system. *Animal Behaviour*, **46**, 23–38.

Favreau, F.-R., Goldizen, A. W. & Pays, O. (2010). Interactions among social monitoring, anti-predator vigilance and group size in eastern grey kangaroos. *Proceedings of the Royal Society B: Biological Sciences*, **277**, 2089–2095.

Fernández-Juricic, E., Erichsen, J. T. & Kacelnik, A. (2004). Visual perception and social foraging in birds. *Trends in Ecology & Evolution*, **19**, 25–31.

Fernández-Juricic, E., Gall, M. D., Dolan, T., Tisdale, V. & Martin, G. R. (2008). The visual fields of two ground-foraging birds, House Finches and House Sparrows, allow for simultaneous foraging and anti-predator vigilance. *Ibis*, **150**, 779–787.

FitzGibbon, C. D. (1994). The costs and benefits of predator inspection behaviour in Thomson's gazelles. *Behavioral Ecology & Sociobiology*, **34**, 139–148.

FitzGibbon, C. D. & Fanshawe, J. (1988). Stotting in Thomson's gazelles: An honest signal of condition. *Behavioral Ecology & Sociobiology*, **23**, 69–74.

Fortin, D., Boyce, M. S., Merrill, E. H. & Fryxell, J. M. (2004). Foraging costs of vigilance in large mammalian herbivores. *Oikos*, **107**, 172–180.

Ge, C., Beauchamp, G. & Li, Z. (2011). Coordination and synchronisation of anti-predation vigilance in two crane species. *Plos One*, **6**, e26447.

Godin, J.-G. J. & Davis, S. A. (1995). Who dares, benefits: Predator approach behaviour in the guppy (*Poecilia reticulata*) deters predator pursuit. *Proceedings of the Royal Society of London. Series B: Biological Sciences*, **259**, 193–200.

Goodale, E., Beauchamp, G., Magrath, R. D., Nieh, J. C. & Ruxton, G. D. (2010). Interspecific information transfer influences animal community structure. *Trends in Ecology & Evolution*, **25**, 354–361.

Grafen, A. (1990). Biological signals as handicaps. *Journal of Theoretical Biology*, **144**, 517–546.

Griesser, M. (2008). Referential calls signal predator behaviour in a group living bird. *Current Biology*, **18**, 69–73.

Hamilton, W. D. (1971). Geometry for the selfish herd. *Journal of Theoretical Biology*, **31**, 295–311.

Kaby, U. & Lind, J. (2003). What limits predator detection in blue tits (*Parus caeruleus*): Posture, task or orientation? *Behavioral Ecology & Sociobiology*, **54**, 534–538.

Kenward, R. E. (1978). Hawks and doves: Factors affecting success and selection in goshawk attacks on woodpigeons. *Journal of Animal Ecology*, **47**, 449–460.

Külling, D. & Milinski, M. (1992). Size-dependent predation risk and partner quality in predator inspection of sticklebacks. *Animal Behaviour*, **44**, 949–955.

Landeau, L. & Terborgh, J. (1986). Oddity and the "confusion effect" in predation. *Animal Behaviour*, **34**, 1372–1380.

Leger, D. W., Owings, D. H. & Gelfand, D. L. (1980). Single-note vocalizations of California ground squirrels: Graded signals and situation-specificity of predator and socially evoked calls. *Zeitscrift fur Tierpsychologie*, **52**, 227–246.

Lima, S. L. (1988). Vigilance during the initiation of daily feeding in dark-eyed juncos. *Oikos*, **53**, 12–16.

Lima, S. L. (1992). Strong preferences for apparently dangerous habitats? A consequence of differential escape from predators. *Oikos*, **64**, 597–600.

Lima, S. L. (1995). Collective detection of predatory attack by social foragers: Fraught with ambiguity? *Animal Behaviour*, **50**, 1097–1108.

Lima, S. L. & Bednekoff, P. A. (1999). Back to the basics of antipredatory vigilance: can nonvigilant animals detect attack? *Animal Behaviour*, **58**, 537–543.

Lima, S. L., Rattenborg, N. C., Lesku, J. A. & Amlaner, C. J. (2005). Sleeping under the risk of predation. *Animal Behaviour*, **70**, 723–736.

Loughry, W. J. & McDonough, C. M. (1988). Calling and vigilance in California ground squirrels: A test of the tonic communication hypothesis. *Animal Behaviour*, **36**, 1533–1540.

Magurran, A. E. (1986). Predator inspection behaviour in minnow shoals: Differences between populations and individuals. *Behavioral Ecology & Sociobiology*, **19**, 267–273.

Magurran, A. E. (1990). The adaptive significance of schooling as antipredator defence in fish. *Annals Zoologi Fennici*, **27**, 51–66.

Manser, M. B., Seyfarth, R. M. & Cheney, D. L.(2002). Suricate alarm calls signal predator class and urgency. *Trends in Cognitive Sciences*, **6**, 55–57.

Mathot, K. J., van den Hout, P. J., Piersma, T. *et al.* (2011). Disentangling the roles of frequency vs. state-dependence in generating individual differences in behavioural plasticity. *Ecology Letters*, **14**, 1254–1262.

McNamara, J. M. & Houston, A. I. (1992). Evolutionarily stable levels of vigilance as a function of group size. *Animal Behaviour*, **43**, 641–658.

Michelena, P. & Deneubourg, J.-L. (2011). How group size affects vigilance dynamics and time allocation patterns: The key role of imitation and tempo. *Plos One*, **6**, e18631.

Milinski, M. (1987). Tit-for-tat in sticklebacks and the evolution of cooperation. *Nature*, **325**, 433–437.

Milinski, M., Lüthi, J. H., Eggler, R. & Parker, G. A. (1997). Cooperation under predation risk: Experiments on costs and benefits. *Proceedings of the Royal Society of London. Series B: Biological Sciences*, **264**, 831–837.

Murphy, T. G. (2006). Predator-elicited visual signal: Why the turquoise-browed motmot wag-displays its racketed tail. *Behavioral Ecology*, **17**, 547–553.

Murphy, T. G. (2007). Dishonest "preemptive" pursuit-deterrent signal? Why the turquoise-browed motmot wags its tail before feeding nestlings. *Animal Behaviour*, **73**, 965–970.

Neill, S. R. S. J. & Cullen, J. M. (1974). Experiments on whether schooling by their prey affects the hunting behaviour of cephalopods and fish predators. *Journal of Zoology*, **172**, 549–569.

Öst, M. & Tierala, T. (2011). Synchronized vigilance while feeding in common eider brood-rearing coalitions. *Behavioral Ecology*, **22**, 378–384.

Owens, N. W. & Goss-Custard, J. D. (1976). The adaptive significance of alarm calls given by shorebirds on their winter feeding grounds. *Evolution*, **30**, 397–398.

Pays, O., Beauchamp, G., Carter, A. J. & Goldizen, A. W. (2013). Foraging in groups allows collective predator detection in a mammal species without alarm calls. *Behavioral Ecology*, **24**, 1229–1236.

Pays, O., Sirot, E. & Fritz, H. (2012). Collective vigilance in the Greater Kudu: Towards a better understanding of synchronization patterns. *Ethology*, **118**, 1–9.

Périquet, S., Valeix, M., Loveridge, A. J. *et al.* (2010). Individual vigilance of African herbivores while drinking: the role of immediate predation risk and context. *Animal Behaviour*, **79**, 665–671.

Pitcher, T. J., Green, D. A. & Magurran, A. E. (1986). Dicing with death: Predator inspection behaviour in minnow shoals. *Journal of Fish Biology*, **28**, 439–448.

Pravosudov, V. V. & Grubb, T. C.(1998). Body mass, ambient temperature, time of day, and vigilance in tufted titmice. *Auk*, **115**, 221–223.

Pulliam, H. R. (1973). On the advantages of flocking. *Journal of Theoretical Biology*, **38**, 419–422.

Quinn, J. L., Whittingham, M. J., Butler, S. J. & Cresswell, W. (2006). Noise, predation risk compensation and vigilance in the chaffinch *Fringilla coelebs*. *Journal of Avian Biology*, **37**, 601–608.

Rattenborg, N. C., Lima, S. L. & Amlaner, C. J. (1999). Half-awake to the risk of predation. *Nature*, **397**, 397–398.

Reale, D., Reader, S. M., Sol, D., McDougall, P. T. & Dingemanse, N. J. (2007). Integrating animal temperament within ecology and evolution. *Biological Reviews*, **82**, 291–318.

Ridgway, S., Carder, D., Finneran, J. *et al.* (2006). Dolphin continuous auditory vigilance for five days. *Journal of Experimental Biology*, **209**, 3621–3628.

Ruxton, G. D., Sherratt, T. N. & Speed, M. P. (2004). *Avoiding Attack: The Evolutionary Ecology of Crypsis, Warning Signals and Mimicry*. Oxford: Oxford University Press.

Seyfarth, R. M., Cheney, D. L. & Marler, P. (1980). Vervet monkey alarm calls: Semantic communication in a free-ranging primate. *Animal Behaviour*, **28**, 1070–1094.

Shelley, E. L. & Blumstein, D. T. (2005). The evolution of vocal alarm communication in rodents. *Behavioral Ecology*, **16**, 169–177.

Sherman, P. W. (1985). Alarm calls of Belding's ground squirrels to aerial predators: Nepotism or self-preservation? *Behavioral Ecology and Sociobiology*, **17**, 313–323.

Shultz, S., Faurie, C. & Noë, R. (2003). Behavioural responses of Diana monkeys to male long-distance calls: Changes in ranging, association patterns and activity. *Behavioral Ecology and Sociobiology*, **53**, 238–245.

Sirot, E. & Pays, O. (2011). On the dynamics of predation risk perception for a vigilant forager. *Journal of theoretical Biology*, **276**, 1–7.

Sirot, E. & Touzalin, F. (2009). Coordination and synchronization of vigilance in groups of prey: The role of collective detection and predators' preference for stragglers. *American Naturalist*, **173**, 47–59.

Stang, A. T. & McRae, S. B. (2009). Why some rails have white tails: The evolution of white undertail plumage and anti-predator signaling. *Evolutionary Ecology*, **23**, 943–961.

Tan, K., Wang, Z., Li, H. *et al.* (2012). An "I see you" prey–predator signal between the Asian honeybee, *Apis cerana*, and the hornet, *Vespa velutina*. *Animal Behaviour*, **83**, 879–882.

Templeton, C. N., Greene, E. & Davis, K. (2005). Allometry of alarm calls: Black-capped chickadees encode information about predator size. *Science*, **308**, 1934–1937.

Thomas, P. O. R., Croft, D. P., Morrell, L. J. **et al.** (2008). Does defection during predator inspection affect social structure in wild shoals of guppies? *Animal Behaviour*, **75**, 43–53.

Tosh, C. R., Jackson, A. L. & Ruxton, G. D. (2006). The confusion effect in predatory neural networks. *American Naturalist*, **167**, E52–E65.

Vega-Redondo, F. & Hasson, O. (1993). A game-theoretic model of predator–prey signaling. *Journal of Theoretical Biology*, **162**, 309–319.

Wallace, D. J., Greenberg, D. S., Sawinski, J. *et al.* (2013). Rats maintain an overhead binocular field at the expense of constant fusion. *Nature*, **498**, 65–69.

Wilson, D. R. & Evans, C. S. (2012). Fowl communicate the size, speed and proximity of avian stimuli through graded structure in referential alarm calls. *Animal Behaviour*, **83**, 535–544.

Zahavi, A. & Zahavi, A. (1997). *The Handicap Principle: A Missing Piece of Darwin's Puzzle*. Oxford: Oxford University Press.

Zuberbühler, K. (2009). Survivor signals: The biology and psychology of animal alarm calling. *Advances in the Study of Behavior*, **40**, 277–322.

Zuberbühler, K., Noë, R. & Seyfarth, R. M. (1997). Diana monkey long-distance calls: Messages for conspecifics and predators. *Animal Behaviour*, **53**, 589–604.

11 Determinants of lizard escape performance: decision, motivation, ability, and opportunity

Kathleen L. Foster, Clint E. Collins, Timothy E. Higham, and Theodore Garland, Jr.

11.1 Introduction

All animal behavior involves movement, and most behavior involves locomotion, i.e., the act of self-propulsion. Arguably, "Locomotion, movement through the environment, is the behavior that most dictates the morphology and physiology of animals" (Dickinson *et al.* 2000). In other words, natural and sexual selection often act on locomotor performance abilities because they are crucial to success in many behaviors, including avoiding or escaping from predators. As Damon Runyon put it, "It may be that the race is not always to the swift nor the battle to the strong, but that is the way to bet" (Runyon 1992). Or, as noted by Woakes and Foster (1991, back cover), "Exercise lies at the heart of the struggle for existence. The exercise abilities of animals are constantly being refined by the relentless process of natural selection." Motivated by this perspective, several artificial selection experiments have targeted aspects of locomotor behavior or performance (Feder *et al.* 2010; Careau *et al.* 2013).

The types of locomotion used while escaping from predators are highly diverse because the animals themselves, both predators and prey, are diverse. Moreover, numerous ecological factors, including gross characteristics of the habitat (e.g., presence of trees, boulders, sand) and environmental characteristics (e.g., temperature, wind, shade) are highly variable. Locomotion and its relationships to such factors ultimately determine whether a potential prey individual escapes from an encounter with a predator (Figure 11.1).

Lizards have been the subject of many studies of both locomotion and antipredator behavior. They provide a rich source for studying the ecology, performance, and biomechanics of escaping, given the disparate ecomorphological adaptations that characterize many lizard groups (Pianka & Vitt 2003). For example, geckos and anoles have adhesive toepads that allow them to escape on vertical and even inverted surfaces

Escaping From Predators: An Integrative View of Escape Decisions, ed. W. E. Cooper and D. T. Blumstein. Published by Cambridge University Press. © Cambridge University Press 2015.

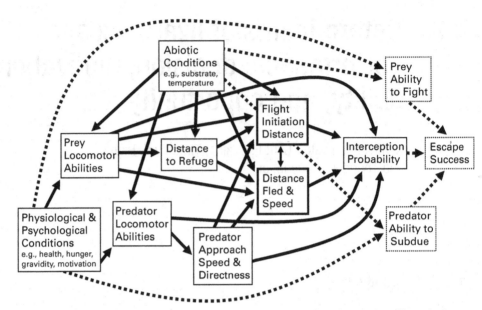

Figure 11.1   Path diagram depicting hypothesized causal relations among various factors that affect whether a
prey is able to escape from a predator (see also Bulova 1994). Note that "prey ability to fight,"
"predator ability to subdue," and "escape success" are beyond the scope of this volume, and so are
depicted in boxes with dotted borders and connected by dotted arrows. Various physiological and
psychological conditions (bottom left) will affect the locomotor abilities of both prey and predator,
and these abilities are also affected by abiotic conditions, especially in ectothermic poikilotherms.
Prey locomotor abilities affect decisions about how far they stray from safe refuge and how closely
they allow a detected predator to approach (i.e., flight initiation distance [FID]). Both FID,
distance fled (DF), and speed affect the probability that the predator intercepts the prey, as do the
locomotor abilities of both predator and prey. Once contact is made, the relative abilities of
predator and prey to subdue or fight (or possibly startle or bluff) determine whether the prey is able
to escape. Physical performance abilities during the "tooth and claw" phase are also affected by
physiological and psychological conditions. A number of other likely effects are depicted but not
discussed in this legend (see text). In addition, several important factors are not depicted, including
predator crypsis and prey ability to detect predators, and prey crypsis and predator ability to
detect prey, all of which are affected by both characteristics intrinsic to the organisms (e.g.,
coloration, visual acuity) and external conditions (e.g., wind, cloud cover, time of day; Bulova
1994). Note also that predator detection abilities, locomotor abilities, and abilities to subdue could
all affect how and when the prey reacts if the prey assess this information prior to making the
decision. Finally, absolute or relative body size of predator and prey can have pervasive effects on
many elements within this network.

(Russell 1975). Chameleons have prehensile feet that allow them to grip thin branches
during escape (Higham & Anderson 2013). In sandy desert habitats, several lizard
species have convergently evolved toe fringes and/or webbed feet that increase surface
area (Carothers 1986; Luke 1986; Bauer & Russell 1991). Basilisks have evolved similar
foot structures to allow them to run across water rather than sand. Flying lizards can
glide using foldable "wings" constructed of skin stretched across their ribs. This
remarkable phenotypic variation should be considered when determining how, where,
and when lizards might escape.

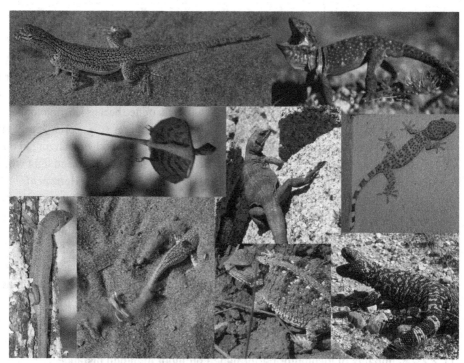

Figure 11.2   Lizards exhibit a great diversity of escape behaviors, including burrowing, sand-swimming, jumping, running, swimming, diving, escaping into crevices, climbing, and even "flying." Shown here are (clockwise from top left) a fringe-toed lizard (*Uma* sp.), collared lizard (*Crotaphytus collaris*), tokay gecko (*Gekko gecko*; photo credit: Lee Grismer), venomous Gila monster (*Heloderma suspectum*; see John-Alder *et al.* 1986), horned lizard after squirting blood from its orbital sinus (*Phrynosoma* sp.), sand lizard shimmying into sand (*Meroles* sp; photo credit: Clint E. Collins), tree lizard (*Lacerta viridis*; photo credit: Robert & Mihaela Vicol), flying lizard in the middle of a glide (*Draco taeniopterus*; see McGuire 2003), and chuckwalla near rock crevices into which it retreats when threatened (*Sauromalus* sp; photo credit: Clint E. Collins). Unless otherwise specified, images were obtained from Wikipedia Commons.

Lizards are diverse and flee by various means, including running, jumping, climbing, gliding (McGuire 2003), swimming, and diving. Aside from fleeing, lizards have alternative ways to avoid or cope with predators, such as crypsis, armor, fighting, blood-squirting, and venom (e.g., John-Alder *et al.* 1986; Sherbrooke & Middendorf 2001). As our experience is mainly with lizards, we focus on them in this chapter although most of the concepts that impact locomotor performance and escape success are more broadly applicable to other terrestrial vertebrates. We will briefly discuss how such concepts as detection of predators, decisions that lizards must make, and flight initiation distance relate to and are determined by locomotor performance (Figure 11.1), but our main focus is the morphological and physiological basis of performance limits in the context of escape success.

11.2   Locomotor performance affects escape decisions

11.2.1   Temperature effects on fight or flight

Once a predator is detected, the prey has to make a decision about whether it will flee or rely on some other mechanism for defense. Temperature is a primary factor that appears to determine whether a lizard will fight or flee because locomotor performance is (up to a point) increased at warmer body temperatures (e.g., sprint speed: Herrel *et al.* 2007; endurance: Garland 1994). Two species of agamid lizards living in open habitats where refuges are scarce attempt to flee when warm, but stand and fight when temperatures are cooler and sprint speed is too slow to permit escape (Hertz *et al.* 1982; see also Crowley & Pietruszka 1983). The physiological basis for this temperature-dependent shift in antipredator behavior appears to center on the differences in temperature dependence of force production in the locomotor and biting muscles of these lizards (Herrel *et al.* 2007). Although locomotor muscles generate peak force under a relatively narrow, warmer range of temperatures, the adductor mandibulae externus superficialis posterior, one of the jaw muscles responsible for producing force during biting, is largely temperature independent, generating near maximal forces over a wide range of temperatures (Herrel *et al.* 2007).

11.2.2   Impacts of locomotor performance on flight initiation distance

Fleeing from predation has largely been understood through the framework of models utilizing economic (cost–benefit) escape theory (Ydenberg & Dill 1986; Cooper & Frederick 2007, Chapter 2). As described in Chapters 1 and 2, an animal detects a predator and then monitors the predator as it approaches, fleeing when the cost of remaining in place equals the cost of fleeing (Ydenberg & Dill 1986) or the expected post-encounter Darwinian fitness is maximized (Cooper & Frederick 2007). The distance between the predator and the prey when the animal initiates its escape is termed the flight initiation distance (FID). Evading predation via locomotion involves complex, high-power movements, including jumping, accelerating, running, and evasive maneuvers (Djawdan 1993; Zehr & Sale 1994; McElroy *et al.* 2007; Higham & Irschick 2013). Therefore, evading predators requires high power output from skeletal muscles while operating within the biomechanical constraints that limit performance. Biomechanical and physiological sources of variation in performance often affect FID in ways consistent with escape theory. For example, individual lizards with cooler body temperatures escape more slowly relative to warmer counterparts (Cooper 2000; Cooper & Frederick 2007; Herrel *et al.* 2007). To compensate for decreased locomotor capacity, cooler lizards increase FID, presumably to prevent their predators from overtaking them (Rand 1964; Chapter 5). Underlying increased FID and reduced locomotor capacity at cooler temperatures is the sensitivity of muscle function to temperature, reduced metabolic rate, and reduced enzymatic activity rate (Adams 1985; Marsh & Bennett 1986a, b; Rome and Bennett 1990; Fitts *et al.* 1991; Dickinson *et al.* 2000; Jayne & Daggy 2000). For example, the frequency of muscle

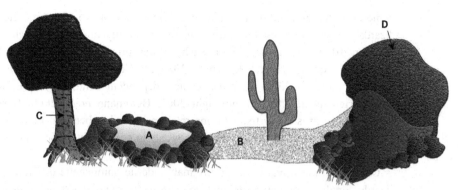

Figure 11.3 Schematic showing the variety of substrate textures or rugosities commonly encountered by lizards. Substrates can be very smooth and/or compliant (e.g., water [A], and sand [B]) or firm with varying degrees of roughness (e.g., tree bark [C] and rock [D]). Many lizards have pedal specializations that assist locomotion on these substrates: geckos have adhesive toe pads that are very effective at clinging to extremely smooth surfaces such as leaves and windows (although they cannot stick to Teflon), sand-dwelling lizards or juvenile basilisks may have toe-fringes or webbed feet to increase surface area for moving on fluid surfaces, and claws help lizards move on rough surfaces.

contraction at which mechanical output is greatest, known as optimal cycling frequency, increases with temperature. However, increasing temperature beyond a certain range may ultimately reduce power output (reviewed in James 2013) and hence locomotor abilities. Thus the interaction between temperature and locomotor physiology can impact not only escape performance, but also decisions about when to initiate escape behaviors.

Variable habitats often contain physical structures that constrain escape behavior and performance, and likely necessitate changes in locomotor kinematics, which could play an important role in determining FID. For example, increases in substrate rugosity or compliance likely constrain a lizard's ability to achieve maximal sprint speeds during escape, thus potentially increasing its FID or requiring an altered trajectory to minimize encounters with substrates that would reduce performance (Figure 11.3; Irschick & Losos 1999; Tulli *et al.* 2012; Collins *et al.* 2013). Given that terrestrial and arboreal environments present a diversity of obstacles, lizards that use highly complex habitats likely have evolved mechanisms for achieving high performance despite structural variability. For example, lizards, including *Anolis carolinensis*, *Callisaurus draconoides*, *Uma scoparia*, and some species of *Varanus*, alter limb posture and/or kinematics to deal with decreases in perch diameter and/or increases in perch incline, and these kinematic changes affect downstream changes in locomotor speed (Irschick & Jayne 1999; Jayne & Irschick 1999; Higham & Jayne 2004a, b; Spezzano & Jayne 2004; Foster & Higham 2012; Clemente 2013). Kinematics also play an important role in enhancing or constraining locomotor performance during escape because postural shifts may alter the ability of elastic tendons to store energy and/or may dictate the operating lengths of muscles (Higham & Irschick 2013). For example, different species of *Anolis* lizards have different levels of elastic energy storage prior to jumps because their femoral protraction differs (Vanhooydonck *et al.* 2006b, c). Further, whereas *Anolis* lizards decrease limb cycling rate to increase stability on narrow perches (Foster & Higham 2012), *Varanus* lizards achieve both high sprint speeds and stability by increasing stride frequency (Marsh & Bennett 1986a, b; Clemente 2013). This highlights the idea that there are likely multiple, context-dependent solutions to predator evasion (Wainwright *et al.* 2005; Wainwright 2007; Bergmann *et al.* 2009; Garland *et al.* 2011). Hence, it is likely that a strong relationship exists between FID and the ability to make kinematic and behavioral adjustments to compensate sufficiently for reduced performance.

Changes in performance capability may underlie ontogenetic differences in FID in lizards. Smaller, younger individuals are slower (Garland 1985), and thus may rely on either longer FID or crypsis to survive. Conversely, adult lizards can increase FID to save the energy that would be expended on a longer, faster run. Nevertheless, the patterns of FID, crypsis, and performance capabilities are nuanced and context specific; for example, in the absence of protective refuges, juveniles flee more frequently than adults (Smith 1997). Future studies should determine how selection acts on the integrated suites of acceleration, agility, sprint speed, and behavior to determine the true modus operandi of selection on locomotion. Finally, to compensate for hypothetically lower performance capabilities, juvenile lizards may use a greater percentage of their maximal sprinting and accelerating capabilities during escape than their adult counterparts (Irschick 2000; Toro *et al.* 2003; Stiller & McBrayer 2013). This variation suggests motivational differences may be key.

11.3   Motivation: how do animals decide what to do?

Motivation can strongly affect the performance exhibited by an individual in a given locomotor event (Astley *et al.* 2013). Performance is defined as the "ability of an individual to conduct a task when maximally motivated" (Careau & Garland 2012, p. 546). We define the motivation of an animal as the sum of factors or conditions that (1) stimulate or arouse an animal to perform a given task and (2) determine the level of persistence and vigor as it performs that task (modified from Beck 1978). Motivation in lizards has been inferred from measures of speed, latency between stimulus and response, and the number of stimuli required to elicit a response (e.g., Sorci *et al.* 1995; Skelton *et al.* 1996). However, these indirect measures may not allow identification of the factor or stimulus that is most important for motivating a lizard to run. Attempts to assess motivation in the field under a variety of natural and ecologically relevant conditions would help identify the situations and motivating factors associated with high performance.

Once a predator has been detected, the motivation of the prey is an integral factor in deciding whether or not to flee and in the subsequent level of locomotor performance during the escape attempt. Interpopulational differences in sprint capacity and/or voluntary running speed have been found within species of *Podarcis, Sceloporus,* and *Tropidurus*: individuals in populations exposed to greater predation risk may have greater sprint speeds (Crowley 1985a, b; Snell *et al.* 1988; Van Damme *et al.* 1998; but see Huey & Dunham 1987; Huey *et al.* 1990). However, many species of lizards do not use their maximum performance capacity when escaping from a predator (Hertz *et al.* 1988; Garland & Adolph 1991; Irschick & Losos 1998; Irschick & Garland 2001; Irschick 2003; Irschick *et al.* 2005; Husak 2006b; Husak & Fox 2006). This may be a function of motivational differences and may help to explain differences between maximum locomotor performance measured in the laboratory and realized field performance (Bennett & Huey 1990; Huey *et al.* 1990; Irschick 2003; Irschick *et al.* 2005). Thus, in some cases, lizards may be more motivated to run away from a human "predator" in a laboratory setting than they are to run from a common natural predator in the wild.

To be successful, prey must be able to effectively forage and attract mates. The conflicting demands imposed by multitasking may contribute to a prey's level of motivation when fleeing. Lizards may be reluctant to escape if their physiological state (e.g., gravidity, injury, tail loss, body size, time since last meal) or the abiotic conditions (e.g., habitat structure, temperature, humidity) are such that their locomotor performance capacity is diminished. Beyond these considerations, personality traits that dispose an animal to take greater or lesser risks may contribute to motivation regarding types and levels of performance during escape (Cooper 2008; Careau & Garland 2012). Unfortunately, intuitive, concrete experimental data supporting the impact of motivation on escape performance in ecologically relevant contexts are scarce.

11.4   Escape ability

The potential level of performance a lizard reaches in a given escape attempt is limited by its ability at that time, which is affected by various morphological and physiological traits (Figure 11.4). All aspects of locomotor ability are likely to be interrelated to some extent because each subcategory of ability is influenced by such factors as body size, limb lengths and proportions, muscle size and composition, innervation, neural control, and tendon characteristics (Garland 1993; Garland & Losos 1994; Christian & Garland 1996; Higham & Irschick 2013; Figure 11.4). Many of these relationships may cause trade-offs or constraints (Garland 2014) on the development or evolution of locomotor abilities (Vanhooydonck *et al.* 2014). Another source of constraint is the conflicting functions of animal phenotypes (Higham & Irschick 2013). This is the case for breathing and running in some lizards, where hypaxial and epaxial muscles drive both the movements of the ribs (for breathing) and of the body (for locomotion) (Carrier 1991; Farmer & Carrier 2000a, b; Brainerd & Owerkowicz 2006). The dual role of these muscles would appear to be one important factor that can limit the endurance capacity of a lizard, and therefore its escape ability in some situations.

11.4.1   Body size and shape

How the evolution of morphological diversity relates to variation in animal performance is a fundamental question in both functional and evolutionary biology. This section will

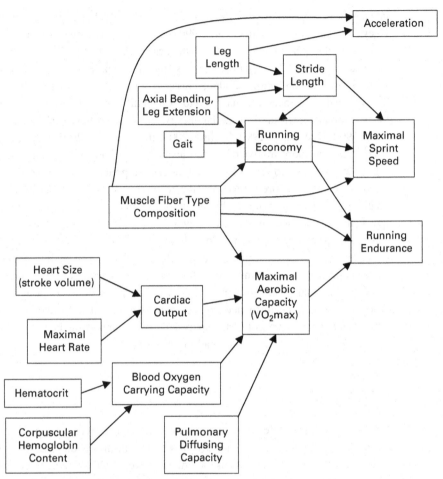

Figure 11.4 Path diagram illustrating interrelationships among some of the phenotypic traits that affect locomotor performance abilities, three of which are depicted (acceleration, sprint speed, and running endurance).

contextualize lizard morphological diversity in relation to escape diversity and attempt to link form with function. An overarching perspective is that body size has pervasive influences because it (1) affects the mass an animal must move and (2) is often allometrically associated with form (e.g., leg length: Christian and Garland 1996; but see McGuire 2003), thus having indirect effects on anything that form affects. Therefore body size strongly impacts lizard locomotor performance and escape behavior (Figure 11.5). Moreover, body size itself often shows complicated evolutionary patterns even within relatively uniform clades of squamates (e.g., McGuire 2003; Collar *et al.* 2011).

Hatchling and juvenile lizards are generally thought to be under relatively strong selection owing to their small size and limited locomotor capacity (Wassersug & Sperry 1977; Carrier 1996; Husak 2006a). However, one advantage smaller, younger lizards

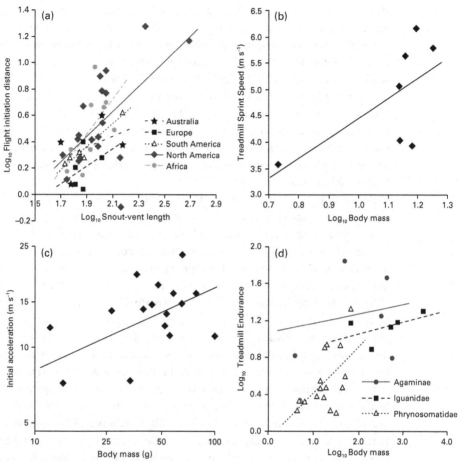

Figure 11.5   Relationships between body size and several traits relevant to escape performance. (A) Snout-vent length vs. flight initiation distance across several lizard taxa from continental Australia, Europe, South America, North America, and Africa (data from Cooper *et al.* 2014). (B) Body mass vs. sprint speed (measured on a treadmill) among seven *Cnemidophorus* species (data from Bonine & Garland 1999). (C) Body mass vs. acceleration (at 0.05 s) in the agamid lizard *Stellio stellio* (redrawn from Huey & Hertz 1984). (D) Body mass vs. endurance (measured on a treadmill) in three groups of iguanian lizards (data from Garland 1994).

may have over adults is the ability to utilize a wider range of habitat structures and to escape into smaller retreats. For example, unlike adults, juvenile basilisks (*Basiliscus basiliscus*) are able to escape by running over water surfaces because the smaller juvenile lizards can generate greater force relative to their body size (Glasheen & McMahon 1996). Similarly, smaller *Anolis* lizard individuals utilize a wider range of habitat structures than their larger counterparts (Irschick & Losos 1999). How juveniles utilize acceleration and agility throughout ontogeny may be of utmost importance, especially given the differential impact of slopes and habitat structure on size. Although larger lizards can sprint and accelerate faster than smaller counterparts

(Huey & Hertz 1984), smaller lizards may have smaller turning radii and thus out-maneuver larger predators, a prediction that deserves empirical testing.

Regardless of the cause of size differences (ontogeny, phylogeny, sexual dimorphism, etc.), steep inclines significantly reduce sprint performance in large animals relative to smaller animals (Jayne & Irschick 2000; Birn-Jeffery & Higham 2014). For example, the striped plateau lizard (*Sceloporus virgatus*) flees shorter distances upslope than horizontally or downslope (Cooper & Wilson 2007). If a larger animal were to chase the lizard upslope, it would have to expend more energy and would be at a disadvantage due to the greater work required to move its larger body uphill, as has been shown in lizards, in both the laboratory and the field (Huey & Hertz 1984; Jayne & Irschick 2000; Birn-Jeffery & Higham 2014).

Sexual differences in escape ability (e.g., sprint performance) are often attributed to the energetic costs of gravidity (Shine 2003a, b). For example, increased body mass alone could cause gravid females to have reduced locomotor abilities (Garland 1985; Garland & Else 1987). However, because reduced locomotor performance likely decreases future opportunities for reproduction, compensating for gravidity-induced impairment would have obvious evolutionary significance (Arnold 1983; Reznick 1985; Brodie 1989; Husak, 2006a, b). When performance and escape differences cannot be attributed to size alone, lower-level physiological differences are often the answer (Shine 2003a, b; Lailvaux 2007; Husak & Fox 2008). Females that are less conspicuous than males can rely relatively more on crypsis compared to males to compensate for lower sprinting capacities (Cooper *et al.* 1990; Cooper & Vitt 1991). In fact, whereas non-gravid female collared lizards (*Crotaphytus collaris*) compensate for reduced locomotor performance by using a greater proportion their lab-tested sprint speed, gravid collared lizards remain closer to refuges relative to non-gravid counterparts. Further, when they do escape, females may use a greater proportion of their maximum sprint capacity to achieve similar escape speeds in the field (Husak 2006b, c; Husak & Fox 2008). Interestingly, although many studies have supported the hypothesis that gravidity temporarily constrains escape capacity due to increased mass (Le Galliard *et al.* 2003), gravid green iguanas (*Iguana iguana*) increase mechanical power, peak forces, step duration, and limb swing speed to compensate for the greater mass (Scales & Butler 2007). Furthermore, differences in escape ability and decisions may be attributed to conflicts between optimal temperatures for eggs and optimal escape temperatures (Lailvaux *et al.* 2003). Finally, Irschick *et al.* (2003) found that at least one gecko, *Hemidactylus garnotii,* actually ran faster with an added load equaling 2% of its body weight (although sprint speed decreased with further increases in load). This non-linear effect suggests that there may be an optimal loading weight that may be related to gravidity. Future studies could compare optimal vs. actual reproductive mass increases.

The evolution of body shape is another important factor in determining escape response and success. In many animals, stockiness constrains flexibility and thus limits the contribution of axial movements to locomotion (Brainerd & Patek 1998; Walker 2000; Bergmann *et al.* 2009). Because many tetrapods, including lizards, rely on axial bending to increase stride length, and thereby sprint speed and endurance, reduced

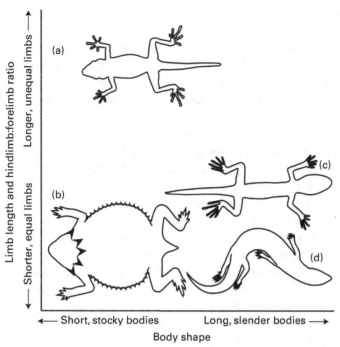

Figure 11.6   Schematic illustrating the relationship between hindlimb to forelimb ratio and body shape among lizards. (A) *Rhoptropus afer* is specialized for higher running speeds and has longer hindlimbs relative to forelimbs. (B) *Phrynosoma cornutum* exemplifies the short-limbed, stocky, and heavily armored phenotype that has reduced mobility. (C) Arboreal *Cnemaspis* species, like many arboreal lizards, tend to have more equal forelimb and hindlimb lengths, reflecting the increased propulsive importance of the forelimbs when climbing, and slender bodies for greater stability on narrower branches. (D) *Scincus scincus* has a hydrodynamic, slender body and short, relatively equal forelimbs and hindlimbs to facilitate sand-swimming.

flexibility of the axial skeleton hypothetically decreases locomotor performance (Reilly & Delancey 1997; Reilly 1998; Walker 2000). Therefore, to evade predators, lizards with relatively stocky bodies should exhibit morphological and behavioral compensations for this locomotor impairment. One clear example is the evolution of stockiness in the genus *Phrynosoma*, which compensates for reduced locomotor capabilities with greater morphological investment in armor (horns) and crypsis, in addition to the unique ability to squirt blood from the orbital sinus (Sherbrooke & Middendorf 2001). Conversely, cursorial sand lizards, such as the zebra-tailed lizard (*Callisaurus draconoides*), have evolved slender bodies with longer legs and tails. Lizards at this end of the spectrum rely on high speeds to evade predators and do not possess armor as *Phrynosoma* does (Figure 11.6A). Furthermore, the medial iliofibularis, a swing phase locomotor muscle, consists primarily of fast-twitch oxidative glycolytic fibers in *Phrynosoma* and fast-twitch glycolytic fibers in the cursorial sand lizards (Bonine & Garland 1999; Bonine *et al.* 2001, 2005). This trade-off indicates that stockier, armored lizards such as *Phrynosoma* rely more on slower, aerobically powered steady locomotion that is unrelated to predation pressure, rather than high-powered, anaerobic bursts (Figure 11.6B).

In contrast with the sand lizards, slender-bodied skinks and alligator lizards have reduced limb lengths (John-Alder *et al.* 1986; Bonine & Garland 1999). Shorter legs and elongate bodies may allow easier navigation through leaf litter, in-ground burrows, and tall grasses. Escape into such microhabitats may confuse predators or prevent them from following (Jaksić & Núñez 1979; Melville & Swain 2000; Melville 2008). Although it is thought this escape behavior enhances the probability of escape (Schall & Pianka 1980), little is known about other axial or appendicular adaptations for increased turning and maneuverability in lizards. Although turning generally decreases sprint speed in some lizards (Jayne & Ellis 1998; Irschick & Jayne 1999; but see Higham *et al.* 2001), it is likely that behavioral and performance responses to turning (Howland 1974) vary by species and habitat type. However, this remains to be explored.

Another body shape modification for escaping in habitats that impose intense functional constraints is body flattening by some saxicolous lizards (Goodman 2007, 2009; Revell *et al.* 2007; Goodman *et al.* 2008). Although some saxicolous species exhibit morphological specializations for highly rugose cliffs and skree, high-speed locomotion on vertical rock faces is difficult, so many saxicolous species hide within narrow crevices to avoid or escape from predators (Revell *et al.* 2007; Goodman *et al.* 2008; Tulli *et al.* 2012; Collins *et al.* 2013).

11.4.2   Limb and muscle morphology

Limb length strongly impacts locomotor performance; lizards with longer hindlimbs and shorter forelimbs achieve greater sprint speeds and jump farther (e.g., Bonine & Garland 1999; Toro *et al.* 2004) although there may be additional advantages to longer limbs that are unrelated to locomotor performance (Iraeta *et al.* 2011). However, longer limbs may not always be optimal for effective escape from a predator. As discussed above, shorter limbs may be advantageous for maneuvering in confined spaces, such as burrows, because they may achieve faster cycling frequencies and are easier to maneuver around obstructions. Shorter limbs may also be beneficial for stability on narrower surfaces. In *Anolis*, although shorter limbed species don't run faster on narrower surfaces than longer limbed species (Irschick & Losos 1999), they may be more effective at escaping if shorter limbs reduce the tendency to fall. This dual requirement of speed and surefootedness in order to achieve effective escape in arboreal situations is illustrated in *Sceloporus occidentalis*, in which terrestrial populations with longer limbs run slower than shorter limbed arboreal populations on narrow substrates (Figure 11.7; Sinervo & Losos 1991).

Differential elongation of limb segments may also affect locomotor performance. Elongation of distal limb segments relative to proximal segments is an indication of cursoriality (Coombs 1978; Hildebrand 1985) and the metatarsal:femur ratio is correlated with maximal sprint speed in mammals (Garland & Janis 1993). However, the effect of different relative limb segment lengths on lizard locomotor performance

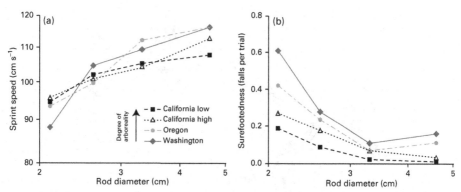

Figure 11.7   Impact of substrate diameter on (A) sprint speed and (B) surefootedness of four populations (California [high and low elevation], Oregon, and Washington) of the western fence lizard, *Sceloporus occidentalis*, that are arboreal to varying degrees. The more arboreal populations sprint faster and are more stable on narrowest perches compared to the more terrestrial populations. (Redrawn from Sinervo & Losos 1991)

remains unclear. Van Damme *et al.* (1998) found a slightly longer foot length in faster species, but this difference was unlikely to have caused the two-fold increase in speed among the species examined (Aerts *et al.* 2000). Similarly, contrary to expectations, limb segment length, independent of total limb length, is not correlated with jumping performance in *Anolis* (Toro *et al.* 2004). In bipedal lizards, the story gets a little more interesting. In addition to longer tails, shorter forelimbs (especially the manus), and longer hindlimbs (except in some agamids), bipedal lizards either have disproportionately longer proximal hindlimb segments (in iguanids) or distal (pes) hindlimb segments (Snyder 1954, 1962). However, although lizards that can run bipedally generally run faster than strictly quadrupedal lizards, these morphological differences may be a function of the different mechanics of the two types of gaits. Based on what we know about mammalian limb morphology and segment ratios, we can hypothesize certain morphologies in lizards specialized for high sprint speeds vs. those with limbs specialized for greater strength (Figure 11.8A). However, more research into the impact of limb morphology and segment length on lizard locomotor performance is necessary to test these hypotheses.

Research into these gross external morphological features should be complemented by examination of internal muscle morphology, as muscles are the functional units responsible for powering locomotion. Muscles are complex and can vary in both morphology and the mechanics of contraction, both of which can have a profound impact on locomotor capacity (Loeb & Gans 1986; Biewener 1998; Lieber & Ward 2011). Here, we will briefly discuss how the morphological aspects of muscle may affect locomotor performance. A discussion of relevant physiological aspects of muscle will follow in section 11.4.4.

The force a muscle can generate is a function of its physiological cross-sectional area (PCSA) because with a greater PCSA, a greater number of sarcomeres in parallel can contract simultaneously to contribute to force, assuming maximal stimulation

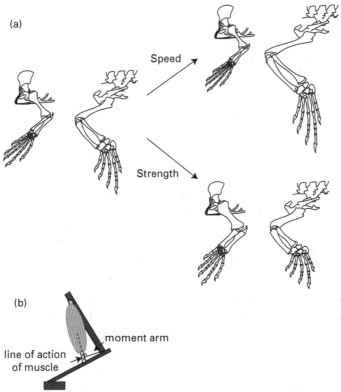

Figure 11.8 (A) Left: forelimb and hindlimb of *Varanus* sp., after Bellairs (1970). Relative size of forelimb and hindlimb approximately scaled to reflect average ratio of forelimb:hindlimb segment length ratio of 22 varanid species from Christian and Garland (1996). Top right: hypothesized morphology of lizard with fast sprint speed. Note elongation of hindlimb segments, especially phalanges, and shortening of forelimb segments, especially manus. Bottom right: hypothesized morphology of lizard specialized for strength, as might be important during digging. Note shortening and thickening of limb segments, lengthening of forelimb, and shortening of hindlimb. (B) Schematic showing calculation of muscle moment arm. The moment arm is the perpendicular distance between the line of action of the muscle and the joint at which the muscle acts.

(Haxton 1944; Alexander 1977; Sacks & Roy 1982; Loeb & Gans 1986; Zaaf *et al.* 1999; Herzog 2000; Allen *et al.* 2010; Lieber & Ward 2011). The length of muscle fibers affects total mechanical power because with longer fibers, more sarcomeres can be arranged in series and greater changes in length (and therefore increases in speed) are possible (Loeb & Gans 1986; Gans & de Vree 1987; Biewener 1998; Biewener & Roberts 2000; Allen *et al.* 2010; Lieber & Ward 2011). The placement of the muscle, i.e., the origin and insertion points of the muscle relative to the joints across which the muscle acts, also can affect locomotor function. When the distance between the joint and the line of action of the muscle is greater, the muscle has a greater moment arm, and this increases the mechanical advantage of the muscle such that less muscular force is required to generate movement about the joint (Figure 11.8B; Gans & de Vree 1987; Richmond 1998; Rassier *et al.* 1999; Zaaf *et al.* 1999; Payne *et al.* 2006;

Wilson & Lichtwark 2011). However, increasing the muscle's moment arm has a negative impact on the angular displacement and velocity that can be achieved about the joint because a given change in muscle length generates a smaller change in joint angle (Rassier *et al.* 1999; Payne *et al.* 2006; Wilson & Lichtwark 2011). These relationships lead to a trade-off between force and velocity such that larger muscle moment arms result in greater force, but lower velocity. Thus we would expect to see smaller moment arms in limbs that need to achieve high angular velocities, as might be beneficial for increasing stride frequency, but larger moment arms in limbs that are built for strength, as might be beneficial in climbing and burrowing species. Although these predictions may hold in small-scale comparisons (Zaaf *et al.* 1999; Herrel *et al.* 2008), broad comparative studies of muscle morphology (in the context of maximum performance) are lacking for lizards. Do lizards that sprint faster (and cycle their limbs faster) exhibit decreased moment arms compared to those lizards that move slower when escaping? Such studies will likely be particularly important because they have the potential to incorporate the ecologically relevant comparison of prey vs. predator morphology and performance.

11.4.3   Escape performance and tail autotomy

Many lizards possess the ability to autotomize (sever) the tail during a predator–prey interaction. The lost tail can provide a meal for the predator. If neither the tail nor the body are captured (Bellairs & Bryant 1985), the autotomized tail may move dramatically, distracting the predator while the lizard flees (Higham & Russell 2010, 2012; Higham *et al.* 2013a, b). Caudal autotomy often enables lizards to survive a predatory attack (e.g., Daniels *et al.* 1986). In some circumstances, the autotomized tail itself evades the predator completely, allowing the lizard to return to the site of autotomy to ingest the lost tail, which contains fat reserves (Clark 1971). Below, we discuss the impact of caudal autotomy on locomotor behaviors critical to escape success: running and jumping.

Although the tail of lizards is critical for locomotor movements, such as running and jumping, losing a tail is beneficial enough to offset the costs associated with modifications of locomotor movements. Running fast is an obvious mechanism for evading a predator, and the tail plays a significant role in locomotor mechanics of terrestrial lizards. A question that has arisen multiple times is whether running speed increases or decreases following autotomy. Skinks and iguanids exhibit a consistent decrease in running speed following autotomy, whereas geckos and lacertids are highly variable, with some geckos exhibiting a drastic increase (Daniels 1983; McElroy & Bergmann 2013). Interestingly, lizards with larger tails tend to exhibit a greater decrease in speed (McElroy & Bergmann 2013).

Jumping is important during escape for many lizards, especially those in arboreal habitats (Losos & Irschick 1996; Higham *et al.* 2001), and tails can be critical for maintaining in-air stability (Gillis *et al.* 2009, 2013). *Anolis* lizards with intact original tails took off and landed with approximately the same body angle. In contrast, tailless anoles underwent significant posterior rotation, up to 90° between take-off and landing (Gillis *et al.* 2009). Further, although lizards often autotomize only a portion of the tail, there was no significant impact of the amount of tail lost on body rotation during jumping (Gillis *et al.* 2013). However, high variation within groups that had autotomized different amounts of the tail may have obscured any effects of the proportion of the tail lost. Lizards that have lost their tail exhibit behavioral shifts to compensate for decreased stability. For anoles, this might mean occupying areas closer to the ground to avoid injury while jumping during an escape or avoiding jumping altogether. Whether such changes result in increased mortality and decreased fitness remains to be tested.

In most cases, the autotomized tail is not lost forever. The ability to regenerate the lost appendage is common, but it is not clear how the ability to escape is impacted by having a regenerated tail. The composition of the regenerated tail is quite different from the original, which suggests that function may be altered (Gilbert *et al.* 2013; Russell *et al.* 2014). It is likely that fine control of tail movements is compromised in the regenerated tail, leading to decreased stabilizing ability during jumping and/or running. Future work should examine how the function of a regenerated tail during locomotion compares with that of the original tail, but also how performance changes immediately after autotomy and during the phase of regeneration. Given that regeneration can take months, loco-motor performance may gradually recover over this period of time. However, it is also possible that performance does not recover at all.

11.4.4   How muscle physiology is related to escape ability

Given that muscles actuate the movements of the limbs during escape, it is expected that muscle physiology correlates with escape performance. Despite this, few studies have linked muscle physiology with running speed in lizards (Gleeson & Harrison 1988; Higham *et al.* 2011a; Kohlsdorf & Navas 2012; Vanhooydonck *et al.* 2014). Additional layers of complexity include a number of physiological and morphological parameters that might be related to locomotor performance, as well as the number of muscles that could be examined. For example, one could quantify the relative proportion of a given fiber type (fast glycolytic [FG], slow oxidative [SO], and fast oxidative glycolytic [FOG]), enzymatic activity, cross-sectional area of the whole muscle, fiber cross-sectional area, mass, moment arm, and other subordinate traits. Both propulsive (stance phase) and recovery (swing phase) muscles could be examined, and each may give a different result. Finally, the ecological context of the locomotor event might impact the relationship between muscle physiology and performance. For example, the morpholo-gical/physiological predictors of performance on a level surface differ from those on a vertical surface in the Florida scrub lizard, *Sceloporus woodi* (Higham *et al.* 2011a). The diameter of FG fibers in the gastrocnemius was correlated with acceleration on a level surface, whereas the percentage of FG fibers in the gastrocnemius predicted acceleration on a vertical surface.

Sprinting fast is commonly associated with increased escape performance. This makes sense, given that faster speeds will potentially increase the distance between the prey and predator over a given period of time. Gleeson and Harrison (1988) linked muscle morphology and physiology (iliofibularis, gastrocnemius, and caudofemoralis) to sprint speed in the desert iguana, *Dipsosaurus dorsalis*. They found that up to 30% of the variation in sprint speed could be explained solely by variation in fiber cross-sectional area; decreased area was associated with faster speeds. In *Tropidurus* lizards, faster sprint speeds were associated with a higher proportion of FG fibers in the iliofibularis muscle (Kohlsdorf & Navas 2012). Although not tested directly, it appears that those phrynosomatid lizards that sprint faster also exhibit a greater proportion of FG fibers in the iliofibularis muscle (Bonine *et al.* 2001). For example, the horned lizards sprint slowly compared to other species of phrynosomatids, and they exhibit the lowest percentage of FG fibers (Bonine *et al.* 2001). Collectively, it appears that increases in the relative proportion of fast-twitch muscle, which is good for power generation, is associated with greater escape performance in lizards.

A key consideration when attempting to quantify escape ability in relation to muscle physiology is which aspect of performance to measure. Although sprint speed is a common metric, and is likely important for escaping, acceleration might be more important in some cases. Indeed, the ability to accelerate maximally may be crucial for initially increasing distance from the predator, whereas maximum sprint speed is likely important for maintaining that distance. Muscle physiology may be linked to acceleration performance, as opposed to sprint speed, given the relatively higher demand that acceleration places on the locomotor system. As noted above, this is true for *Sceloporus woodi* moving on level and inclined surfaces (Higham *et al.* 2011a). Muscle mass-specific power during acceleration in *Sceloporus woodi* approaches the maximum power output measured for lizard hindlimb muscles, 90 W kg^{-1} (McElroy & McBrayer 2010). Future work should tease apart the relative importance of acceleration and maximum sprint speed in determining the outcome of predator–prey interactions in lizards. In addition to sprint speed and acceleration, endurance capacity may play a critical role in escaping from predators. This type of performance is likely enhanced by having a greater proportion of SO muscle fibers, which are ideal for powering behaviors requiring endurance. We know very little about the links between endurance and escape success in lizards, so studying this would be a logical first step.

Overall, the relationship between muscle and escape performance is incredibly complex, depending on the type of muscle measurement, the muscle being measured, the species being examined, the ecological context, and the performance variable being quantified. Future work that illuminates the key variables would propel our understanding of escape performance.

11.5 Opportunity: escaping in different habitats

Habitat structure and substrate characteristics can profoundly impact the successful negotiation of an animal through its environment. In this section we discuss the interesting challenges posed by sandy, arboreal and saxicolus habitats, and the potential consequences for escape performance.

11.5.1   Sandy habitats

Although sandy habitats are often considered relatively simple, they make physical demands that impose selection on many psammophilous lizards. Two well-studied challenges common to many deserts are substrate compliance and incline. Here, we will discuss the challenges and compensatory mechanisms related to substrate compliance, leaving discussion of the effects of incline for the following arboreal section.

Compliant surfaces, such as sandy flats and dunes, dissipate greater amounts of energy than non-compliant surfaces such as rocks. Consequently, escaping on compliant surfaces requires increased energy expenditure (Zamparo *et al.* 1992; Lejeune *et al.* 1998). One reason for this is the decreased ability to employ elastic elements as energy-saving mechanisms because the greater compliance interferes with effective loading of structures such as tendons. However, various adaptations, such as specialized external morphological features (e.g., toe fringes) and modified kinematics (e.g., foot posture and movement) enable effective, high-speed locomotion on compliant surfaces (Glasheen & McMahon 1996; Hsieh & Lauder 2004; Tulli *et al.* 2009; Li *et al.* 2012). Nonetheless, maximal speeds and/or acceleration of lizards running on sand may be reduced as compared with the same species running on a surface that provides good traction and is less compliant (Carothers 1986).

Laterally projected, elongated toe fringes increase toe surface area, and thus traction, on substrates such as sand and water (Carothers 1986; Luke 1986). The benefits of toe fringes were discovered through an experiment that demonstrated that ablating toe fringes reduced acceleration and sprint speed on sandy surfaces, but not on rigid surfaces (Carothers 1986). Interestingly, whereas some lizards have toe fringes to increase surface area, secondarily terrestrial geckos exhibit digit modifications that reduce surface area. Many arboreal and saxicolous pad-bearing geckos achieve adhesion by increasing their subdigital surface area to form microscopic setae, which bond with surfaces through van der Waals interactions (Autumn & Peattie 2002), but can become clogged with sand (Hansen & Autumn 2005). Thus secondarily terrestrial geckos have lost or reduced these adhesive structures, which likely allows them to perform better on flat, sandy surfaces (Lamb & Bauer 2006).

When lizards traverse non-solid surfaces, their hindlimb kinematics and foot use change to accommodate slipping and energy dissipation (Li *et al.* 2012). On solid surfaces the zebra-tailed lizard, *Callisaurus draconoides*, employs digitigrade foot posture and spring-mass mechanics, whereas on granular surfaces they use plantigrade foot posture and paddle-like foot rotation (Li *et al.* 2012). In addition to these kinematic modifications, sand-swimming lizards can employ unusual locomotor mechanisms to propel themselves beneath the sand surface. For example, high-speed x-ray cinematography of sand-swimming revealed that the sandfish (*Scincus scincus*) retracts its limbs to the sides of its body and propagates a wave down its body through lateral undulation to propel itself through the sand (Maladen *et al.* 2009). This study highlights the importance of integrating natural history, morphology, and biomechanical techniques to understand how evolution has acted upon integrated suites of locomotor traits.

In special cases, lizards, such as the plumed basilisk (*Basiliscus plumifrons*), can escape across water, which is also a compliant surface. Much like running across soft sand, elastic energy storage capacity is compromised when escaping across water since the foot actually breaches the water's surface during the stance phase (Hsieh & Lauder 2004). Thus the limb acts like a piston, doing work throughout the stride, which is in contrast with typical terrestrial legged mechanics.

11.5.2   Arboreal habitats

The arboreal habitat may be one of the more challenging habitats; it is often highly heterogeneous in incline, perch diameter, clutter, and substrate texture and compliance. How many of these characteristics impact escape performance and/or escape behavior is poorly understood. However, the impact on locomotor performance has been identified for a few of these conditions.

Climbing up inclines not only poses a challenge for stability, but it also increases the cost of locomotion because a greater proportion of gravity acts to resist forward locomotion, leaving a smaller proportion of gravity to help hold the animal against the surface (Taylor *et al.* 1972; Cartmill 1985; Farley & Emshwiller 1996; Roberts *et al.* 1997; Preuschoft 2002; Daley & Biewener 2003; Autumn *et al.* 2006; Birn-Jeffery & Higham, 2014). This leads to a decrease in locomotor performance on steeper inclines. However, as discussed above, the magnitude of this decrease in performance is size dependent, permitting smaller animals to use inclines to facilitate escape from larger predators (Taylor *et al.* 1972; Irschick & Jayne 1999; Irschick 2003). One way to offset the challenges of moving up an incline is to increase muscle mass-specific power output. A recent examination of ten species of *Anolis* lizards found that the evolution toward a higher incidence of escaping upward (based on behavioral observation) has been paralleled by the evolution toward higher mass-specific power output (Vanhooydonck *et al.* 2006a). It is important to note that the degree of arboreality does not necessarily imply that a lizard will escape up an incline when confronted by a predator. In fact, some species of *Anolis* will escape up (e.g., *A. valencienni*), whereas others will not (e.g., *A. lineatopus*; Vanhooydonck *et al.* 2006a). Thus it is critical to match morphological and physiological measurements with natural behavior.

Narrower perches cause a reduction in locomotor performance primarily through their effects on stability. As substrate diameter decreases, so does the base of support, since foot placement is constrained to positions closer to the midline of the body. This increases the toppling moment about the perch, and thus decreases stability because a greater proportion of gravitational force acts tangentially to the perch surface (Cartmill 1985; Preuschoft 2002). The resulting decrease in locomotor performance (Losos & Sinervo 1989; Losos & Irschick 1996; Vanhooydonck *et al.* 2006b; but see Schmidt & Fischer 2010) presumably occurs because stability must be increased via postural changes (Figure 11.7; Peterson 1984; Higham & Jayne 2004b; Foster & Higham 2012), which, in turn, may affect muscle function (Foster & Higham 2014). As with increases in incline, smaller animals may benefit from retreating to a narrow perch during an escape, since larger animals would suffer a larger decrease in stability for a given perch diameter.

Despite these challenges, the arboreal habitat may offer some advantages in terms of refuge availability. The abundance of higher order branching and leaves, especially in the canopy, may obstruct locomotion by impeding limb movement, but it may also help reduce detectability of the prey by the predator, thereby reducing both frequency of escape events and necessary distance fled (Irschick & Garland 2001; Irschick 2003; Husak & Fox 2006). Further, obstruction due to clutter may also be size dependent, with larger predators unable to negotiate the barriers as effectively as smaller prey.

Complex branching patterns may also restrict either escape trajectory or escape behavior because a fleeing lizard will be forced to either execute sharp turns or jump to bridge gaps. In *Anolis*, locomotor speed decreases with increasing turning angle, regardless of escape strategy, because prey must pause to arrange limbs for jumping (Higham *et al.* 2001). However, the magnitude of this decrease differs among species (Higham *et al.* 2001).

The effect of perch compliance on lizard locomotion has been largely neglected. Its effect on jump performance in *Anolis carolinensis* suggests that increasing perch compliance decreases both take-off velocity and jump distance and alters jump trajectory due to recoil (Gilman *et al.* 2012). This species preferentially selects more rigid perches as take-off points for jumping in the field (Gilman & Irschick 2013). The effect of perch compliance on other locomotor behaviors and in other lizard species is unknown.

Finally, it is important to note that these challenges do not occur in isolation. Rather, fleeing lizards must encounter various combinations of these factors, some of which may have greater impacts on escape success than others. In some cases, the ability to rapidly alter locomotor behavior (through changes in kinematics) several times as various types of surfaces are encountered might determine the outcome of a predator–prey interaction. This ability to modulate locomotion, rather than the ability to move on any single perch, could be subject to strong selection. Although the relative importance of these challenges is poorly understood, *Anolis* lizards may select broader substrates, even if this requires sharper turning angles. This may reflect avoidance of instability caused by narrower surfaces to facilitate increased escape speeds (even if this reduces effective distance fled; Figure 11.7; Mattingly & Jayne 2005).

11.5.3   Saxicolous habitats

Many of the physical constraints of climbing described for arboreal lizards apply to saxicolous (rock-dwelling) lizards because steeply inclined surfaces are prevalent in rocky habitats. However, some rocky habitats also have the additional challenges of unsteady surfaces with variable rugosity (Figure 11.3; Revell *et al.* 2007 Goodman *et al.* 2008) that may lead to strong selection on locomotor morphology and performance (Taylor *et al.* 1972; Farley & Emshwiller 1996; Goodman *et al.* 2008; Collins *et al.* 2013). Interestingly, support for this hypothesis is equivocal. For example, whereas *Liolaemus* lizards exhibit no apparent ecomorphological or performance associations related to habitat use, Collins *et al.* (2013) found that saxicolous lizards, with longer tails, broader body shapes, and longer distal limb elements were less sensitive to substrate rugosity than their arboreal and psammophilous counterparts. Furthermore, in some lizards, saxicoly is tightly linked with increased jumping, clinging, and sprint performance (Goodman *et al.* 2008). The evolution of fast sprinting may be directly related to the distance an animal has to run to escape predation, which may be comparatively greater in rocky habitats than in other terrestrial habitats (Revell *et al.* 2007; Goodman 2009). Another possibility is that exposure to predators might be greater when a lizard is on top of a rock surface, as compared to being on an inclined branch of a tree (within clutter) or on the ground (with vegetation). However, conflicting hypotheses regarding how lizards deal with rocky habitats suggest that the three-dimensional structure of rocks, and how they are used during escape (e.g., jumping from rock to rock vs. climbing), may determine the morphological "fit" to the environment. Biomechanical studies, combined with corresponding behavioral studies in the field, would clarify how morphology is used under various circumstances.

Clinging and adhering are important in saxicolous habitats. In general, lizards with shorter, highly curved claws and short toes have a comparative clinging advantage relative to other lizards (Zani 2000). This is likely important for lizards that need to prevent detachment during predation attempts, though it does conflict with the need to attain high speeds or execute long jumps (Goodman *et al.* 2007, 2008; Collins *et al.* 2013). The toe pad of geckos is a key innovation that allows geckos to climb on the vertical and inverted surfaces of rocks and trees through friction and van der Waals interactions (Russell 1975, 1986; Autumn & Peattie 2002; Tian *et al.* 2006). Setae, the micro-structures comprising the toe pads, are hair-like structures ranging from 20 to 110 micrometers in length. Setae are pushed into the substrate and loaded in tension, thereby creating the intermolecular bonds that allow them to adhere (Autumn *et al.* 2000). If variation in micro-rugosity is high, only a percentage of setae may be able to engage with the surface at any given time, yet no evidence of morphological specialization for particular rugosities has been found. Instead, toe pads accommodate adhesion on a wide variety of unpredictable and highly variable structures (Russell & Johnson 2007, 2014). Collins *et al.* (2015) found that the morphology of the adhesive structures varies depending on the incline of the habitat. Those species that move on surfaces with relatively low inclines exhibit a reduction in the adhesive system.

11.5.4   Intermittent locomotion and habitat structure

As outlined above, habitat structure can profoundly impact escape behavior and performance. During an escape, pausing can be beneficial for avoiding fatigue and enhancing endurance in lizards (Weinstein & Full 1999), but can also be detrimental if it allows the predator to approach closer. Inclines and branching are two additional aspects of habitat structure that can increase intermittent locomotion (Higham *et al.* 2001, 2011b). On a vertical surface (compared to a level), *Sceloporus woodi* exhibits decreased running speeds, increased maximum acceleration, and increased pausing (Figure 11.9; Higham *et al.*

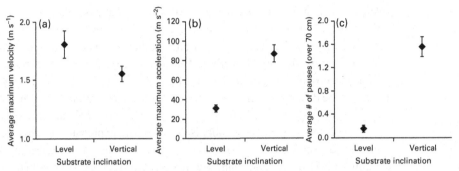

Figure 11.9   The average maximum velocity (A), acceleration (B), and number of pauses (C) in *Sceloporus woodi* moving along horizontal and vertical surfaces. Although the average acceleration was higher on the vertical surface compared to the horizontal surface, the average velocity was lower because the number of pauses was greater on the more energetically demanding vertical surface. However, greater acceleration in this condition may partially offset, and indeed may be possible because of, the effects of frequent pausing. (Redrawn from Higham *et al.* 2011b)

2011b). Thus it appears that either the enhanced acceleration may offset the costs associated with pausing or pausing facilitates increased acceleration by giving the propulsive muscles a chance to recover. With increasing turning angles, *Anolis* lizards pause more frequently to orient themselves before jumping across a turn (Higham *et al.* 2001), but these pauses may take valuable time during escapes, increasing the likelihood of predation. In addition to these potential benefits of intermittent locomotion, pausing may be beneficial for evaluating the continued need to escape, thus permitting an earlier return to activities such as foraging, courtship, and thermoregulation. Regardless, negotiating complex escape paths should be studied in greater detail because selection may act primarily on these demanding behaviors. We expect that there will be a trade-off between escaping into demanding areas of a habitat (steep inclines, narrow perches, areas with sharp turns, more compliant perches, etc.) and the ability to escape at high speeds, but we need to discover the context dependence of these strategies.

11.6   Conclusions and future directions

The extraordinary diversity of behavior, morphology, and ecology among lizards makes them an ideal system for addressing many questions in biology, including those related to escape behavior and performance. Nevertheless, a number of facets contributing to lizard escape performance remain poorly understood.

Both temperature and motivation impact not only the decision of whether to escape, but the level of performance that is achieved during escape. To better understand how motivation affects the common measures of locomotor performance, we must improve our understanding of how such factors as personality traits, conflicting priorities (e.g., foraging, mating, defending territories), physiological state, and abiotic conditions contribute to motivation in ecologically relevant contexts (see also Careau & Garland 2012). Although a daunting prospect, such studies have the potential to profoundly affect our understanding of organismal biology.

Although performance measures may increase as motivation increases, the maximal level of performance during escape is limited by the prey's locomotor ability. Numerous morphological and physiological traits interact to determine locomotor performance. Despite extensive research relating limb length and body size and shape to locomotor performance, there remains a paucity of data on the impact of differences in relative limb segment lengths and muscle morphology and physiology on locomotor capacity. Beyond this, however, it is essential that we establish the ecological relevance of such performance measures as acceleration and maximum sprint speed in order to ensure we are correctly characterizing and predicting the outcome of predator–prey interactions.

The impacts of hormones on locomotion in non-human vertebrates have received surprisingly little attention, despite their potential importance (O'Connor *et al.* 2011; Careau & Garland 2012; Higham & Irschick 2013). Although circulating levels of testosterone have been positively linked to increased performance in lizards (Husak *et al.* 2007), few significant impacts after experimentally elevating testosterone levels have been found. In the northern fence lizard, *Sceloporus undulatus hyacinthinus*, sprint speed and burst stamina were greater in individuals with experimentally elevated plasma testosterone (Klukowski *et al.* 1998). However, testosterone supplementation did not affect locomotor performance (burst distance and treadmill endurance) in *Aspidoscelis sexlineata* (O'Connor *et al.* 2011), leading to additional questions rather than answers. The conflicting results in the literature are likely a consequence of confounding factors associated with the experiments and natural differences among species and among populations within species (Crowley 1985a, b; Garland & Adolph 1991; Sinervo & Losos 1991; Bulova 1994; Snell *et al.* 1988; Van Damme *et al.* 1998; Iraeta *et al.* 2011).

Finally, lizards must interact with their habitat when escaping from predators. Thus the opportunities or challenges of aspects of substrates have the potential to impact performance capacity, resulting in the realized level of performance that the lizard achieves. However, the impact and relative importance of habitat characteristics on escape performance, rather than simply locomotor performance, is poorly understood. Biomechanical studies of ecologically relevant behaviors and interactions in the field are becoming increasingly feasible and are necessary to improve our understanding of escape performance in lizards.

Escaping from predators involves an integrated suite of behavioral, physiological, and morphological phenotypes, all of which may experience varying levels of selection in the wild. In addition, escape behavior and performance can be modulated depending on motivation. To fully understand when, how, and why lizards escape, future research should aim to integrate decision, motivation, ability, and opportunity. Only when we consider all of these categories simultaneously within a single lineage can we gain an appreciation for how they interact and interconnect to produce the observed escape performance and behavior.

References

Adams, B. (1985). The thermal-dependence of muscle membrane constants in 2 iguanid lizards (*Dipsosaurus dorsalis, Sceloporus occidentalis*). *Federation Proceedings*, **44**, 1377–1377.

Aerts, P., Van Damme, R., Vanhooydonck, B., Zaaf, A. & Herrel, A. (2000). Lizard locomotion: How morphology meets ecology. *Netherlands Journal of Zoology*, **50**, 261–277.

Alexander, R. M. (1977). Allometry of the limbs of antelopes (Bovidae). *Journal of Zoology*, **183**, 125–146.

Allen, V., Elsey, R. M., Jones, N., Wright, J. & Hutchinson, J. R. (2010). Functional specialization and ontogenetic scaling of limb anatomy in *Alligator mississippiensis*. *Journal of Anatomy*, **216**, 423–445.

Arnold, S. J. (1983). Morphology, performance and fitness. *American Zoologist*, **23**, 347–361.

Astley, H. C., Abbott, E. M., Azizi, E., Marsh, R. L. & Roberts, T. J. (2013). Chasing maximal performance: a cautionary tale from the celebrated jumping frogs of Calaveras County. *Journal of Experimental Biology*, **216**, 3947–3953.

Autumn, K. & Peattie, A. M. (2002). Mechanisms of adhesion in geckos. *Integrative and Comparative Biology*, **42**, 1081–1090.

Autumn, K., Liang, Y. A., Hsieh, S. T., *et al.* (2000). Adhesive force of a single gecko foot-hair. *Nature*, **405**, 681–685.

Autumn, K., Hsieh, S. T., Dudek, D. M., *et al.* (2006). Dynamics of geckos running vertically. *Journal of Experimental Biology*, **209**, 260–272.

Bauer, A. M. & Russell, A. P. (1991). Pedal specializations in dune-dwelling geckos. *Journal of Arid Environments*, **20**, 43–62.

Beck, R. C. (1978). *Motivation: Theories and Principles*. Englewood Cliffs: Prentice-Hall, Inc.

Bellairs, A. d. A. (1970). *The Life of Reptiles*. New York: Universe Books.

Bellairs, A. d. A. & Bryant, S. V. (1985). Autotomy and regeneration in reptiles. In Gans, C. & Billett, F. (eds.) *Biology of the Reptilia*. New York: John Wiley and Sons, **15**, 301–410.

Bennett, A. F. & Huey, R. B. (1990). Studying the evolution of physiological performance. In Futuyma, D. J. & Antonovics, J. (eds.) *Oxford Surveys in Evolutionary Biology, Vol. 6*. Oxford: Oxford University Press, pp. 251–284.

Bergmann, P. J., Meyers, J. J. & Irschick, D. J. (2009). Directional evolution of stockiness coevolves with ecology and locomotion in lizards. *Evolution*, **63**, 215.

Biewener, A. A. (1998). Muscle function *in vivo*: A comparison of muscles used for elastic energy savings *versus* muscles used to generate mechanical power. *American Zoologist*, **38**, 703–717.

Biewener, A. A. & Roberts, T. J. (2000). Muscle and tendon contributions to force, work, and elastic energy savings: a comparative perspective. *Exercise and Sport Sciences Reviews*, **28**, 99–107.

Birn-Jeffery, A. & Higham, T. E. (2014). The scaling of uphill and downhill locomotion in legged animals. *Integrative and Comparative Biology*, **54**, 1159–1172.

Bonine, K. E. & Garland, T., Jr. (1999). Sprint performance of phrynosomatid lizards, measured on a high-speed treadmill, correlates with hindlimb length. *Journal of Zoology*, **248**, 255–265.

Bonine, K. E., Gleeson, T. T. & Garland, T., Jr. (2001). Comparative analysis of fiber-type composition in the iliofibularis muscle of phrynosomatid lizards (Squamata). *Journal of Morphology*, **250**, 265–280.

Bonine, K. E., Gleeson, T. T. & Garland, T., Jr. (2005). Muscle fiber-type variation in lizards (Squamata) and phylogenetic reconstruction of hypothesized ancestral states. *Journal of Experimental Biology*, **208**, 4529–4547.

Brainerd, E. L. & Owerkowicz, T. (2006). Functional morphology and evolution of aspiration breathing in tetrapods. *Respiratory Physiology & Neurobiology*, **154**, 73–88.

Brainerd, E. L. & Patek, S. N. (1998). Vertebral column morphology, C-start curvature, and the evolution of mechanical defenses in tetraodontiform fishes. *Copeia*, **1998**, 971–984.

Brodie, E. D., III. (1989). Behavioral modification as a means of reducing the cost of reproduction. *American Naturalist*, **134**, 225–238.

Bulova, S. J. (1994). Ecological correlates of population and individual variation in antipredator behavior of two species of desert lizards. *Copeia*, **1994**, 980–992.

Careau, V. & Garland, T., Jr. (2012). Performance, personality, and energetics: Correlation, causation, and mechanism. *Physiological and Biochemical Zoology*, **85**, 543–571.

Careau, V., Wolak, M. E., Carter, P. A. & Garland, T., Jr. (2013). Limits to behavioral evolution: The quantitative genetics of a complex trait under directional selection. *Evolution*, **67**, 3102–3119.

Carothers, J. H. (1986). An experimental confirmation of morphological adaptation: Toe fringes in the sand-dwelling lizard *Uma scoparia*. *Evolution*, **40**, 871–874.

Carrier, D. R. (1991). Conflict in the hypaxial musculo-skeletal system: Documenting an evolutionary constraint. *American Zoologist*, **31**, 644–654.

Carrier, D. R. (1996). Ontogenetic limits on locomotor performance. *Physiological Zoology*, **69**, 467–488.

Cartmill, M. (1985). Climbing. In Hildebrand, M., Bramble, D. M., Liem, K. F. & Wake, D. B. (eds.) *Functional Vertebrate Morphology*. Cambridge: Harvard University Press, pp. 73–88.

Christian, A. & Garland, T., Jr. (1996). Scaling of limb proportions in monitor lizards (Squamata: Varanidae). *Journal of Herpetology*, **30**, 219–230.

Clark, D. R., Jr. (1971). The strategy of tail-autotomy in the ground skink, *Lygosoma laterale*. *Journal of Experimental Zoology*, **176**, 295–302.

Clemente, C. J., Withers, P. C., Thompson, G., & Loyd, D. (2013). Lizard tricks: Overcoming conflicting requirements of speed versus climbing ability by altering biomechanics of the lizard stride. *Journal of Experimental Biology*, **216**, 3854–3862.

Collar, D. C., Schulte, J. A., II, & Losos, J. B. (2011). Evolution of extreme body size disparity in monitor lizards (*Varanus*). *Evolution*, **65**, 2664–2680.

Collins, C. E., Russell, A. P. & Higham, T. E. (2015). Subdigital adhesive pad morphology varies in relation to structural habitat use in the Namib Day Gecko, *Rhoptropus afer*. *Functional Ecology*. **29**, 66–77.

Collins, C. E., Self, J. D., Anderson, R. A. & McBrayer, L. D. (2013). Rock-dwelling lizards exhibit less sensitivity of sprint speed to increases in substrate rugosity. *Zoology*, **116**, 151–158.

Coombs, W. P., Jr. (1978). Theoretical aspects of cursorial adaptations in dinosaurs. *Quarterly Review of Biology*, **53**, 393–418.

Cooper, W. E., Jr. (2000). Effect of temperature on escape behaviour by an ectothermic vertebrate, the keeled earless lizard (*Holbrookia propinqua*). *Behaviour*, **137**, 1299–1315.

Cooper, W. E., Jr. (2008). Visual monitoring of predators: Occurrence, cost and benefit for escape. *Animal Behaviour*, **76**, 1365–1372.

Cooper, W. E., Jr. & Frederick, W. G. (2007). Optimal flight initiation distance. *Journal of Theoretical Biology*, **244**, 59–67.

Cooper, W. E., Jr. & Vitt, L. J. (1991). Influence of detectability and ability to escape on natural selection of conspicuous autonomous defenses. *Canadian Journal of Zoology*, **69**, 757–764.

Cooper, W. E., Jr. & Wilson, D. S. (2007). Beyond optimal escape theory: Microhabitats as well as predation risk affect escape and refuge use by the phrynosomatid lizard Sceloporus virgatus. *Behaviour*, **144**, 1235–1254.

Cooper, W. E., Jr., Vitt, L. J., Hedges, R. & Huey, R. B. (1990). Locomotor impairment and defense in gravid lizards (*Eumeces laticeps*): Behavioral shift in activity may offset costs of reproduction in an active forager. *Behavioral Ecology and Sociobiology*, **27**, 153–157.

Cooper, W. E., Jr., Pyron, R. A. & Garland, T., Jr. (2014). Island tameness: Living on islands reduces flight initiation distance. *Proceedings of the Royal Society B*, **281**, 20133019.

Crowley, S. R. (1985a). Thermal sensitivity of sprint-running in the lizard *Sceloporus undulatus*: support for a conservative view of thermal physiology. *Oecologia*, **66**, 219–225.

Crowley, S. R. (1985b). Insensitivity to desiccation of sprint running performance in the lizard, *Sceloporus undulatus*. *Journal of Herpetology*, **19**, 171–174.

Crowley, S. R. & Pietruszka, R. D. (1983). Aggressiveness and vocalization in the leopard lizard. (*Gambelia wislizennii*): The influence of temperature. *Animal Behaviour*, **31**, 1055–1060.

Daley, M. A. & Biewener, A. A. (2003). Muscle force-length dynamics during level versus incline locomotion: A comparison of in vivo performance of two guinea fowl ankle extensors. *Journal of Experimental Biology*, **206**, 2941–2958.

Daniels, C. B. (1983). Running: An escape strategy enhanced by autotomy. *Herpetologica*, **39**, 162–165.

Daniels, C. B., Flaherty, S. P. & Simbotwe, M. P. (1986). Tail size and effectiveness of autotomy in a lizard. *Journal of Herpetology*, **20**, 93–96.

Dickinson, M. H., Farley, C. T., Full, R. J., *et al.* (2000). How animals move: An integrative view. *Science*, **288**, 100–106.

Djawdan, M. (1993). Locomotor performance of bipedal and quadrupedal heteromyid rodents. *Functional Ecology*, **7**, 195–202.

Farley, C. & Emshwiller, M. (1996). Efficiency of uphill locomotion in nocturnal and diurnal lizards. *Journal of Experimental Biology*, **199**, 587–592.

Farmer, C. G. & Carrier, D. R. (2000a). Pelvic aspiration in the American alligator (*Alligator mississippiensis*). *Journal of Experimental Biology*, **203**, 1679–1687.

Farmer, C. G. & Carrier, D. R. (2000b). Ventilation and gas exchange during treadmill locomotion in the American alligator (*Alligator mississippiensis*). *Journal of Experimental Biology*, **203**, 1671–1678.

Feder, M. E., Garland, T., Jr., Marden, J. H. & Zera, A. J. (2010). Locomotion in response to shifting climate zones: Not so fast. *Annual Review of Physiology*, **72**, 167–190.

Fitts, R. H., McDonald, K. S. & Schluter, J. M. (1991). The determinants of skeletal muscle force and power: Their adaptability with changes in activity pattern. *Journal of Biomechanics*, **24**, 111–122.

Foster, K. L. & Higham, T. E. (2012). How fore- and hindlimb function changes with incline and perch diameter in the green anole, *Anolis carolinensis*. *Journal of Experimental Biology*, **215**, 2288–2300.

Foster, K. L. & Higham, T. E. (2014). Context-dependent changes in motor control and kinematics during locomotion: Modulation and decoupling. *Proceedings of the Royal Society B*, **281**, 20133331.

Gans, C. & de Vree, F. (1987). Functional bases of fiber length and angulation in muscle. *Journal of Morphology*, **192**, 63–85.

Garland, T., Jr. (1985). Ontogenetic and individual variation in size, shape and speed in the Australian agamid lizard *Amphibolurus nuchalis*. *Journal of Zoology*, **207**, 425–439.

Garland, T., Jr. (1993). Locomotor performance and activity metabolism of *Cnemidophorus tigris* in relation to natural behaviors. In Wright, J. W. & Vitt, L. J. (eds.) *Biology of Whiptail Lizards (Genus Cnemidophorus)*. Norman: Oklahoma Museum of Natural History, pp. 163–210.

Garland, T., Jr. (1994). Phylogenetic analyses of lizard endurance capacity in relation to body size and body temperature. In Vitt, L. J. & Pianka, E. R. (eds.) *Lizard Ecology: Historical and Experimental Perspectives*. Princeton: Princeton University Press, pp. 237–259.

Garland, T., Jr. (2014). Quick guide: Trade-offs. *Current Biology*, **24**, R60–R61.

Garland, T., Jr. & Adolph, S. C. (1991). Physiological differentiation of vertebrate populations. *Annual Review of Ecology and Systematics*, **22**, 193–228.

Garland, T., Jr. & Else, P. L. (1987). Seasonal, sexual, and individual variation in endurance and activity metabolism in lizards. *American Journal of Physiology-Regulatory, Integrative and Comparative Physiology*, **252**, R439–R449.

Garland, T., Jr. & Janis, C. M. (1993). Does metatarsal/femur ratio predict maximal running speed in cursorial mammals? *Journal of Zoology*, **229**, 133–151.

Garland, T., Jr. & Losos, J. B. (1994). Ecological morphology of locomotor performance in squamate reptiles. In Wainwright, P. C. & Reilly, S. M. (eds.) *Ecological Morphology: Integrative Organismal Biology*. Chicago: University of Chicago Press, pp. 240–302.

Garland, T., Jr., Kelly, S. A., Malisch, J. L. *et al.* (2011). How to run far: Multiple solutions and sex-specific responses to selective breeding for high voluntary activity levels. *Proceedings of the Royal Society B: Biological Sciences*, **278**, 574–581.

Gilbert, E. A. B., Payne, S. L. & Vickaryous, M. K. (2013). The anatomy and histology of caudal autotomy and regeneration in lizards. *Physiological & Biochemical Zoology*, **86**, 631–644.

Gillis, G. B., Bonvini, L. A. & Irschick, D. J. (2009). Losing stability: Tail loss and jumping in the arboreal lizard *Anolis carolinensis*. *Journal of Experimental Biology*, **212**, 604–609.

Gillis, G. B., Kuo, C.-Y. & Irschick, D. J. (2013). The impact of tail loss on stability during jumping in green anoles (*Anolis carolinensis*). *Physiological & Biochemical Zoology*, **86**, 680–689.

Gilman, C. A. & Irschick, D. J. (2013). Foils of flexion: The effects of perch compliance on lizard locomotion and perch choice in the wild. *Functional Ecology*, **27**, 374–381.

Gilman, C. A., Bartlett, M. D., Gillis, G. B. & Irschick, D. J. (2012). Total recoil: Perch compliance alters jumping performance and kinematics in green anole lizards (*Anolis carolinensis*). *Journal of Experimental Biology*, **215**, 220–226.

Glasheen, J. W. & McMahon, T. A. (1996). Size-dependence of water-running ability in basilisk lizards (*Basiliscus basiliscus*). *Journal of Experimental Biology*, **199**, 2611–2618.

Gleeson, T. T. & Harrison, J. M. (1988). Muscle composition and its relation to sprint running in the lizard *Dipsosaurus dorsalis*. *American Journal of Physiology*, **255**, R470–R477.

Goodman, B. A. (2007). Divergent morphologies, performance, and escape behaviour in two tropical rock-using lizards (Reptilia: Scincidae). *Biological Journal of the Linnean Society*, **91**, 85–98.

Goodman, B. A. (2009). Nowhere to run: The role of habitat openness and refuge use in defining patterns of morphological and performance evolution in tropical lizards. *Journal of Evolutionary Biology*, **22**, 1535–1544.

Goodman, B. A., Miles, D. B. & Schwarzkopf, L. (2008). Life on the rocks: Habitat use drives morphological and performance evolution in lizards. *Ecology*, **89**, 3462–3471.

Hansen, W. R. & Autumn, K. (2005). Evidence for self-cleaning in *Gecko setae*. *Proceedings of the National Academy of Sciences*, **102**, 385–389.

Haxton, H. A. (1944). Absolute muscle force in the ankle flexors of man. *Journal of Physiology*, **103**, 267–273.

Herrel, A., James, R. S. & Van Damme, R. (2007). Fight versus flight: Physiological basis for temperature-dependent behavioral shifts in lizards. *Journal of Experimental Biology*, **210**, 1762–1767.

Herrel, A., Vanhooydonck, B., Porck, J. & Irschick, D. J. (2008). Anatomical basis of differences in locomotor behavior in *Anolis* lizards: A comparison between two ecomorphs. *Bulletin of the Museum of Comparative Zoology*, **159**, 213–238.

Hertz, P. E., Huey, R. B. & Nevo, E. (1982). Fight versus flight: Body temperature influences defensive responses of lizards. *Animal Behaviour*, **30**, 676–679.

Hertz, P. E., Huey, R. B. & Garland, T., Jr. (1988). Time budgets, thermoregulation, and maximal locomotor performance: Are reptiles olympians or boy scouts? *American Zoologist*, **28**, 927–938.

Herzog, W. (2000). Muscle properties and coordination during voluntary movement. *Journal of Sports Science*, **18**, 141–152.

Higham, T. E. & Anderson, C. V. (2013). Function and adaptation. In Tolley, K. A. & Herrel, A. (eds.) *The Biology of Chameleons*. Berkeley: University of California Press, pp. 63–83.

Higham, T. E. & Irschick, D. J. (2013). Springs, steroids, and slingshots: The roles of enhancers and constraints in animal movement. *Journal of Comparative Physiology B*, **183**, 583–595.

Higham, T. E. & Jayne, B. C. (2004a). *In vivo* muscle activity in the hindlimb of the arboreal lizard, *Chamaeleo calyptratus*: General patterns and the effects of incline. *Journal of Experimental Biology*, **207**, 249–261.

Higham, T. E. & Jayne, B. C. (2004b). Locomotion of lizards on inclines and perches: Hindlimb kinematics of an arboreal specialist and a terrestrial generalist. *Journal of Experimental Biology*, **207**, 233–248.

Higham, T. E. & Russell, A. P. (2010). Flip, flop and fly: Modulated motor control and highly variable movement patterns of autotomized gecko tails. *Biology Letters*, **6**, 70–73.

Higham, T. E. & Russell, A. P. (2012). Time-varying motor control of autotomized leopard gecko tails: Multiple inputs and behavioral modulation. *Journal of Experimental Biology*, **215**, 435–441.

Higham, T. E., Davenport, M. S. & Jayne, B. C. (2001). Maneuvering in an arboreal habitat: The effects of turning angle on the locomotion of three sympatric ecomorphs of *Anolis* lizards. *Journal of Experimental Biology*, **204**, 4141–4155.

Higham, T. E., Korchari, P. G. & McBrayer, L. M. (2011a). How muscles define maximum locomotor performance in lizards: An analysis using stance and swing phase muscles. *Journal of Experimental Biology*, **214**, 1685–1691.

Higham, T. E., Korchari, P. G. & McBrayer, L. M. (2011b). How to climb a tree: Lizards accelerate faster, but pause more, when escaping on vertical surfaces. *Biological Journal of the Linnean Society*, **102**, 83–90.

Higham, T. E., Lipsett, K. R., Syme, D. A. & Russell, A. P. (2013a). Controlled chaos: Three-dimensional kinematics, fiber histochemistry and muscle contractile dynamics of autotomized lizard tails. *Physiological and Biochemical Zoology*, **86**, 611–630.

Higham, T. E., Russell, A. P. & Zani, P. A. (2013b). Integrative biology of tail autotomy in lizards. *Physiological and Biochemical Zoology*, **86**, 603–610.

Hildebrand, M. (1985). Walking and running. In Hildebrand, M., Bramble, D. M., Liem, K.F. & Wake, D. B. (eds.) *Functional Vertebrate Morphology*. Cambridge: Harvard University Press, pp. 38–57.

Howland, H. C. (1974). Optimal strategies for predator avoidance: The relative importance of speed and manoeuvrability. *Journal of Theoretical Biology*, **47**, 333–350.

Hsieh, S. T. & Lauder, G. V. (2004). Running on water: Three-dimensional force generation by basilisk lizards. *Proceedings of the National Academy of Sciences*, **101**, 16784–16788.

Huey, R. B. & Dunham, A. E. (1987). Repeatability of locomotor performance in natural populations of the lizard *Sceloporus merriami*. *Evolution*, **41**, 1116–1120.

Huey, R. B. & Hertz, P. E. (1984). Effects of body size and slope on acceleration of a lizard (*Stellio stellio*). *Journal of Experimental Biology*, **110**, 113–123.

Huey, R. B., Dunham, A. E., Overall, K. L. & Newman, R. A. (1990). Variation in locomotor performance in demographically known populations of the lizard *Sceloporus merriami*. *Physiological Zoology*, **63**, 845–872.

Husak, J. F. (2006a). Does speed help you survive? A test with collared lizards of different ages. *Functional Ecology*, **20**, 174–179.

Husak, J. F. (2006b). Does survival depend on how fast you can run or how fast you do run? *Functional Ecology*, **20**, 1080–1086.

Husak, J. F. (2006c). Do female collared lizards change field use of maximal sprint speed capacity when gravid? *Oecologia*, **150**, 339–343.

Husak, J. F. & Fox, S. F. (2006). Field use of maximal sprint speed by collared lizards (*Crotaphytus collaris*): Compensation and sexual selection. *Evolution*, **60**, 1888–1895.

Husak, J. F. & Fox, S. F. (2008). Sexual selection on locomotor performance. *Evolutionary Ecology Research*, **10**, 213–228.

Husak, J. F., Irschick, D. J., Meyers, J. J., Lailvaux, S. P. & Moore, I. T. (2007). Hormones, sexual signals, and performance of green anole lizards (*Anolis carolinensis*). *Hormones and Behavior*, **52**, 360–367.

Iraeta, P., Monasterio, C., Salvador, A. & Díaz, J. A. (2011). Sexual dimorphism and interpopulation differences in lizard hind limb length: Locomotor performance or chemical signalling? *Biological Journal of the Linnean Society*, **104**, 318–329.

Irschick, D. J. (2000). Effects of behaviour and ontogeny on the locomotor performance of a West Indian lizard, *Anolis lineatopus*. *Functional Ecology*, **14**, 438–444.

Irschick, D. J. (2003). Measuring performance in nature: implications for studies of fitness within populations. *Integrative and Comparative Biology*, **43**, 396–407.

Irschick, D. J. & Garland, T. (2001). Integrating function and ecology in studies of adaptation: Investigations of locomotor capacity as a model system. *Annual Review of Ecology and Systematics*, **32**, 367–396.

Irschick, D. J. & Jayne, B. C. (1999). A field study of the effects of incline on the escape locomotion of a bipedal lizard, *Callisaurus draconoides*. *Physiological & Biochemical Zoology*, **72**, 44–56.

Irschick, D. J. & Losos, J. B. (1998). A comparative analysis of the ecological significance of maximal locomotor performance in Caribbean *Anolis* lizards. *Evolution*, **52**, 219–226.

Irschick, D. J. & Losos, J. B. (1999). Do lizards avoid habitats in which performance is submaximal? The relationship between sprinting capabilities and structural habitat use in Caribbean anoles. *American Naturalist*, **154**, 293–305.

Irschick, D. J., Vanhooydonck, B., Herrel, A. & Andronescu, A. (2003). Effects of loading and size on maximum power output and gait characteristics in geckos. *Journal of Experimental Biology*, **206**, 3923–3934.

Irschick, D. J., Herrel, A., Vanhooydonck, B., Huyghe, K. & van Damme, R. (2005). Locomotor compensation creates a mismatch between laboratory and field estimates of escape speed in lizards: A cautionary tale for performance-to-fitness studies. *Evolution*, **59**, 1579–1587.

Jaksić, F. M. & Núñez, H. (1979). Escaping behavior and morphological correlates in two *Liolaemus* species of central Chile (Lacertilia: Iguanidae). *Oecologia*, **42**, 119–122.

James, R. S. (2013). A review of the thermal sensitivity of the mechanics of vertebrate skeletal muscle. *Journal of Comparative Physiology B*, **183**, 723–733.

Jayne, B. C. & Daggy, M. W. (2000). The effects of temperature on the burial performance and axial motor pattern of the sand-swimming of the Mojave fringe-toed lizard *Uma scoparia*. *Journal of Experimental Biology*, **203**, 1241–1252.

Jayne, B. C. & Ellis, R. V. (1998). How inclines affect the escape behaviour of a dune-dwelling lizard, *Uma scoparia*. *Animal Behavior*, **55**, 1115–1130.

Jayne, B. C. & Irschick, D. J. (1999). Effects of incline and speed on the three-dimensional hindlimb kinematics of a generalized iguanian lizard (*Dipsosaurus dorsalis*). *Journal of Experimental Biology*, **202**, 143–159.

Jayne, B. C. & Irschick, D. J. (2000). A field study of incline use and preferred speeds for the locomotion of lizards. *Ecology*, **81**, 2969–2983.

John-Alder, H. B., Garland, T., Jr. & A. F., Bennett, (1986). Locomotory capacities, oxygen consumption, and the cost of locomotion of the shingle-back lizard (*Trachydosaurus rugosus*). *Physiological Zoology*, **59**, 523–531.

Klukowski, M., Jenkinson, N. M. & Nelson, C. E. (1998). Effects of testosterone on locomotor performance and growth in field-active northern fence lizards, *Sceloporus undulatus hyacinthinus*. *Physiological Zoology*, **71**, 506–514.

Kohlsdorf, T. & Navas, C. (2012). Evolution of form and function: Morphophysiological relationships and locomotor performance in tropidurine lizards. *Journal of Zoology*, **288**, 41–49.

Lailvaux, S. P. (2007). Interactive effects of sex and temperature on locomotion in reptiles. *Integrative and Comparative Biology*, **47**, 189–199.

Lailvaux, S. P., Alexander, G. J. & Whiting, M. J. (2003). Sex-based differences and similarities in locomotor performance, thermal preferences, and escape behaviour in the lizard *Platysaurus intermedius wilhelmi*. *Physiological & Biochemical Zoology*, **76**, 511–521.

Lamb, T. & Aaron, M. B. (2006). Footprints in the sand: Independent reduction of subdigital lamellae in the Namib-Kalahari burrowing geckos. *Proceedings of the Royal Society, B.*, **273**, 855–864.

Le Galliard, J. F., Le Bris, M. & Clobert, J. (2003). Timing of locomotor impairment and shift in thermal preferences during gravidity in a viviparous lizard. *Functional Ecology*, **17**, 877–885.

Lejeune, T. M., Willems, P. A. & Heglund, N. C. (1998). Mechanics and energetics of human locomotion on sand. *Journal of Experimental Biology*, **201**, 2071–2080.

Li, C., Hsieh, S. T. & Goldman, D. I. (2012). Multi-functional foot use during running in the zebra-tailed lizard (*Callisaurus draconoides*). *Journal of Experimental Biology*, **215**, 3293–3308.

Lieber, R. L. & Ward, S. R. (2011). Skeletal muscle design to meet functional demands. *Philosophical Transactions of the Royal Society B*, **366**, 1466–1476.

Loeb, G. E. & Gans, C. (1986). The organization of muscle. In *Electromyography for Experimentalists*. London: University of Chicago Press, pp. 25–43.

Losos, J. B. & Irschick, D. J. (1996). The effect of perch diameter on escape behaviour of *Anolis* lizards: Laboratory predictions and field tests. *Animal Behaviour*, **51**, 593–602.

Losos, J. B. & Sinervo, B. (1989). The effects of morphology and perch diameter on sprint performance of *Anolis* lizards. *Journal of Experimental Biology*, **145**, 23–30.

Luke, C. (1986). Convergent evolution of lizard toe fringes. *Biological Journal of the Linnean Society*, **27**, 1–16.

Maladen, R. D., Ding, Y., Li, C. & Goldman, D. I.(2009). Undulatory swimming in sand: Subsurface locomotion of the sandfish lizard. *Science*, **325**, 314–318.

Marsh, R. L. & Bennett, A. F. (1986a). Thermal-dependence of contractile properties of skeletal-muscle from the lizard *Sceloporus occidentalis* with comments on methods for fitting and comparing force-velocity curves. *Journal of Experimental Biology*, **126**, 63–77.

Marsh, R. L. & Bennett, A. F. (1986b). Thermal-dependence of sprint performance of the lizard *Sceloporus occidentalis*. *Journal of Experimental Biology*, **126**, 79–87.

Mattingly, W. B. & Jayne, B. C. (2005). The choice of arboreal escape paths and its consequences for the locomotor behaviour of four species of *Anolis* lizards. *Animal Behaviour*, **70**, 1239–1250.

McElroy, E. & Bergmann, P. J. (2013). Tail autotomy, tail size and locomotor performance in lizards. *Physiological & Biochemical Zoology*, **86**, 669–679.

McElroy, E. J. & McBrayer, L. D. (2010). Getting up to speed: Acceleration strategies in the Florida scrub lizard, Sceloporus woodi. *Physiological & Biochemical Zoology*, **83**, 643–653.

McElroy, E. J., Meyers, J. J., Reilly, S. M. & Irschick, D. J. (2007). Dissecting the effects of behaviour and habitat on the locomotion of a lizard (*Urosaurus ornatus*). *Animal Behaviour*, **73**, 359–365.

McGuire, J. A. (2003). Allometric prediction of locomotor performance: An example from Southeast Asian flying lizards. *American Naturalist*, **161**, 337–349.

Melville, J. (2008). Evolutionary correlations between microhabitat specialisation and locomotor capabilities in the lizard genus *Niveoscincus*. *Australian Journal of Zoology*, **55**, 351–355.

Melville, J. & Swain, R. (2000). Evolutionary relationships between morphology, performance and habitat openness in the lizard genus *Niveoscincus* (Scincidae : Lygosominae). *Biological Journal of the Linnean Society*, **70**, 667–683.

O'Connor, J. L., McBrayer, L. M., Higham, T. E. *et al.* (2011). Effects of training and testosterone on muscle fiber types and locomotor performance in male six-lined racerunners (*Aspidoscelis sexlineata*). *Physiological and Biochemical Zoology*, **84**, 394–405.

Payne, R. C., Crompton, R. H., Isler, K., *et al.* (2006). Morphological analysis of the hindlimb in apes and humans. II. Moment arms. *Journal of Anatomy*, **208**, 725–742.

Peterson, J. A. (1984). The locomotion of *Chamaeleo* (Reptilia: Sauria) with particular reference to the forelimb. *Journal of Zoology*, **202**, 1–42.

Pianka, E. R. & Vitt, L. J. (2003). *Lizards: Windows to the Evolution of Diversity*. Berkeley, CA: University of California Press.

Preuschoft, H. (2002). What does "arboreal locomotion" mean exactly and what are the relationships between "climbing", environment and morphology? *Zeitschrift fur Morphologie und Anthropologie*, **83**, 171–188.

Rand, A. S. (1964). Ecological distribution in anoline lizards of Puerto Rico. *Ecology*, **45**, 745–752.

Rassier, D. E., MacIntosh, B. R. & Herzog, W. (1999). Length dependence of active force production in skeletal muscle. *Journal of Applied Physiology*, **86**, 1445–1457.

Reilly, S. M. (1998). Sprawling locomotion in the lizard *Sceloporus clarkii*: speed modulation of motor patterns in a walking trot. *Brain, Behavior & Evolution*, **52**, 126–138.

Reilly, S. M. & Delancey, M. J. (1997). Sprawling locomotion in the lizard *Sceloporus clarkii:* the effects of speed on gait, hindlimb kinematics, and axial bending during walking. *Journal of Zoology*, **243**, 417–433.

Revell, L. J., Johnson, M. A., Schulte, J. A., II, Kolbe, J. J. & Losos, J. B. (2007). A phylogenetic test for adaptive convergence in rock-dwelling lizards. *Evolution*, **61**, 2898–2912.

Reznick, D. (1985). Costs of reproduction: An evaluation of the empirical evidence. *Oikos*, **44**, 257–267.

Richmond, F. J. R. (1998). Elements of style in neuromuscular architecture. *American Zoologist*, **38**, 729–742.

Roberts, T. J., Marsh, R. L., Weyand, P. G. & Taylor, C. R. (1997). Muscular force in running turkeys: the economy of minimizing work. *Science*, **275**, 1113–1115.

Rome, L. C. & Bennett, A. F. (1990). Influence of temperature on muscle and locomotor performance. *American Journal of Physiology-Regulatory, Integrative and Comparative Physiology*, **259**, R189–R190.

Runyon, D. (1992). *Guys and Dolls*. New York: Penguin Books, Ltd.

Russell, A. P. (1975). A contribution to the functional analysis of the foot of the Tokay, *Gekko gecko* (Reptilia: Gekkonidae). *Journal of Zoology*, **176**, 437–476.

Russell, A. P. (1986). The morphological basis of weight-bearing in the scansors of the tokay gecko (Reptilia: Sauria). *Canadian Journal of Zoology*, **64**, 948–955.

Russell, A. P. & Johnson, M. K. (2007). Real-world challenges to, and capabilities of, the gekkotan adhesive system: contrasting the rough and the smooth. *Canadian Journal of Zoology*, **85**, 1228–1238.

Russell, A. P. & Johnson, M. K. (2014). Between a rock and a soft place: Microtopography of the locomotor substrate and the morphology of the setal fields of Namibian day geckos (Gekkota: Gekkonidae: Rhoptropus). *Acta Zoologica*, **95**, 295–318.

Russell, A. P., Lai, E. K., Powell, G. L. & Higham, T. E. (2014). Density and distribution of cutaneous sensilla on tails of leopard geckos (Eublepharis macularius) in relation to caudal autotomy. *Journal of Morphology*, **275**, 961–979.

Sacks, R. D. & Roy, R. R. (1982). Architecture of the hind limb muscles of cats: Functional significance. *Journal of Morphology*, **173**, 185–195.

Scales, J. & Butler, M. (2007). Are powerful females powerful enough? Acceleration in gravid green iguanas (*Iguana iguana*). *Integrative and Comparative Biology*, **47**, 285–294.

Schall, J. J. & Pianka, E. R. (1980). Evolution of escape behavior diversity. *American Naturalist*, **115**, 551–566.

Schmidt, A. & Fischer, M. S. (2010). Arboreal locomotion in rats. The challenge of maintaining stability. *Journal of Experimental Biology*, **213**, 3615–3624.

Sherbrooke, W. C., George, A. & Middendorf, G. A., III. (2001). Blood-squirting variability in horned lizards (*Phrynosoma*). *Copeia*, **2001**, 1114–1122.

Shine, R. (2003a). Effects of pregnancy on locomotor performance: An experimental study on lizards. *Oecologia*, **136**, 450–456.

Shine, R. (2003b). Locomotor speeds of gravid lizards: Placing "costs of reproduction" within an ecological context. *Functional Ecology*, **17**, 526–533.

Sinervo, B. & Losos, J. B.(1991). Walking the tight rope: arboreal sprint performance among *Sceloporus occidentalis* lizard populations. *Ecology*, **72**, 1225–1233.

Skelton, T. M., Waran, N. K. & Young, R. J. (1996). Assessment of motivation in the lizard, *Chalcides ocellatus*. *Animal Welfare*, **5**, 63–69.

Smith, D. G. (1997). Ecological factors influencing the antipredator behaviors of the ground skink, *Scincella lateralis*. *Behavioral Ecology*, **8**, 622–629.

Snell, H. L., Jennings, R. D., Snell, H. M. & Harcourt, S. (1988). Intrapopulation variation in predator-avoidance performance of Galápagos lava lizards: The interaction of sexual and natural selection. *Evolutionary Ecology*, **2**, 353–369.

Snyder, R. C. (1954). The anatomy and function of the pelvic girdle and hindlimb in lizard locomotion. *American Journal of Anatomy*, **95**, 1–45.

Snyder, R. C. (1962). Adaptations for bipedal locomotion of lizards. *American Zoologist*, **2**, 191–203.

Sorci, G., Swallow, J. G., Theodore, G., Jr. & Clobert, J. (1995). Quantitative genetics of locomotor speed and endurance in the lizard *Lacerta vivipara*. *Physiological Zoology*, **68**, 698–720.

Spezzano, L. C. & Jayne, B. C. (2004). The effects of surface diameter and incline on the hindlimb kinematics of an arboreal lizard (*Anolis sagrei*). *Journal of Experimental Biology*, **207**, 2115–2131.

Stiller, R. B. & McBrayer, L. D. (2013). The ontogeny of escape behavior, locomotor performance, and the hind limb in *Sceloporus woodi*. *Zoology*, **116**, 175–181.

Taylor, C. R., Caldwell, S. L. & Rowntree, V. J. (1972). Running up and down hills: Some consequences of size. *Science*, **178**, 1096–1097.

Tian, Y., Pesika, N., Zeng, H. *et al.* (2006). Adhesion and friction in gecko toe attachment and detachment. *Proceedings of the National Academy of Sciences*, **103**, 19320–19325.

Toro, E., Herrel, A., Vanhooydonck, B. & Irschick, D. J. (2003). A biomechanical analysis of intra- and interspecific scaling of jumping and morphology in Caribbean *Anolis* lizards. *Journal of Experimental Biology*, **206**, 2641–2652.

Toro, E., Herrel, A. & Irschick, D. J. (2004). The evolution of jumping performance in Caribbean *Anolis* lizards: Solutions to biomechanical trade-offs. *American Naturalist*, **163**, 844–856.

Tulli, M. J., Cruz, F. B., Herrel, A., Vanhooydonck, B. & Abdala, V. (2009). The interplay between claw morphology and microhabitat use in neotropical iguanian lizards. *Zoology*, **112**, 379–392.

Tulli, M. J., Abdala, V. & Cruz, F. B. (2012). Effects of different substrates on the sprint performance of lizards. *Journal of Experimental Biology*, **215**, 774–784.

Van Damme, R., Aerts, P. & Vanhooydonck, B. (1998). Variation in morphology, gait characteristics and speed of locomotion in two populations of lizards. *Biological Journal of the Linnean Society*, **63**, 409–427.

Vanhooydonck, B., Aerts, P., Irschick, D.J. & Herrel, A. (2006a). Power generation during locomotion in *Anolis* lizards: An ecomorphological approach. In Herrel, A., Speck, T. & Rowe, N.P. (eds.) *Ecology and Biomechanics: A Mechanical Approach to the Ecology of Animals and Plants*. Boca Raton, FL: CRC Press, pp. 253–269.

Vanhooydonck, B., Herrel, A. & Irschick, D. J. (2006b). Out on a limb: the differential effect of substrate diameter on acceleration capacity in *Anolis* lizards. *Journal of Experimental Biology*, **209**, 4515–4523.

Vanhooydonck, B., Herrel, A., Van Damme, R. & Irschick, D. J. (2006c). The quick and the fast: The evolution of acceleration capacity in *Anolis* lizards. *Evolution*, **60**, 2137–2147.

Vanhooydonck, B., James, R. S., Tallis, J., *et al.* (2014). Is the whole more than the sum of its parts? Evolutionary trade-offs between burst and sustained locomotion in lacertid lizards. *Proceedings of the Royal Society B: Biological Sciences*, **281**, 20132677.

Wainwright, P. C. (2007). Functional versus morphological diversity in macroevolution. *Annual Review of Ecology, Evolution, and Systematics*, **38**, 381–401.

Wainwright, P. C., Alfaro, M. E., Bolnick, D. I. & Hulsey, C. D. (2005). Many-to-one mapping of form to function: A general principle in organismal design? *Integrative and Comparative Biology*, **45**, 256–262.

Walker, J. A. (2000). Does a rigid body limit maneuverability? *Journal of Experimental Biology*, **203**, 3391–3396.

Wassersug, R. J. & Sperry, D. G. (1977). The relationship of locomotion to differential predation on *Pseudacris triseriata* (Anura: Hylidae). *Ecology*, **58**, 830–839.

Weinstein, R. B. & Full, R. J. (1999). Intermittent locomotion increases endurance in a gecko. *Physiological and Biochemical Zoology*, **72**, 732–739.

Wilson, A. & Lichtwark, G. (2011). The anatomical arrangement of muscle and tendon enhances limb versatility and locomotor performance. *Philosophical Transactions of the Royal Society B*, **366**, 1540–1553.

Woakes, A. J. & Foster, W. A. (eds.) (1991). The comparative physiology of exercise. *Journal of Experimental Biology*, **160**, 1–340.

Ydenberg, R. C. & Dill, L. M. (1986). The economics of fleeing from predators. In Rosenblatt, J. S., Beer, C., Busnel, M.-C. & Slater, P. J. B. (eds.) *Advances in the Study of Behavior*, Vol. 16. pp. 229–249.

Zaaf, A., Herrel, A., Aerts, P. & De Vree, F. (1999). Morphology and morphometrics of the appendicular musculature in geckoes with different locomotor habits (Lepidosauria). *Zoomorphology*, **119**, 9–22.

Zamparo, P., Perini, R., Orizio, C., Sacher, M. & Ferretti, G. (1992). The energy cost of walking or running on sand. *European Journal of Applied Physiology*, **65**, 183–187.

Zani, P. A. (2000). The comparative evolution of lizard claw and toe morphology and clinging performance. *Journal of Evolutionary Biology*, **13**, 316–325.

Zehr, E. P. & Sale, D. G. (1994). Ballistic movement: muscle activation and neuromuscular adaptation. *Canadian Journal of Applied Physiology*, **19**, 363–378.

12 Sensory systems and escape behavior

Luke P. Tyrrell and Esteban Fernández-Juricic

12.1 Sensory systems are at the center of predator–prey interactions

Despite being on opposite sides of the arms race, predators and prey share a common goal: detecting each other as early as possible. Early detection is important for prey so they can initiate their escape behavior and increase their chances of survival. Early detection is also important for predators so they can take advantage of the surprise factor and enhance the chances of prey capture. We can then expect selection pressures on the predator and prey sensory systems to enhance the chances of mutual detection (Cronin 2005). For example, the sand cricket filiform hairs, which detect air movements, are especially sensitive to the frequencies and velocities that its predators produce (Magal *et al*. 2006).

We review, from a mechanistic perspective, how sensory system configuration can influence antipredator behavior. For the sake of space, we focus on the visual system of vertebrate prey (see also the electronic supplementary material for a discussion on other sensory modalities), but some of the fundamental ideas can be extended to other sensory modalities (e.g., Phelps 2007). Within the visual system, several dimensions have been implicated in the responses of prey to predators: configuration of the visual fields (the degree of visual coverage around the prey's head), spatial visual resolution (visual acuity), temporal visual resolution (how fast the retina can process temporal changes in visual stimuli), the type and number of centers of acute vision in the retina (retinal specialization), visual contrast (ability to resolve a stimulus against the background), motion detection, etc. We will discuss the role of many of these visual dimensions in affecting the decision-making of prey under the risk of predation. This approach will allow us to draw attention to some sensory aspects that behavioral ecologists tend to inadvertently omit when designing and interpreting studies on antipredator behavior.

12.2 Steps involved in predator–prey interactions from a sensory perspective

Before prey can escape from a predator, they must first use their sensory systems to gather information about the presence of the predator as well as its behavior. Decisions

Escaping From Predators: An Integrative View of Escape Decisions, ed. W. E. Cooper and D. T. Blumstein. Published by Cambridge University Press. © Cambridge University Press 2015.

to eventually escape are based on the trade-off between staying in the patch to enhance foraging/breeding benefits and leaving to reduce the risks of mortality (Krause & Ruxton 2002). Not all decisions are correct, as they may lead to false alarms, where the detected stimulus is not a predator, or it is a predator that is not in a position to attack (i.e., the predator is not hunting, has not detected the prey, is attacking a different individual, or has already captured prey). Sensory systems are expected to be configured to work in conditions that would reduce the probability of false alarms, if false alarms are costly (Beauchamp & Ruxton 2007). Consequently, sensory systems can be particularly relevant in reducing uncertainty, and thus improve escape decisions, in the following key steps of the sequence of predator–prey interactions: scanning, detection, assessment of risk, alert, and finally fleeing to cover (Figure 12.1).

12.2.1   Scanning

From a theoretical perspective, scanning or vigilance behavior is a key parameter in antipredator behavior models (reviewed in Beauchamp 2014). An increase in scanning effort is expected to raise the probability of predator detection (e.g., Lima 1987), an assumption that has received empirical support (e.g., Cresswell et al. 2003). However, the sensory basis of scanning behavior has been less studied (Fernández-Juricic et al. 2004; Fernández-Juricic 2012).

Old models (and some new ones) make the simplistic assumption, from a purely behavioral perspective, that scanning is restricted to some body postures (Fernández-Juricic et al. 2004). More specifically, animals can only scan when head-up, but not when head-down searching for food or pecking (i.e., mutual exclusivity assumption). From a sensory perspective, this assumption does not apply to those species with laterally placed eyes (most vertebrates). The reason is because the large degree of visual coverage (i.e., wide lateral visual fields) would allow vertebrates with laterally placed eyes to engage in scanning behavior even when head down (e.g., Fernández-Juricic et al. 2008; Figure 12.2). Even more compelling is the fact that in some bird species, the center of acute vision in the retina projects laterally in head-down postures (Dolan & Fernández-Juricic 2010; Figure 12.2). Actually, there is empirical evidence in at least three bird species that the probability of predator detection in head-down body postures is not 0%, as assumed, but actually around 30% in pecking postures and 75% in food-searching postures (Lima & Bednekoff 1999; Tisdale & Fernández-Juricic 2009).

Some may argue that even though this sensory assumption is not realistic, it may be valid enough for modeling purposes. However, model predictions can change substantially when this assumption is relaxed. For instance, the frequency of different group foraging strategies (producers, scroungers, opportunists) changes depending on the degree of visual coverage of a species (Fernández-Juricic et al. 2004). This is relevant because there is substantial variation between species in visual coverage (e.g., Martin 2014). Overall, modeling with assumptions that do not reflect the sensory systems of study species largely constrains our ability to develop predictions that can be tested empirically and makes our interpretations of the empirical results more challenging.

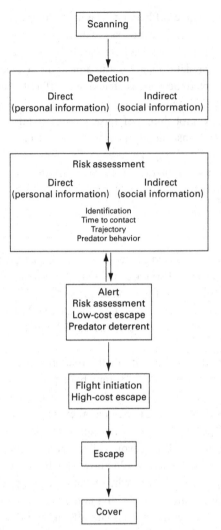

Figure 12.1   Sequence of events, from the perspective of prey, to avoid predation.

The mutual-exclusivity assumption has deeply shaped the way in which behavioral biologists measure scanning behavior (Caro 2005). The most commonly recorded parameters have been (a) the rate at which an animal goes head-up from a head-down position (e.g., scanning rate), and (b) the duration of time (raw or proportional) the animal stays in the head-up position (e.g., scan bout length). However, while the animal is head-up, it cannot gather information 360° around its head due to the constraints imposed by its visual field configuration (i.e., blind area at the rear of the head; Figure 12.2). For instance, in some studies comparing two species, the one with a wider blind area allocated more time to head-up scanning (Guillemain et al. 2002; Tisdale & Fernández-Juricic 2009) likely to compensate for the lower detection ability

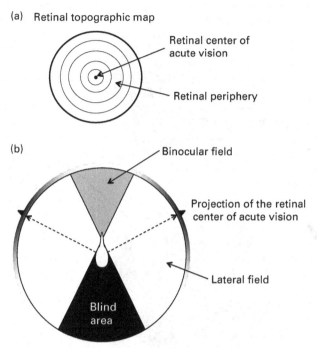

(a) Retinal topographic map

Retinal center of
acute vision

Retinal periphery

(b)

Binocular field

Projection of the retinal
center of acute vision

Lateral field

Blind
area

Figure 12.2 Retinal and visual field configuration. (a) Retinal topographic map showing changes in retinal cell density (photoreceptors, ganglion cells) with isoclines. In this schematic representation, cell density increases from the retinal periphery toward the center of the retina where the spot of highest cell density lies (i.e., center of acute vision). The center of acute vision will provide higher visual resolution than the retinal periphery (see Figure 12.3 for an example). (b) Top-view schematic representation of the visual field configuration of a bird. The binocular field represents the overlap of the lateral fields of the right and left eyes and the blind area at the rear of the head provides no visual input. The center of acute vision projects into the lateral fields but not into the binocular field. Also shown in grayscale are the changes in retinal cell density (photoreceptors, ganglion cells) around the visual field (darker values indicate higher cell densities).

at the back of its head (Kaby & Lind 2003; Devereux *et al.* 2006). A new scanning metric has been proposed, head movement rate, which is more sensory based because it captures the process of using vision for information gathering while head-up, particularly in species with laterally-placed eyes (Jones *et al.* 2007; Fernández-Juricic *et al.* 2011a; Fernández-Juricic 2012). To better interpret the variation in head-movement behavior, we need to understand some basic properties of the vertebrate eye.

From a visual perspective, scanning while head-up (i.e., through head movements) is similar to a visual search task that involves searching for an object of interest (a predator) in the visual background when that object is not detectable (Land 1999). Visual search is akin to taking a sequence of snapshots (one per each head or eye position) around the head with each retina. Every snapshot, however, is not like a regular picture with high definition throughout it (Figure 12.3). The retina is configured in such a way that there is usually (at least) one area of acute vision (e.g., a fovea) surrounded by areas that

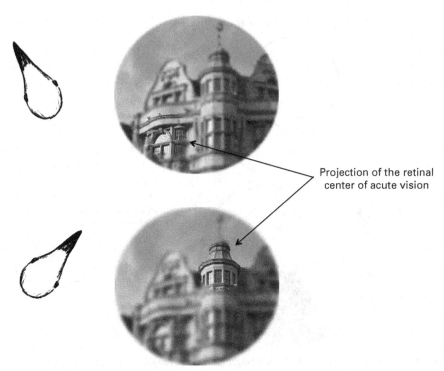

Projection of the retinal
center of acute vision

Figure 12.3   Schematic representation of how changes in head position vary the spatial position of the
projection of the retinal center of acute vision for right lateral visual field. The center of acute
vision provides high-quality visual information, but the retinal periphery provides lower quality
information due to variations in the cell density (photoreceptors, ganglion cells) across the retina
(see Figure 12.2).

provide less acute vision (the retinal periphery; Figure 12.2). The center of acute vision
generally has a high density of cones (which work under daylight conditions) and a low
density of rods (which work at night) (McIlwain 1996). The periphery of the retina
usually has the reversed pattern of cone vs. rod photoreceptor density. Cones and rods
transfer the information from the retina to the visual centers of the brain through the
retinal ganglion cells, whose nuclei are part of the retina and whose axons form the optic
nerve (McIlwain 1996).

In general, the relative size of the retinal center of acute vision is much smaller than
the rest of the retina (Figure 12.2). This means that at each snapshot obtained by the
retina, a small proportion of the visual space is at high resolution, but most of it is at low
resolution (Figure 12.3). The behavioral implication is that animals need to move the
retinas around to get a sufficient number of snapshots with high visual resolution per unit
time to cover the visual space around their heads (Figure 12.3). The retinas are moved
around through eye and/or head movements. In general, head-movement rates increase
when the perceived risk of predation increases, likely to visually search more actively for
the position of the potential threat (Fernández-Juricic *et al.* 2011a; Randolet *et al.* 2014).

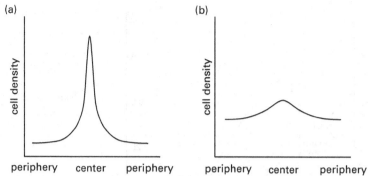

Figure 12.4 Schematic representation of cell density profiles across the retina (i.e., photoreceptors/ganglion cells). (a) Steep cell-density profiles have high peak cell densities within the center of acute vision, but decrease rapidly toward the retinal periphery. At a given eye size, steep cell-density profiles are expected to provide high visual resolution in a small retinal area, but lower resolution in the periphery. (b) Shallow cell-density profiles generally have relatively lower peak cell densities within the center of acute vision, but cell densities decrease slowly toward the retinal periphery. At a given eye size, shallow cell-density profiles are expected to provide high visual resolution over a relatively larger retinal area, with a comparatively lower change in visual resolution from the periphery to the center of acute vision.

Recent studies have suggested that variation in the density of photoreceptors and retinal ganglion cells from the retinal periphery to the retinal center of acute vision (Figure 12.2) could influence scanning behavior (Dolan & Fernández-Juricic 2010). These changes in cell density across the retina are known as cell density profiles, and can take different shapes (Figure 12.4). For instance, a steep change in cell density (Figure 12.2a) would make individuals rely mostly on their retinal center of acute vision (rather than the periphery) to gather information, which could increase the rate of eye/head movements to gather sufficient high-quality visual information per unit time. On the other hand, a shallow change in cell density (Figure 12.2b) would allow individuals to rely not only on their center of acute vision, but also partly on the retinal periphery, providing a larger proportion of retina with high-quality visual information, thereby reducing the rate of eye/head movements. For instance, California towhees *Melozone crissalis*, with relatively steeper cell density profiles, have been shown to have higher head movement rates than white-crowned sparrows *Zonotrichia leucophrys*, which have relatively shallower cell density profiles (Fernández-Juricic *et al.* 2011b). This type of variation in retinal configuration could have implications for head-up scanning and hence predator detection. For instance, if a species with a steep retinal cell density profile reduces its eye/head movement rate, it could decrease the chances of predator detection because of the fewer retinal snapshots collected per unit time and the smaller retinal area with high visual resolution within each snapshot (Fernández-Juricic 2012; Figure 12.3).

12.2.2   Detection

The sensory capabilities of an animal are likely to influence three aspects of predator detection: (1) the probability of early predator detection; (2) the maximum detection

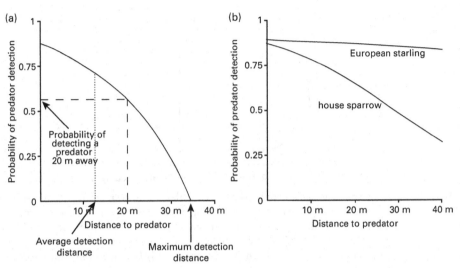

Figure 12.5   Probability of predator detection as a function of distance to predator. (a) The probability of detecting a predator (y) can be calculated for any given distance (x). The non-linear nature of the relationship is due to the non-linear decrease in visual contrast over distance. When the area under the curve is equal on both sides of the dotted line, the dotted line represents the average detection distance. (b) Empirical data showing higher detection probabilities over greater distances in the European starling (high overall visual resolution) than the house sparrow (low overall visual resolution). (Figure adapted from Tisdale & Fernández-Juricic 2009).

distance; and (3) the average detection distance (Figure 12.5a). Maximum detection distance refers to the distance at which prey could detect a given predator with its acute center of vision (high-quality information), whereas average detection distance refers to the average distance at which prey could detect a given predator with any part of the retina (high- and low-quality information pooled together). There are two relevant visual resolution dimensions that may affect these three aspects of predator detection, but not necessarily in the same way. First, detection has been proposed to depend on *overall* visual resolution (Tisdale & Fernández-Juricic 2009), which refers to the average resolution across the whole visual field as determined by the size of the eye (i.e., larger eyes have higher acuity, Pettigrew *et al.* 1988) and the average density of photoreceptors/ganglion cells across the whole retina. Second, detection has been proposed to depend on cell-density profiles, which are determined by the variation in relative cell density between the retinal center of acute vision and the retinal periphery (Dolan & Fernández-Juricic 2010, Fernández-Juricic *et al.* 2011b; Fernández-Juricic 2012; Figure 12.4).

We propose a novel way of representing in space how the visual configuration can influence detection behavior with *spatial detection maps*, which can be particularly useful to predict spatial variations in perceived predation risk for different species (Figure 12.6). Spatial detection maps provide a top-view schematic representation of the areas around the animal where the probabilities of predator detection are higher as a function of (a) the configuration of the visual fields; (b) the position of the centers of

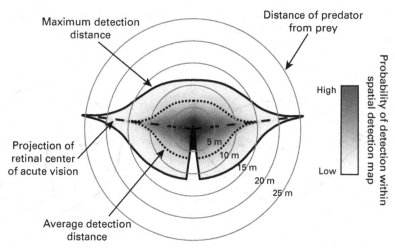

Figure 12.6 Spatial detection map. The solid gray lines provide a scale for the distance from the prey. The maximum detection distance a prey (center) is capable of, for a given predator, is bounded by the solid black line. The grayscale within the detection map represents the probability of detection at any given location within the detection map. The dotted line corresponds to the average detection distance around the prey, and the dashed line represents the projection of the prey's retinal center of acute vision.

acute vision; (c) the cell-density profiles; and (d) the variation in visual contrast and resolution with distance. Spatial detection maps are bounded by the maximum detection distance for any given area of the visual field (black continuous line in Figure 12.6), which is estimated based on the limits of visual resolution by eye size and cell density. The maximum detection distance is expected to vary in different parts of the visual field (binocular, lateral, blind areas), reflecting changes in cell density across the retina (Figures 12.2, 12.4). The highest values of the maximum detection distance (farthest detection point from the prey) are constrained in space and given by the projections of the centers of acute vision into visual space (Figure 12.6). Average detection distance for any given position in the visual field is represented by the dotted line inside the detection map. The probability of detection at any given point *within* the spatial detection map is represented by grayscale shading (Figure 12.6) and represents the decrease in visual contrast and visual resolution with increasing distances (Tisdale & Fernández-Juricic 2009). The probability of detection within a given distance range is represented by the proportional area of that range within the spatial detection map weighted by the average probability of detection within that distance range.

We can make predictions on the variations in the shape of spatial detection maps based on some of the visual properties discussed in the previous section (Figure 12.7). For the sake of clarity, we present different scenarios, but without considering changes in the probability of detection within the spatial detection maps (grayscale in Figure 12.6).

Species with higher overall visual resolution are expected to have greater probability of predator detection and greater maximum and average detection distances because

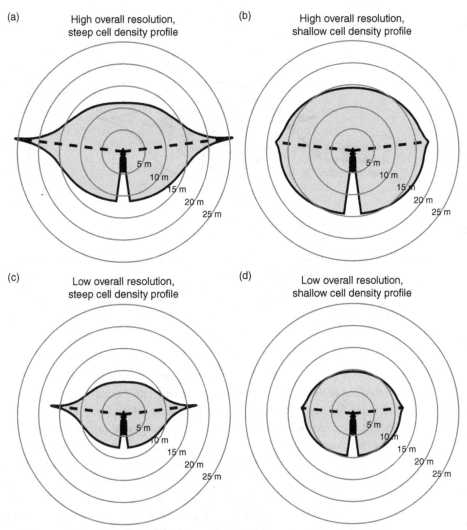

Figure 12.7 Hypothetical spatial detection maps for animals with (a) high overall visual resolution and steep cell-density profile; (b) high overall resolution and shallow cell-density profile; (c) low overall resolution and steep profile; and (d) low overall resolution and shallow profile. Blind areas were kept constant for clarity purposes.

they can see predators from farther away (Kiltie 2000; Tisdale & Fernández-Juricic 2009). For example, Tisdale and Fernández-Juricic (2009) found that European starlings *Sturnus vulgaris* (overall visual resolution = 5.9 cycles/degree; Dolan & Fernández-Juricic 2010) have higher probabilities of detection and greater detection distances than house sparrows *Passer domesticus* (overall visual resolution = 4.5 cycles/degree; Dolan & Fernández-Juricic 2010; Figure 12.5b). Differences in overall visual resolution between species can be translated into spatial detection maps. For instance, consider scenarios (b) and (d) in Figure 12.7. Scenario (b) represents an individual with higher overall visual resolution than that in scenario (d), which translates into maximum detection distances around 18 m and average detection distances around 15 m for (b) and 12 m and 10 m, respectively, for (d). Likewise, the detection map in (b) covers 92% of the area between 10 and 15 m, suggesting a high probability of detecting a predator that appears anywhere between 10 and 15 m. In scenario (d), on the other hand, the detection map only covers 8% of the area between 10 and 15 m, giving the individual a much lower probability of predator detection.

Species with steep cell-density profiles are expected to have greater maximum detection distances than species with shallow cell-density profiles, but similar average detection distances assuming that species do not vary in overall (or average) visual resolution. To illustrate these predictions, Figure 12.7a shows a species with a steep cell-density profile and Figure 12.7b one with a shallow density profile. Scenario (a) portrays a maximum detection distance greater than 25 m, whereas in scenario (b) maximum detection distance is around 18 m. Both (a) and (b) have average detection distances around 15 m, but those averages come about in very different ways. In scenario (b), the detection distance is relatively consistent throughout the visual field, whereas in scenario (a) detection distance is higher in the parts of the visual field subtended by the centers of acute vision and lower in the parts of the visual field subtended by the retinal periphery. The inconsistency in detection distances could lead to the species in scenario (a) actually having lower probability of early detection. While the species in scenario (a) could potentially detect a predator from greater than 25 m away, it only has a 56% probability of detecting a predator that appears 10 to 15 m away, compared to 92% for the species in scenario (b). Therefore prey with steep cell-density profiles (Figure 12.7a) are expected to become more reliant on their centers of acute vision for predator detection. This retinal configuration may be most advantageous in environments where predators approach from predictable locations that can be consistently monitored. For example, many predators attack from cover (Lima et al. 1987; Roth & Lima 2007), and therefore prey in habitats with limited cover can focus on monitoring only the most likely areas of attack. On the other hand, shallow cell-density profiles may be more advantageous for detecting predators that could come from anywhere (Hughes 1977).

Prey with wider visual fields, and thus smaller blind areas, are expected to have higher probabilities of predator detection because they can see more of their environment at any given time than prey with narrower visual fields (Fernández-Juricic et al. 2004; Tisdale & Fernández-Juricic 2009). For instance, blue tits, Cyanistes cyaneus, have a lower probability of detection when a predator appears in their blind areas (Kaby & Lind 2003). Figure 12.8 shows why prey with narrower blind areas would be able to detect a predator in more different head orientations than a prey with wider blind areas.

Prey that are more sensitive to motion are also expected to be better able to detect predator movements and thus have higher probabilities of early detection. There are two independent mechanisms that each could yield greater motion detection ability: temporal visual resolution and the abundance of photoreceptors associated with motion vision. A higher temporal visual resolution is the result of shorter photoreceptor integration times yielding more frequent updating of the visual image on the retina (Legge 1978). Therefore

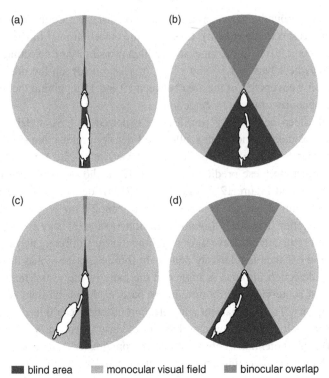

blind area   monocular visual field   binocular overlap

Figure 12.8 Eyes in the back of the head. The circles in this figure represent the visual field parameters, as viewed from above, of two hypothetical hares (at center of the circle) when being chased by a lynx (at bottom of the circle). (a) A hare with a small blind area can partially see a predator directly behind it. (b) A hare with a large blind area cannot see a predator directly behind. (c) A hare with a small blind area can see a predator in a more lateral position. (d) A hare with a large blind area cannot always see the predator, even when the predator is not directly behind it.

temporal visual resolution plays a major role in motion detection, especially in detecting fast moving objects (Lappin *et al.* 2009) such as predators. Avian double cone photoreceptors have been associated with motion-detection ability in studies using physiological (von Campenhausen & Kirschfeld 1998) and behavioral approaches (Goldsmith & Butler 2005). Double cones are abundant in most vertebrate retinas (Walls 1942; Bowmaker 1990; Hart 2001a). In European starlings, for example, double cones outnumber all four types of single cones combined (Hart *et al.* 1998). More double cones in the retina would confer more acute motion detection ability because a moving image would pass across more double cone photoreceptors per unit time. For example, bird species that have unobstructed overhead vision (in open habitats) have more double cones in the ventral retina, which projects upward, where aerial predators are likely to come from; whereas species with obstructed overhead vision (e.g., arboreal species with branches overhead) have more double cones in the dorsal retina, which projects downward, where ground predators would initiate attacks (Hart 2001b). We expect visual systems with higher temporal visual resolution or more double cones to be more sensitive to motion and increase the probability of early predator detection.

Ultimately, the brain prioritizes how the different components of the information gathered by the visual system are processed through attention mechanisms, which involve selectively allocating cognitive resources to a specific portion of visual field with specific stimuli. Attention is limited because the amount of information received by the sensory systems is greater than the amount of information that can be processed by the brain (Milinski 1990; Kastner & Ungerleider 2000; Dukas 2002). The probability of detection is expected to decrease when an individual is not allocating attention to the sensory modality or region of sensory space within the modality where the predator becomes detectable (Dukas 2002). Interestingly, there are two main attention mechanisms that occur in different parts of the retina (center of acute vision vs. retinal periphery). Overt visual attention takes place with the center of acute vision, whereas covert visual attention occurs in the retinal periphery (Bisley 2011). Animals often use overt visual attention; for instance, if a moving stimulus is detected with the retinal periphery, the eye/head will move very quickly to align the center of acute vision with that stimulus to obtain an image with higher visual resolution (hence, higher information quality; Zani & Proverbio 2012; Yorzinski & Platt 2014; Figure 12.3). For example, peafowl, *Pavo cristatus*, appear to inspect model predators with their centers of acute vision after detection with the retinal periphery (Yorzinski & Platt 2014).

The allocation of cognitive resources between overt and covert attention could also vary with the nature of the task, and ultimately influence predator detection. For instance, blue jays, *Cyanocitta cristata,* focused on solving a complex task (e.g., discriminating prey from a visually complex background) have more difficulty detecting predators elsewhere in their visual fields (Dukas & Kamil 2000). This effect could be the result of an increase in overt attention at the expense of covert attention. Additionally, in species with laterally placed eyes, individuals appear to attend to only one eye at a time and simultaneously suppress input from the unattended eye. However, information processing still occurs in the retina of the unattended eye because suppression acts on specific visual centers in the brain (tectofugal pathway), not on the retina itself (Engelage & Bischof 1988; Voss & Bischof 2003). Therefore the appearance of a salient object in the visual field of the unattended eye may be able to override the central suppression and redirect attention to the previously unattended eye (Voss & Bischof 2003). If this is the case, a predator moving across the visual field of an unattended eye is more likely to override attentional suppression if the prey species has a greater abundance of motion sensitive photoreceptors because the predator's movement will stimulate more photoreceptors.

12.2.3   Assessing predation risk

After a stimulus has been detected, the sensory systems are far from done. Prey continue gathering information with their sensory systems to assess the risk of a potential threat. Prey modify their perception of risk depending on predator identity, predator behavior, how long they have before the predator can strike, and if detected through conspecifics/heterospecifics, whether a predator is even present (Lima & Dill 1990). Escape behaviors are energetically costly and, perhaps more importantly, reduce foraging and mating opportunities. Fitness-wise, it would be in an animal's best interest to only flee when the probability of mortality is high. To that end, sensory systems that gather information more accurately are expected to reduce the incidence of mistakes when deciding on an escape response, and sensory systems that gather information more quickly or from greater distances are expected to give prey more time to respond to a predator.

From a sensory perspective, it is not totally clear how assessment translates into behavioral changes. One of the reasons is that an individual may be engaged in both sensory assessment and other activities (e.g., foraging) simultaneously without necessarily modifying its behavior. For instance, given the wide visual field of birds and the lateral projection of the foveae in many species (Fernández-Juricic 2012), it is likely that birds could assess a potential threat from a head-down body posture if the risk is not too high. Consequently, we could consider different levels of sensory assessment: low quality and high quality. Low-quality sensory assessment is expected to occur when the animal is in a body posture not intended for gaining a large amount of information about the threat (e.g., head down) and/or using portions of the visual field that do not provide high visual resolution (e.g., retinal periphery). High-quality assessment, on the other hand, is expected in head-up body postures and/or using the centers of acute vision as individuals can enhance the amount and quality of visual information obtained. For example, *Sceloporus* lizards that detect predators with the peripheral retina flee a short distance to put space between themselves and the predator, then stop and assess the predation risk with high-quality information before seeking cover (Cooper 2008). The implication is that establishing the duration of assessment (and consequently its costs) would require measurements that go beyond classic behavioral responses (Cresswell *et al.* 2009) and consider the sensory systems of the study species (e.g., eye-tracking for birds; Yorzinski & Platt 2014; Tyrrell *et al.* 2014).

A major step in assessing predation risk is the identification of a detected stimulus as a predator or a non-predator. Identification requires a sufficient level of sensory acuity to distinguish certain characteristics of the stimulus. For example, mallards *Anas platyrhynchos* characterize a silhouette with a short neck and long tail as a predator (e.g., a hawk) and a silhouette with a long neck and short tail as a non-predator (e.g., a goose) (Green *et al.* 1968). Identification of predators is likely to be dependent on the centers of acute vision because prey orient them toward predators (after detection) rather than assessing the predator with the retinal periphery (Yorzinski & Platt 2014). Therefore, species with higher localized visual resolution are expected to have higher identification distances. Additionally, because predators that are farther away take more time to reach prey, higher localized visual resolution would allow prey to gather information for longer times before making decisions to flee. The distance at which an animal detects a stimulus (hereafter, detection distance) will be greater than the distance at which it can identify the stimulus (hereafter, identification distance). Prey may not react to a predator until it is close enough to identify, or prey may actually approach the predator to identify it (Magurran & Girling 1986).

In addition to identification, prey estimate time to contact (the amount of time it will take the predator to reach the prey's current position), trajectory (whether the predator is approaching the prey directly or tangentially), and the motivational state of the predator to assess the actual risk of predation (Lima & Dill 1990). Time to contact informs the prey how long it has before it can no longer safely flee to cover (Regan & Vincent 1995). In the visual system, time to contact and predator trajectory appear to be estimated by the rate and symmetry of image expansion on the retina, respectively (looming; Regan & Vincent 1995). As an object approaches the viewer, the image of that object will expand on the retina. Faster rates of image expansion correspond to objects that will come in contact with the viewer more quickly. If the image expands symmetrically, the object can be interpreted as approaching the viewer directly. If the image expands asymmetrically, the object is approaching at an angle, and it is moving slightly sideways in the direction of greater expansion rather than directly toward the viewer. There is evidence across many taxa that animals associate looming stimuli with predation (Schaller & Emlen 1962; Schiff 1965; Hassenstein & Hustert 1999; Carlile *et al.* 2006).

12.2.4   Alert and escape

Most animals display some kind of alert behavior (e.g., cease foraging, head movement, extended neck) after detection, but before fleeing. Alert distance has been associated with the detection of a threat (Fernández-Juricic & Schroeder 2003; Blumstein *et al.* 2005). The rationale is that prey are expected to switch to an alert posture (i.e., from foraging head-down to scanning head-up) immediately after detection. This leads to the prediction that alert distance (AD) would be similar to detection distance. However, a recent study considering the visual system of prey has challenged this view. Blackwell *et al.* (2009) estimated detection distances of brown-headed cowbirds and mourning doves *Zenaida macroura* based on eye size and the density of retinal ganglion cells as 1012 m and 1363 m, respectively (under optimal light conditions). The authors also measured ADs behaviorally toward a vehicle approaching them directly, and found that they were an order of magnitude smaller (71 m and 105 m, respectively). This suggests that animals detect early but do not show alert behaviors until later in the approach sequence. The two implications are that (a) sensory detection is difficult to measure behaviorally, and (b) detection and alert distances are not necessarily identical.

Another metric that has been linked to detection and alert is starting distance (SD). Some papers have explicitly assumed that SD is higher than AD (i.e., prey do not exhibit alert before the approach begins; Dumont *et al.* 2012). Such assumptions consider that SD is higher than detection distance. However, as mentioned before, detection distance may be greater than SD and different sensory configurations could lead to different probabilities of detection after the approach begins. Violating these assumptions may lead to erroneous interpretations of the decision-making processes involved in antipredator responses.

Alert behaviors themselves may function as an assessment phase (Cresswell *et al.* 2009), but for the most part, the sensory functions of alert have not been empirically tested. We do not know when the prey gathers much of the information used for assessment, but it is possible that such information is gathered before becoming alert, after becoming alert, or both. The timing of risk assessment in relation to alert behavior could lead to different functions and costs of alert behavior, as well as differences in the expected slopes of the positive relationship observed between AD and FID (Blumstein *et al.* 2005; Dumont *et al.* 2012).

If risk assessment occurs after prey display overt alert behaviors, then the function of alert may be stabilization of gaze to visually track the predator and gather information to estimate risk. In this case, alert becomes a costly activity as it diverts attention and time from foraging. If assessment requires a certain amount of time, then we would predict a shallower slope in the positive relationship between AD and FID (Blumstein *et al.* 2005; Dumont *et al.* 2012), all else being equal. The reason is because the time invested in alert would constrain the time the individual has to flee.

The opposite scenario is that an individual assesses risk before becoming overtly alert. In this case, alert behavior might not serve a sensory function at all, but rather it is simply a signal to the predator reflecting that the prey is aware of its presence (e.g., pursuit detterence; Hasson 2000; Caro 2005) or a low-cost escape attempt (e.g., becoming stationary to reduce movement cues about its position; Misslin 2003) before the individual resorts to a high-cost escape attempt. This scenario would lead to a steeper slope in the positive relationship between AD and FID (Blumstein *et al.* 2005; Dumont *et al.* 2012), all else being equal. Individuals would be able to quickly flee right after alert, if the situation is risky enough, without investing time in assessment at that point.

A third scenario is that prey have acquired some limited measure of risk assessment before displaying alert behavior. For instance, before becoming alert, an individual could gather some low-quality information while in a head-down posture or with the periphery of the retina. This initial low-quality stage will have low attention costs, allowing the individual to continue with other important tasks (e.g., foraging). By having some limited information available before devoting a large amount of sensory resources to the predator, individuals would be able to make an initial decision as to whether the predator was threatening enough to become alert or not. After making the decision to become alert, individuals would then be able to gather higher quality information while head-up and with the centers of acute vision (Yorzinski & Platt 2014). The higher quality assessment phase would obviously have higher attention costs (Blumstein 2010), but would allow for a more accurate estimation of the level of risk before escaping or resuming foraging. This scenario would lead to an intermediate slope in the positive relationship between AD and FID (Blumstein *et al.* 2005; Dumont *et al.* 2012), all else being equal, because low- and high-quality assessment may require certain amounts of time.

12.3   Implications for predator–prey interactions

From a sensory perspective, the prey's ultimate goal is to detect predators before being detected and to assess their level of risk to determine if they are (1) in danger and should flee, or (2) safe from predation and should resume other activities. However, there appears to be variability between prey species in detection distances due to the configuration of the sensory systems (Kiltie 2000). Prey with greater long-distance

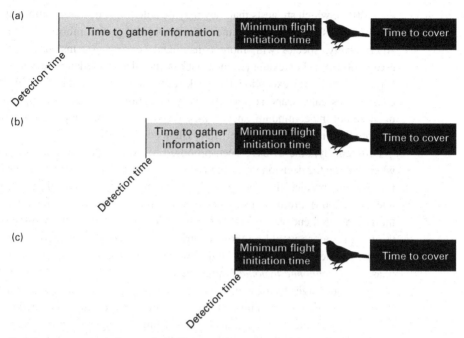

Figure 12.9   Sensory systems can influence the ability to make correct decisions when assessing predation risk. In this figure, detection time refers to the moment the prey first detects a potential predator. The length of the black bar to the right of the bird represents the amount of time it will take for the bird to flee to cover. The black bar to the left of the bird (minimum flight initiation time) represents the last possible moment in time that the bird can safely flee to cover. The length of the gray bar represents the amount of time the bird has to assess the likelihood of an attack. Species with more sensitive or acute sensory organs (a) can detect potential predators sooner, and therefore have more time to gather additional information than prey whose sensory organs have lower detection ranges (b). For a prey whose sensory organs do not detect the predator until close to minimum flight initiation time (e.g., surprise predator attack), detection time must be only slightly greater than or equal to minimum flight initiation time if the prey is to escape (c).

sensory detection abilities can gather information for a longer period of time before making a decision to flee (Figure 12.9a). However, prey with short-distance sensory detection abilities will have less time to gather the same information (Figure 12.9b), potentially leading to a scenario where time to contact is shorter than the time it takes to identify and flee from a predator (Figure 12.9c). This brings up an interesting question: how do species with more constrained sensory systems successfully avoid predators? There is a continuum of potential (non-mutually exclusive) explanations that should be investigated in the future. On one end of the continuum, prey with more constrained sensory systems and thus less time to engage in assessment may trade-off with other sensory modalities (or dimensions within a given modality) or components of the antipredator behavior sequence (Figure 12.1). For instance, species with smaller body mass tend to have lower spatial visual resolution because of smaller eye sizes (Kiltie 2000), reducing detection distances, and hence detection times (Figure 12.9b). However, a recent study found that smaller species have higher temporal visual resolution (Healy *et al.* 2013), which suggests that they may be able to get necessary information about a predator in a shorter period of time because they can gather information at a faster rate. Alternatively, species with more constrained sensory systems may have enhanced escape abilities. For example, cockroaches that detect predators at very close range (Figure 12.9c) have exceptionally quick response times (Camhi *et al.* 1978). Because cockroaches can escape so quickly, early detection becomes less important. On the other end of the continuum, species may forgo assessment completely and flee as soon as a predator is detected (Figure 12.9c; Blumstein, 2010).

Different hypotheses have been proposed to explain the rules animals may follow when making the decision to stay and assess or to flee. The *perceptual limits hypothesis*, for example, predicts that species will detect a predator and immediately flee (Quinn & Cresswell 2005). From a sensory perspective, the perceptual limits hypothesis excludes the risk-assessment phase. Therefore, the relevant sensory dimensions that influence the prey response would be those contributing to detection of predators (see above). Other hypotheses, however, make different predictions but consider a risk-assessment phase. The *economic hypothesis* predicts that prey will delay fleeing until the risk of predation outweighs the benefits of continuing other tasks (Ydenberg & Dill 1986). The *optimality hypothesis* is similar to the economic hypothesis, but predicts that prey will flee when the accrued fitness gains from staying are optimized, whereas the economic hypothesis predicts flight when fitness gains and losses break even (Cooper and Frederick 2007). The *flush early and avoid the rush* (FEAR) *hypothesis* predicts that prey will only delay fleeing for a short time because the attention costs of tracking a predator can outweigh the costs of fleeing early and losing foraging time (Blumstein 2010). Therefore the major difference between the optimality and FEAR hypotheses is the cost of attention associated with the risk-assessment phase (Cooper & Blumstein 2014). From a sensory perspective, we could expect species that can minimize the attention costs associated with risk assessment (e.g., wide visual fields that can take advantage of tracking the predator with the periphery of the retina through lateral vision while simultaneously engaging in other tasks) to fall on the optimality hypothesis end of the spectrum. Conversely, species with very high attention costs (e.g., narrow visual fields that require ceasing other tasks to track the predator with the centers of acute vision) would fall on the FEAR hypothesis end of the spectrum.

Overall, many of the sensory mechanisms underlying predator–prey interactions remain poorly understood, presenting a largely unexplored avenue to investigate many proximate as well as ultimate questions about the sensory basis for escape behavior. Future studies could also benefit from a comparative approach to understand the important environmental factors that drive differences in the sensory ecology and antipredator behaviors across taxa.

References

Beauchamp, G. (2014). *Social Predation: How Group Living Benefits Predators and Prey.* London: Academic Press.

Beauchamp, G. & Ruxton, G. D. (2007). False alarms and the evolution of antipredator vigilance. *Animal Behaviour*, **74**, 1199–1206.

Bisley, J. W. (2011). The neural basis of visual attention. *Journal of Physiology*, **589**, 49–57.

Blackwell, B. F., Fernández-Juricic, E., Seamans, T. W. & Dolan, T. (2009). Avian visual system configuration and behavioural response to object approach. *Animal Behaviour*, **77**, 673–684.

Blumstein, D. T. (2010). Flush early and avoid the rush: a general rule of antipredator behavior? *Behavioral Ecology*, **21**, 440–442.

Blumstein, D. T., Fernández-Juricic, E., Zollner, P. A. & Garity, S. C. (2005). Interspecific variation in avian responses to human disturbance. *Journal of Applied Ecology*, **42**, 943–953.

Bowmaker, J. K. (1990). Visual pigments of fishes. In Douglas, R. H. & Djamgoz, M. B. A. (eds.) *The Visual System of Fish*. London: Chapman and Hall, pp. 81–104.

Camhi, J. M., Tom, W. & Volman, S. (1978). The escape behavior of the cockroach *Periplaneta americana*. *Journal of Comparative Physiology A*, **12**, 203–212.

Carlile, P. A., Peters, R. A. & Evans, C. S. (2006). Detection of a looming stimulus by the Jacky dragon: Selective sensitivity to characteristics of an aerial predator. *Animal Behaviour*, **72**, 553–562.

Caro, T. (2005). *Antipredator Defenses in Birds and Mammals*. Chicago, IL: University of Chicago Press.

Cooper, W. E. Jr. (2008). Visual monitoring of predators: occurrence, cost and benefit for escape. *Animal Behaviour*, **76**, 1365–1372.

Cooper, W. E. Jr. & Blumstein, D. T. (2014). Novel effects of monitoring predators on costs of fleeing and not fleeing explain flushing early in economic escape theory. *Behavioral Ecology*, **25**, 44–52.

Cooper, W. E. Jr. & Frederick, W. G. (2007). Optimal flight initiation distance. *Journal of Theoretical Biology*, **244**, 59–67.

Cresswell, W., Quinn, J. L., Whittingham, M. J. & Butler, S. (2003). Good foragers can also be good at detecting predators. *Proceedings of the Royal Society of London B*, **270**, 1069–1076.

Cresswell, W., Butler, S., Whittingham, M. J. & Quinn, J. L. (2009). Very short delays prior to escape from potential predators may function efficiently as adaptive risk-assessment periods. *Behaviour*, **146**, 795–813.

Cronin, T. W. (2005). The visual ecology of predator–prey interactions. In Barbosa, P. & Castellanos, I. (eds.) *Ecology of Predator–prey Interactions*. Oxford: Oxford University Press, pp. 105–138.

Devereux, C. L., Whittingham, M. J., Fernández-Juricic, E., Vickery, J. A. & Krebs, J. R. (2006). Predator detection and avoidance by starlings under differing scenarios of predation risk. *Behavioral Ecology*, **17**, 303–309.

Dolan, T. & Fernández-Juricic, E. (2010). Retinal ganglion cell topography of five species of ground-foraging birds. *Brain, Behavior and Evolution*, **75**, 111–121.

Dukas, R. (2002). Behavioural and ecological consequences of limited attention. *Philosophical Transactions of the Royal Society B: Biological Sciences*, **357**, 1539–1547.

Dukas, R. & Kamil, A. C. (2000). The cost of limited attention in blue jays. *Behavioral Ecology*, **11**, 502–506.

Dumont, F., Pasquaretta, C., Réale, D., Bogliani, G. & von Hardenberg, A. (2012). Flight initiation distance and starting distance: Biological effect or mathematical artefact? *Ethology*, **118**, 1051–1062.

Engelage, J. & Bischof, H.-J. (1988). Enucleation enhances ipsilateral flash evoked respones in the ectostriatum of the zebra finch (*Taeniopyia guttata castanotis* Gould). *Experimental Brain Research*, **70**, 79–89.

Fernández-Juricic, E. (2012). Sensory basis of vigilance behavior in birds: Synthesis and future prospects. *Behavioural Processes*, **89**, 143–152.

Fernández-Juricic, E. & Schroeder, N. (2003). Do variations in scanning behavior affect tolerance to human disturbance? *Applied Animal Behaviour Science*, **84**, 219–234.

Fernández-Juricic, E., Erichsen, J. T. & Kacelnik, A. (2004). Visual perception and social foraging in birds. *Trends in Ecology & Evolution*, **19**, 25–31.

Fernández-Juricic, E., Gall, M. D., Dolan, T., Tisdale, V. & Martin, G. R. (2008). The visual fields of two ground-foraging birds, house finches and house sparrows, allow for simultaneous foraging and anti-predator vigilance. *Ibis*, **150**, 779–787.

Fernández-Juricic, E., Gall, M. D., Dolan, T. *et al.* (2011a). Visual systems and vigilance behaviour of two ground-foraging avian prey species: White-crowned sparrows and California towhees. *Animal Behaviour*, **81**, 705–713.

Fernández-Juricic, E., Beauchamp, G., Treminio, R. & Hoover, M. (2011b). Making heads turn: Association between head movements during vigilance and perceived predation risk in brown-headed cowbird flocks. *Animal Behaviour*, **82**, 573–577.

Goldsmith, T. H. & Butler, B. K. (2005). Color vision of the budgerigar (*Melopsittacus undulatus*): Hue matches, tetrachromacy, and intensity discrimination. *Journal of Comparative Physiology A*, **191**, 933–951.

Green, R., Carr, W. J. & Green, M. (1968). The hawk-goose phenomenon: Further confirmation and a search for the releaser. *Journal of Psychology*, **69**, 271–276.

Guillemain, M., Martin, G. R. & Fritz, H. (2002). Feeding methods, visual fields and vigilance in dabbling ducks (Anatidae). *Functional Ecology*, **16**, 522–529.

Hart, N. S. (2001a). The visual ecology of avian photoreceptors. *Progress in Retinal and Eye Research*, **20**, 675–703.

Hart, N. S. (2001b). Variations in cone photoreceptor abundance and the visual ecology of birds. *Journal Of Comparative Physiology A*, **187**, 685–698.

Hart, N., Partridge, J. & Cuthill, I. (1998). Visual pigments, oil droplets and cone photoreceptor distribution in the European starling (*Sturnus vulgaris*). *Journal of Experimental Biology*, **201**, 1433–1446.

Hassenstein, B. & Hustert, R. (1999). Hiding responses of locusts to approaching objects. *Journal of Experimental Biology*, **202**, 1701–1710.

Hasson, O. (2000). Knowledge, information, biases and signal assemblages. In Espmark, Y., Amundsen, T. & Rosenqvist, G. (eds.) *Animal Signals: Signalling and Signal Design in Animal Communication*. Trondheim: Tapir Academic Press, pp. 445–463.

Healy, K., McNally, L., Ruxton, G. D., Cooper, N. & Jackson, A. L. (2013). Metabolic rate and body size are linked with perception of temporal information. *Animal Behaviour*, **86**, 685–696.

Hughes, A. (1977). The topography of vision in mammals of contrasting life style: Comparative optics and retinal organisation. In Crescittelli, F. (ed.) *Handbook of Sensory Physiology*. New York: Springer, pp. 613–756.

Jones, K. A., Krebs, J. R. & Whittingham, M. J. (2007). Vigilance in the third dimension: Head movement not scan duration varies in response to different predator models. *Animal Behaviour*, **74**, 1181–1187.

Kaby, U. & Lind, J. (2003). What limits predator detection in blue tits (*Parus caeruleus*): Posture, task or orientation? *Behavioral Ecology and Sociobiology*, **54**, 534–538.

Kastner, S. & Ungerleider, L. G. (2000). Mechanisms of visual attention in the human cortex. *Annual Review of Neuroscience*, **23**, 315–341.

Kiltie, R. A. (2000). Scaling of visual acuity with body size in mammals and birds. *Functional Ecology*, **14**, 226–234.

Krause, J. & Ruxton, G. D. (2002). *Living in Groups*. Oxford: Oxford University Press.

Land, M. F. (1999). Motion and vision: Why animals move their eyes. *Journal of Comparative Physiology A*, **185**, 341–352.

Lappin, J. S., Tadin, D., Nyquist, J. B. & Corn, A. L. (2009). Spatial and temporal limits of motion perception across variations in speed, eccentricity, and low vision. *Journal of Vision*, **9**, 1–14.

Legge, G. E. (1978). Sustained and transient mechanisms in human vision: Temporal and spatial properties. *Vision Research*, **18**, 69–81.

Lima, S. L. (1987). Vigilance while feeding and its relation to the risk of predation. *Journal of Theoretical Biology*, **124**, 303–316.

Lima, S. L. & Bednekoff, P. A. (1999). Back to the basics of antipredatory vigilance: Can nonvigilant animals detect attack? *Animal Behaviour*, **58**, 537–543.

Lima, S. L. & Dill, L. M. (1990). Behavioral decisions made under the risk of predation: a review and prospectus. *Canadian Journal of Zoology*, **68**, 619–634.

Lima, S. L., Wiebe, K. L. & Dill, L. M. (1987). Protective cover and the use of space by finches: is closer better? *Oikos*, **50**, 225–230.

Magal, C., Dangles, O., Caparroy, P. & Casas, J. (2006). Hair canopy of cricket sensory system tuned to predator signals. *Journal of Theoretical Biology*, **241**, 459–66.

Magurran, A. E. & Girling, S. L. (1986). Predator model recognition and response habituation in shoaling minnows. *Animal Behaviour*, **34**, 510–518.

Martin, G. R. (2014). The subtlety of simple eyes: The tuning of visual fields to perceptual challenges in birds. *Philosophical Transactions of the Royal Society B*, **369**, 20130040.

McIlwain, J. T. (1996). *An Introduction to the Biology of Vision*. Cambridge: Cambridge University Press.

Milinski, M. (1990). Information overload and food selection. In Hughes, R. N. (ed.) *Behavioural Mechanisms of Food Selection*. Berlin: Springer, pp. 721–737.

Misslin, R. (2003). The defense system of fear: behavior and neurocircuitry. *Clinical Nerophysiology*, **33**, 55–66.

Pettigrew, J. D., Dreher, B., Hopkins, C. S., McCall, M. J. & Brown, M. (1988). Peak density and distributions of ganglion cells in the retinae of microchiropteran bats: Implications for visual acuity. *Brain, Behavior and Evolution*, **32**, 39–56.

Phelps, S. M. (2007). Sensory ecology and perceptual allocation: New prospects for neural networks. *Philosophical Transactions of the Royal Society B*, **362**, 355–367.

Quinn, J. & Cresswell, W. (2005). Escape response delays in wintering redshank, *Tringa totanus*, flocks: Perceptual limits and economic decisions. *Animal Behaviour*, **69**, 1285–1292.

Randolet, J., Lucas, J. R. & Fernández-Juricic, E. (2014). Non-redundant social information use in avian flocks with multisensory stimuli. *Ethology*, **120**, 375–387.

Regan, D. & Vincent, A. (1995). Visual processing of looming and time to contact throughout the visual field. *Vision Research*, **35**, 1845–1857.

Roth, T. C. & Lima, S. L. (2007). The predatory behavior of wintering *Accipiter* hawks: Temporal patterns in activity of predators and prey. *Oecologia*, **152**, 169–178.

Schaller, G. B. & Emlen, J. T. (1962). The ontogeny of avoidance behaviour in some precocial birds. *Animal Behaviour*, **10**, 370–381.

Schiff, W. (1965). Perception of impending collision: A study of visual directed avoidant behavior. *Psychological Monographs*, **79**, 1–26.

Tisdale, V. & Fernández-Juricic, E. (2009). Vigilance and predator detection vary between avian species with different visual acuity and coverage. *Behavioral Ecology*, **20**, 936–945.

Tyrrell, L. P., Butler, S. R., Yorzinski, J. L. & Fernández-Juricic, E. (2014). A novel system for bi-ocular eye-tracking in vertebrates with laterally placed eyes. *Methods in Ecology and Evolution*, **5**, 1070–1077.

Von Campenhausen, M. & Kirschfeld, K. (1998). Spectral sensitivity of the accessory optic system of the pigeon. *Journal of Comparative Physiology A*, **183**, 1–6.

Voss, J. & Bischof, H.-J. (2003). Regulation of ipsilateral visual information within the tectofugal visual system in zebra finches. *Journal of Comparative Physiology A*, **189**, 545–553.

Walls, G. L. (1942). *The Vertebrate Eye and its Adaptive Radiation*. New York: Hafner.

Ydenberg, R. C. & Dill, L. M. (1986). The economics of fleeing from predators. *Advances in the Study of Behaviour*, **16**, 229–249.

Yorzinski, J. L. & Platt, M. L. (2014). Selective attention in peacocks during predator detection. *Animal Cognition*, **17**, 767–777.

Zani, A. & Proverbio, A. M. (2012). Is that a belt or a snake? Object attentional selection affects the early stages of visual sensory processing. *Behavioral and Brain Functions*, **8**, 6.

13 The physiology of escape

Yoav Litvin, D. Caroline Blanchard, and Robert J. Blanchard

13.1 Introduction

In this chapter we review physiological mechanisms and correlates of flight or escape behavior. Although aspects of the physiology of flight have been studied in many prey taxa, our knowledge of physiological mechanisms has largely been obtained in studies of rodents. In much of this book, the focus is on decisions to flee, especially the decision about how close to allow a predator to approach before beginning to flee. In a typical field study, this is measured as flight initiation distance (FID), the distance between an approaching predator and the prey when the prey starts to flee. In part because the vast majority of studies of the physiology of escape have been done in laboratories in small spaces, very little is known about physiological influences on FID. However, flight is one component of a complex array of defensive behaviors to predators and other threat stimuli that has been intensively investigated in recent years, and a substantial body of information has accumulated about the endocrine, pharmacological, and neuroanatomical systems involved in defense. These findings are outlined here.

13.2 Defensive behaviors and physiology

13.2.1 Defensive behaviors (see Figure 13.1 for summary)

Defensive behaviors comprise a group of immediate and direct behavioral reactions to threats to life and bodily safety (Blanchard *et al.* 2009). Many defensive behaviors are evolved responses to the types of stimuli and situations that were frequent dangers in the evolutionary histories of a species, evolving as a result of the survival/reproductive success that they afforded to individuals displaying them appropriately. In this context "appropriately" means not only that the defenses be well executed, but also that each individual defensive behavior is one that has been particularly successful in response to that particular type of threat, and in that particular type of situation. Flight, avoidance, freezing, defensive threat, defensive attack, and risk assessment to threatening stimuli have been characterized in a variety of species, as have some other behaviors, e.g.,

Escaping From Predators: An Integrative View of Escape Decisions, ed. W. E. Cooper and D. T. Blumstein. Published by Cambridge University Press. © Cambridge University Press 2015.

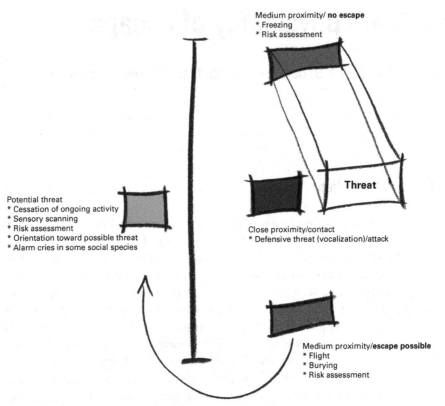

Medium proximity/ no escape
* Freezing
* Risk assessment

Threat

Potential threat
* Cessation of ongoing activity
* Sensory scanning
* Risk assessment
* Orientation toward possible threat
* Alarm cries in some social species

Close proximity/contact
* Defensive threat (vocalization)/attack

Medium proximity/escape possible
* Flight
* Burying
* Risk assessment

Figure 13.1   Fear- and anxiety-like defensive behaviors are modulated by subject–threat distance and context. Notably, the availability of escape enables flight, while its absence promotes freezing. (Used with permission from Litvin & Pfaff 2013)

burying of novel, aversive, or potentially dangerous objects, or alarm cries, that may be functional in particular threat situations (Blanchard 1997; Litvin *et al.* 2008).

13.2.2   Endocrine roles in defense

Evolution has shaped organisms that are adequately adapted to a dynamic, at times hostile, environment. The brain detects a stimulus from the environment, integrates it with internal states, and in response potentiates appropriate physiology and behavior. The process of maintaining a constant, stabile internal milieu in a changing setting is termed "allostasis" and the ability to continually adapt by learning appropriate behaviors indicates "resilience" (Karatsoreos & McEwen 2013). Chronic stress leads to wear and tear on the body and brain and is thus termed "allostatic load" (McEwen 2007). In situations when an organism is faced with a threat, correctly executed escape behaviors are essential for survival and future propagation of the species. Further, after an escape is successful a quick return to non-defensive behaviors, e.g., territorial defense, foraging, or copulation, promotes rank within a social hierarchy and reproductive success (Blanchard & Blanchard 1989).

W. B. Cannon and P. Bard were the first to systematically examine the physiology of escape in the first half of the twentieth century (Cannon 1915, 1927; Bard 1928). Cannon and Bard's findings linked activity in the brain stem and hypothalamus with behavioral and peripheral manifestations of emotions. Their studies provided the first associations between secretion of epinephrine from the adrenal medulla, peripheral mobilization, and emotional responses, indicating that the adrenals play a role in activation of the muscles and promote sugar metabolism. This "fight-or-flight" response facilitates increases in heart rate, circulation rate and depth, rate of respiration to facilitate oxygenation of necessary muscles, sweating for temperature regulation, increases in glucose metabolism for energy, redirection of blood from the skin and gut to muscles, and increases in blood clotting in preparation for bodily injury. In addition, the sympathetic branch of the autonomic nervous system facilitates the cognitive enhancement due to epinephrine release from the adrenal medulla.

Autonomic activation begins at the central nucleus of the amygdala, wherein corticotropin-releasing factor (CRF) is synthesized and subsequently released into the locus coeruleus, stimulating the release of norepinephrine and epinephrine into the general circulation, which in turn activate the peripheral autonomic response including cardiovascular responses (heart rate and blood pressure), body temperature regulation, perspiration, and bronchiole dilation (Cannon 1915, 1927).

The endocrine stress response also involves activation of the hypothalamic–pituitary–adrenal (HPA) axis. This process commences when neuroendocrine cells in the medial parvocellular division of the paraventricular nucleus of the hypothalamus (PVN) release the 41 amino acid neuropeptide CRF (Spiess et al. 1981; Vale et al. 1981) as well as oxytocin and arginine vasopressin (Turner et al. 1951; Tuppy 1953; Du Vigneaud et al. 1953). CRF travels axonally to the median eminence and is subsequently released into the hypophysial portal system, which leads to the anterior pituitary. At this location it binds to corticotrophs to stimulate the release of adrenocorticotropin hormone (ACTH). As a result, ACTH is released into the bloodstream where it causes the secretion of glucocorticoids from the adrenal cortex: cortisol in humans and corticosterone (CORT) in rodents. The HPA axis is tightly controlled by a number of central negative feedback sites; specifically, the hypothalamus, pituitary, and hippocampus have been identified as major brain targets of glucocorticoid-mediated regulation (see Herman et al. 2005 for a review). Glucocorticoids mobilize energy by promoting catabolism of proteins, glycogen, and triglycerides, stimulating gluconeogenesis in the liver and kidneys, and augmenting cardiovascular effects of catecholamines at target tissues by enhancing epinephrine release and sharpening cognition. Glucocorticoids also inhibit physiological and biochemical processes in the body that are either unnecessary in times of danger or can interfere with appropriate escape. These include suppression of systems related to digestion, reproduction, and immunity. Although both CRF and glucocorticoids aid in the facilitation of an appropriate response to stressors that ultimately enhances chances of survival, chronic release of these hormones has been shown to produce deleterious effects on a number of bodily processes, such as immunity, digestion, learning and memory, and reproduction (McEwen 2007).

The level of HPA activation, i.e., glucocorticoid release, is used as a valid measure of the health of an individual and of a population within an ecological system (Romero 2004). As such it is important to notice the factors that affect glucocorticoid release in response to a stressor when examining physiology of defensive behaviors such as flight. These include genetic influences on the HPA axis as well as epigenetic factors. Genetic factors determine glucocorticoid receptor distribution, which in turn affect rate of termination/recovery from HPA activation, while epigenetic factors include early-life experience (trauma/enrichment), subjugation to chronic stressors during the lifetime of the animal, all of which can alter expression of genes relevant to a stress response (McEwen 2007).

Stress produces structural remodeling in the hippocampus, amygdala, and prefrontal cortex with these changes altering behavioral and physiological responses to subsequent stressors (McEwen 2007). For example, stress-induced activation of adrenergic and glucocorticoid receptors modulates memory-enhancing effects that facilitate resilience by regulating defensive behavior (escape, among others) toward a learned stimulus (Lupien & McEwen 1997; McGaugh & Roozendaal 2002; Karatsoreos & McEwen 2013). Glucocorticoids are also involved in neuronal excitability and long-term potentiation in the hippocampus, consistent with a role in memory storage (Diamond *et al.* 1992; Joels & de Kloet 1992). The hippocampus is a major target of adrenal steroids and is said to modulate memory processes via intracellular cascades that result from glucocorticoid and adrenergic receptor activation. The putative molecular mechanisms involve glucocorticoid-mediated expression of neural cell adhesion molecules, which in turn cause synaptic structural changes (McGaugh & Roozendaal 2002). In fact, post-training injections of corticosterone, the principal rat glucocorticoid, or other specific glucocorticoid agonists, into the hippocampus enhance memory consolidation in an inverted-U fashion, with lesions of the basolateral nucleus of the amygdala blocking this type 2-glucocorticoid receptor (GR)-mediated effect (Micheau *et al.* 1984; Roozendaal *et al.* 1997, 2004).

A single study suggests that glucocorticoids affect flight initiation distance (FID) in the field. In the lizard *Sceloporus undulatus*, FID increases during a series of successive approaches by a predator (Thaker *et al.* 2010). However, following injection of metapyrone, which blocks synthesis of corticosterone, FID failed to increase during repeated approaches (Thaker *et al.* 2010). This study suggests that some of the physiological mechanisms influencing escape and related behaviors in laboratory tests may apply as well to FID and related behaviors in the field.

13.2.3   Anatomy/neurochemistry of flight-relevant defense systems

Several excellent reviews (e.g., Johnson *et al.* 1995; Carrasco & Van de Kar 2003; Quintino-dos-Santos *et al.* 2014) have documented the history of attempts to describe the brain circuitry involved in defensive behaviors. A major difficulty in relating these unequivocally to flight is that there may be quite different brain systems underlying defensiveness to different types of threat stimuli, even though most or all of these stimuli can elicit flight as a consistent and substantial component of the defense pattern. Canteras and Graeff (2014), provide information, and indeed schematics, of focal neuroanatomic components of the defense systems, for defensiveness to stimuli conditioned to painful experiences; and to fear based on predator exposure or on social defeat. In addition, Canteras and Graeff (2014) describe neural systems underlying fear to interoceptive challenges such as cardiac arrhythmias, visceral pain, and hypoxia, all of which represent threat to the organism. None of the latter is associated with a substantial range of potentially effective defensive behaviors – indeed no behavior is likely to remedy an acute cardiac arrhythmia – but it is notable that hypoxia, associated with suffocation, might be expected to involve behavioral attempts to deal with the cause of the suffocation, potentially including fight or flight responses (Klein 1993). These different types of threat stimuli and how they may be differentially involved in activity in specific sites in the brain are discussed extensively in Gross and Canteras (2012).

Predator stimuli, to this date more often used than any natural threats in analyses of the neuroanatomy of defensiveness, typically involve a cat, or cat fur/skin odor, or odors derived from another predator, e.g., trimethylthiazoline (TMT), a component of fox feces (Apfelbach *et al.* 2005). These predator stimuli all elicit some elements of defense, but there are striking differences among the specific behaviors seen: cat exposure typically involves confrontation of the (usually rat) subject with a cat that is caged or otherwise restrained from actual contact with the subject. In most such situations, flight is limited by the dimensions of the test cage, and freezing is by far the predominant response seen: for example, Motta *et al.* (2009) reported that about 97% of a five-minute test period involving confrontation of a rat with a caged cat involved freezing. While it is plausible that the motivation to flee was definitely present for these rat subjects, flight itself, and the neural circuitry supporting the actual behaviors involved in flight, would be expected to be less activated in these tests. Similarly, cat odor tends to involve freezing, but this may be mixed with some approach – investigational activities (risk assessment) that are typically associated with more ambiguous threat stimuli (Blanchard *et al.* 2011). Trimethylthiazoline, while it does not robustly support fear learning (Blanchard *et al.* 2003b) and produces a brain activation pattern rather different than cat odor (Staples *et al.* 2008), is also used extensively for studies of the physiology of defense (Rosen 2004). Freezing rather than more active defense is the actual behavior associated with the brain activation in most of these studies. However, it is clear that confrontation with a predator does indeed elicit flight when this is possible, so these studies are nonetheless relevant to analyses of the neural systems involved in flight/escape. In keeping with the focus of this book, findings from the predator exposure model(s) will be the center of attention here.

Predator odors activate olfactory pathways projecting to the medial amygdala, and after predator (cat) odor exposure activation of the immediate early gene c-Fos is seen specifically in the posteroventral part of the medial amygdala (MeApv; Dielenberg *et al.* 2001), with additional high-level expression (compared to that seen with a strong but non-predator odor) in the dorsomedial part of the ventromedial nucleus of the hypothalamus (VMHdm), the hypothalamic dorsal premammillary nucleus (PMd), and the

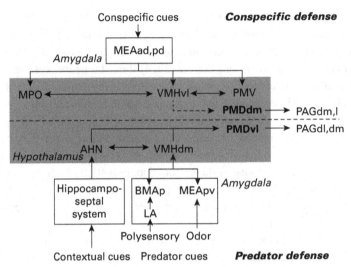

Figure 13.2 A schematic diagram showing the putative brain systems involved in processing predatory and conspecific threats and in organizing predator and conspecific defense. Abbreviations: AHN, anterior hypothalamic nucleus; BMAp, basomedial amygdalar nucleus, posterior part; LA, lateral amygdalar nucleus; MEAad, -pd, and -pv, medial amygdalar nucleus, anterodorsal, posterodorsal, and posteroventral parts; MPO, medial preoptic area; PAGdl, -dm, and -l, periaqueductal gray, dorsolateral, dorsomedial, and lateral parts; PMDdm and -vl, dorsal premammillary nucleus, dorsomedial, and ventrolateral parts; PMV, ventral premammillary nucleus; VMHdm and -vl, ventromedial nucleus, dorsomedial and ventrolateral parts. (Used with permission from Motta *et al.* 2009)

dorsomedial, dorsolateral (and more caudal levels), and the ventrolateral periaqueductal gray matter of the midbrain (PAGdm, PAGdl, and PAGvl, respectively). These findings are in agreement with reports from Canteras *et al.* (2002) of the organization of hypothalamic nuclei activated in exposure of a rat to a live cat (see Figure 13.2 for summary). Notably, these findings implicated the basolateral and lateral nuclei of the amygdala as well as the MeA. The former receive inputs from a number of sensory systems, likely reflecting additional sensory information about the cat, rather than the cat odor alone that was provided in Dielenberg *et al.* (2001).

With reference to this core set of hypothalamic nuclei, the medial amygdala, projects via the bed nucleus of the stria terminalis, to the VMHdm (Cezario *et al.* 2008). In addition, the MeA projects to the ventral hippocampus and in turn information from the hippocampus projects via the septum to the anterior hypothalamic nucleus (AHN), and the lateral hypothalamic area (LHA) (Petrovich *et al.* 2001). Lesions of the ventral hippocampus reduced freezing and enhanced non-defensive behaviors to cat presentation (Pentkowski *et al.* 2006). Strong involvement of the hippocampus in spatial representation (O'Keefe & Nadel 1978) suggests that these projections may carry information relative to the context in which the predator stimuli appear (a crucial feature in the choice of defensive behaviors, especially the balance between freezing and flight (Blanchard & Blanchard 2008). The latter areas are interconnected, and connect also to the VMHdm, and all three of these project to the PMD (Cezario *et al.* 2008), that, in turn, projects to dorsal parts of the PAG.

Cytotoxic lesions or muscimol (GABAA agonist-induced) blockade of the PMd produced profound reductions in defensive responding to cat-related stimuli and also a reduction in Fos activation of the dorsal PAG (Cesario *et al.* 2008). These relationships are schematized in Cesario *et al.* (2008), including an additional connection of the PMd to the ventral part of the anteromedial nucleus of the thalamus. This area provides a connection to a component of the cingulate cortex that may be involved in eye/head movements associated with attention (Risold & Swanson 1995). Canteras *et al.* (2008) reported that the NMDA antagonist AP5, injected into the PMd, also reduced conditioning to a coffee-odor stimulus associated with footshock, consonant with a view that the PMd, through its connections to the cingulate cortex, may be accessing attentional and associational mechanisms for defensive behavior.

A number of recent studies have outlined differences in the neural circuitry of defensive behaviors elicited by different types of threat stimuli (Motta *et al.* 2009; Gross & Canteras 2012; Canteras & Graeff 2014), finding substantial differences for systems associated with responsivity to predators, conspecifics, and conditioned threat stimuli associated with pain. However, in contrast to its immediate responsivity to predator stimuli, defensiveness to conspecifics in laboratory rats tends to require contact, and the pain of biting attack (Blanchard & Blanchard 1989). A bitten animal quickly displays defensive behaviors that have been differentially evaluated, in one recent study of associated neural activation (Motta *et al.* 2009), as active responses (flight, boxing, and an upright defense of pushing off the attacker) vs. passive responses (freezing and lying on the back – the so-called "submissive" posture). The Motta *et al.* (2009) studies thus provide the possibility to differentiate passive and active defenses in terms of areas activated during these behaviors, and to determine behavior changes when relevant areas are inactivated. They report that while predator exposure produces Fos upregulation in the ventrolateral portions of the PMd, conspecific threat/attack results in enhanced Fos in the dorsomedial PMd (Motta *et al.* 2009). Lesions that affect the entire PMd strikingly disrupt defensive behaviors to a cat, but when conspecific threat is used such lesions reduce only passive defenses, with active defenses showing a non-significant but substantial increase.

While this pattern of results does indicate a differentiation of PMd inactivation effects on active vs. passive defenses, suggesting that the PMd may be less involved with the former than with the latter, an alternative explanation is that it is consonant with the interpretation of a general decrease in the intensity of defensiveness after PMd lesions. In particular, lying on the back or "submission" is a high-intensity response to threat, with accompanying signs of autonomic and glucocorticoid arousal (e.g., Fokkema & Koolhaas 1985; Huhman *et al.* 1990), whereas active defenses such as upright pushing away of the opponent and flight may under some circumstances actually reduce stress responsivity (Viken *et al.* 1989). Thus a reduction of "passive" in favor of more active defensive responses may reflect a change in the intensity of the threat motivation rather than alteration of a system underlying a specific type of defensive behavior.

13.2.4   Systemic drug effects on defensive behaviors, including flight

Preclinical animal models are utilized in the study of unconditioned and conditioned behaviors potentially related to fear and anxiety, with a view to understanding their neural and endocrine correlates, and their underlying etiology, and to screen novel pharmaceuticals aimed at alleviating these conditions. Such assays include high-throughput models; for example, the elevated plus-maze (EPM), open field, elevated T-maze (ETM), light/dark box, social interaction test, and separation-induced ultrasonic vocalizations. They also include more ethologically relevant models such as seminatural visible burrow systems (VBS) and other situations where rats or mice are confronted by predators or predator-related stimuli (Blanchard & Blanchard 1989; Litvin *et al.* 2008; Motta *et al.* 2009).

Two animal models: the elevated T-maze (ETM) and the mouse defense test battery (MDTB) are particularly relevant to flight/escape behaviors. The MDTB was created specifically to enable evaluation of the magnitude of a range of defensive behaviors of mice (*Mus musculus*) to a hand-held, anesthetized rat. Because rats are predators of mice (Blanchard *et al.* 2003a), they elicit strong defensive behaviors in mice, with the form or type of defense varying with the movements of the rat and features of the threat situation (Blanchard *et al.* 2003a). In the MDTB, in which features of the threat stimulus and situation are varied in order to elicit a number of different defensive behaviors in succession, profiles of changes in various defensive responses to a given drug manipulation can be obtained in a single test session.

Results of pharmacological manipulations of mice assessed using the MDTB suggest that a number of neuroactive chemicals may enhance or reduce defensive behaviors in a relatively non-specific fashion. Intracerebroventricular administration of CRF tends to enhance the predominant defensive behavior elicited by each stimulus combination of threat and situation utilized in the MDTB (Yang *et al.* 2006). Blanchard *et al.* (2001) reported that a number of benzodiazepines (BZPs) alter flight in the MDTB. However, for most BZPs there was no selective effect on flight with doses that did not impair motor function. However, two benzodiazepines, alprazolam given on a chronic, but not acute, basis (Griebel *et al.* 1995b) and clonazepam (Griebel *et al.* 1996) selectively impaired mouse escape responses. In addition, chronic administration of the selective serotonin reuptake inhibitors (SSRIs) fluoxetine and paroxetine both robustly reduced flight (Griebel *et al.* 1995a; Beijamini & Andreatini 2003). In contrast, cocaine and yohimbine substantially and selectively increase flight compared to other aspects of defensiveness (Blanchard *et al.* 1993, 1999). As the drugs selectively reducing flight are clinically effective against panic, while cocaine and yohimbine may precipitate or enhance panic (Cox *et al.* 1990; Bourin *et al.* 1998), these findings suggest that flight may serve as a relatively selective animal model for panic disorder (Blanchard *et al.* 1993; Griebel *et al.* 1996).

The elevated T-maze (ETM) has been used even more extensively in the analysis of flight/escape responses. The ETM consists of three elevated arms – one enclosed and two open, forming a "T". To assess inhibitory avoidance, a subject is placed at the end of the enclosed arm and the latency to exit this arm is recorded in three consecutive trials.

Inhibitory avoidance learning is indicated by the increase in withdrawal latency across trials. Thirty seconds after the completion of avoidance training, the second behavioral task (one-way escape) is measured. For this, the animal is placed at the end of one of the open arms of the maze and the withdrawal latency from this arm is similarly registered in three consecutive trials.

The ETM was designed specifically to separate these defensive behaviors (Deakin & Graeff 1991) with the underlying premise that inhibitory avoidance and escape responses are differentially regulated by serotonin (5-HT) released from fibers in the dorsal raphe nucleus (DRN), a midbrain structure that innervates neural substrates particularly involved in defensive behaviors (e.g., amygdala, frontal cortex, dorsal periaqueductal gray (dPAG), among others) (Graeff et al. 1993; Viana et al. 1994). This emphasis on the separation of inhibitory avoidance of the open arms of the ETM and escape from the same open arms was associated with interpretation of the former as a model of generalized anxiety, while the latter, escape, was viewed as an animal model for panic. Zangrossi and Graeff (2014) have conducted a number of experiments to behaviorally validate the ETM. Their results showed that rats trained on an ETM with three enclosed arms did not show the increase in withdrawal latency along three consecutive trials that is often observed in the standard ETM procedure. Therefore, open arm experience seems to be critical for inhibitory avoidance learning. Moreover, over repeated trials in an open arm, animals left at increasingly higher speeds. Both findings are consonant with a view that the open arms are aversive, and that repeated placement in the closed arm or an open arm does elicit avoidance, or escape, respectively. Indeed, repeated open arm experience appears to enhance the sensitivity of the resulting escape response to drug effects.

Zangrossi and Graeff (2014) also summarize the effects of systemic drugs on escape from the open arms of the ETM. Briefly, reduction of escape from the open arms was produced by acute administration of the benzodiazepine alprazolam, and the SSRI paroxetine, with no effect from acute treatment of a number of additional benzodiazepines and 5-HT-acting drugs. Similarly, chronic treatment (9–14 days) with the benzodiazepine diazepam, and the 5-HT1A receptor partial agonist buspirone failed to alter escape. However, chronic treatment with a number of SSRIs, including sertraline, paroxetine, escitalopram, fluoxetine, and clomipramine all reduced escape, as did chronic treatment with the tricyclic imipramine. Moreover, most of these positive effects on escape were obtained in tests in which there was no alteration of the inhibitory avoidance effect, indicting a relatively selective effect of these treatments. Finally, as SSRIs are frequently the first choice drugs for treatment of panic, with effects that usually appear after chronic administration, while alprazolam is the only benzodiazepine with antipanic efficacy at non-sedative doses, this pattern of results is very supportive of a view that escape measured in the ETM can serve as an animal model of panic (Mochcovitch & Nardi 2010).

Additional evidence of involvement of serotonin in flight-escape is suggested by findings that injection into the dorsomedial hypothalamic nucleus (DMH) of the pre-ferential 5-HT2a agonist, 2,5-dimethoxy-4-iodoamphetamine (DOI), or of the 5-HT1a receptor agonist 8-OH-DPAT, raised the threshold for escape responses (running or jumping reactions) elicited by electrical stimulation of the DMH. Both of these effects were enhanced by chronic systemic administration of imipramine, a strong inhibitor of serotonin reuptake that also affects several other neurotransmitters, and the DOI effect was enhanced by chronic fluoxetine, which inhibits serotonin reuptake (de Bortoli *et al.* 2006). As noted earlier, the relationship between these findings and antipredator flight is complicated, in that the DMH is not part of what is currently regarded as the antipredator circuitry of the hypothalamus, although it is prominently featured in neural responsivity to conspecific threat (Canteras & Graeff 2014). However, this difference in circuitry may be at least partly the result of a methodological difference between the use of predators and conspecifics as threat stimuli, with the latter, alone, being allowed to actually attack (and cause pain) to the subject in such experiments: this possibility requires additional investigation.

The same caveat, that the relevant locale may not be part of the antipredator circuitry of the brain, applies to orexins/hypocretins, which are hypothalamic peptides located preferentially in the perifornical area, that may also affect escape responses. Orexin is co-localized with glutamate and is involved in regulation of a number of neurovegetative activities (see Johnson *et al.* 2012 for review). Afferent connections to orexin neurons originate in a host of sites such as the septohippocampal system (Hahn & Swanson 2012) and involve neurochemicals such as GABA and serotonin (Johnson *et al.* 2012) that are important for defensiveness. In turn, orexin neurons project to a variety of putative defense areas. One of these, the dorsal raphe (Lowry *et al.* 2005), is of particular interest (see below).

Glutamate receptors, including the n-methyl-d-aspartic acid (NMDA) type, within the dorsal or dorsolateral PAG play a major role in the initiation of PAG-evoked defensive behaviors, specifically escape. Microinjection of NMDA into this area produced flight-related behaviors (galloping, jumping) in a dose-dependent manner, thus mimicking the response to electrical stimulation in this region (Bittencourt *et al.* 2004). In fact, NMDA-induced excitation of the dorsal PAG elicits a range of defensive behaviors, from freezing to escape, with freezing evoked at lower doses and escape, at higher levels (Cardoso *et al.* 1994).

The dorsal PAG expresses high levels of GABA (Ferreira-Netto *et al.* 2005). GABAergic fibers from the substantia nigra and the pars reticulata exert an inhibitory effect on aversive behavior induced by dorsolateral PAG stimulation (Coimbra & Brandao 1993). These GABA receptors are modulated in a dose-dependent manner by benzodiazepines (Bovier *et al.* 1982). Further evidence for GABA involvement in this region is that microinjection of GABA antagonists, such as bicuculline, into the mid-brain tectum induce flight and autonomic reactions similar to those of the defense response (Brandao *et al.* 1982; Melo *et al.* 1992). As with NMDA agonists, escalating doses of GABA antagonists produce freezing and escape, respectively (Graeff 1990). In addition, prior treatment with chlordiazepoxide (a benzodiazepine hypnotic and muscle relaxant) inhibits escape induced by bicuculline, an antagonist of GABA receptors (Borelli *et al.* 2005) and prior bicuculline injection abolishes the inhibitory effect of benzodiazepines (Brandao *et al.* 1982). Collectively, these findings implicate a GABA-benzodiazepine system in the midbrain tectum as an inhibitor of escape.

The dorsal raphe nuclei of the midbrain receive input from orexin neurons in the hypothalamic perifornical area and provide an inhibitory serotonergic input to the dorsal PAG (Lowry *et al.* 2005). Drug injections into the dorsal raphe that enhance serotonin release from the PAG tend to inhibit flight in the ETM (Graeff 1997). Roncon *et al.* (2013) demonstrated an opioid effect in this area: morphine in the dPAG increased escape latency in the ETM. Moreover, both the 5-HT1a agonist 8-OH-DPAT and the 5-HT2a agonist DOI produced anti-escape effects, but only the first of these was antagonized by naloxone. Additional studies in this series (Roncon *et al.* 2013) supported an interaction of serotonergic and opioidergic mechanisms in the dPAG.

The SSRIs fluoxetine and paroxetine (as well as alprazolam) reduced flight-like escape behavior produced in rats by electrical stimulation of the dPAG (Hogg *et al.* 2006). These data are in agreement with ETM findings for dPAG injections of the same agonists, again in rats (Zanoveli *et al.* 2003; de Paula Soares & Zangrossi 2004). Connecting this escape measure to the flight seen in the MDTB and providing considerable evidence of consistency across rat and mouse subjects, injections of the 5-HT1A agonist 8-OH-DPAT, and the preferential 5-HT2A receptor agonist DOI into the dPAG, consistently reduced flight speed and distance run during escape in the MDTB, and increased contacts of the mouse subjects with an anesthetized rat (Pobbe & Zangrossi 2005). However, the 5-HT1a antagonist WAY-100635, which impaired escape in the ETM (Pobbe & Zangrossi 2005), did not affect defensive behaviors in the MDTB (Pobbe *et al.* 2011).

In summary, these findings suggest that flight is modulated by some relatively specific neurotransmitter mechanisms involving particular brain circuitry. They indicate relatively good agreement among the several measures of flight that have been devised to differentiate flight from other defensive behaviors or specifically to measure responsiveness of flight to drugs and other variables that affect the modulation of panic. These findings also support the concept of a specific link between flight and panic.

13.3   Conclusions

Nearly a century of research using increasingly sophisticated and multifaceted neuroscience methodologies has produced a great deal of information on endocrine, neuroanatomic, and neurochemical systems involved in defensive behaviors, including flight/escape. The components of these systems that specifically control flight/panic, as distinct from other defensive behaviors, have received a great deal of recent attention and analysis due to an increasingly well-established association of flight/escape with panic. However, research on escape decisions based on costs and benefits of fleeing such as flight initiation distance, distance fled, and hiding time in refuge, are also needed to determine the physiological underpinnings of escape decisions that are the foci of economic models of escape (see Chapter 2).

References

Apfelbach, R., Blanchard, C. D., Blanchard, R. J., Hayes, R. A. & Mcgregor, I. S. (2005). The effects of predator odors in mammalian prey species: A review of field and laboratory studies. *Neuroscience Biobehavioral Reviews*, **29**, 1123–1144.

Bard, P. (1928). A diencephalic mechanism for the expression of rage with special reference to the sympathetic nervous system. *American Journal Physiology*, **84**, 490–410.

Beijamini, V. & Andreatini, R. (2003). Effects of *Hypericum perforatum* and paroxetine in the mouse defense test battery. *Pharmacology Biochemistry and Behavior*, **74**, 1015–1024.

Bittencourt, A. S., Carobrez, A. P., Zamprogno, L. P., Tufik, S. & Schenberg, L. C. (2004). Organization of single components of defensive behaviors within distinct columns of periaqueductal gray matter of the rat: Role of N-methyl-D-aspartic acid glutamate receptors. *Neuroscience*, **125**, 71–89.

Blanchard, D. C. (1997). Stimulus, environmental and pharmacological control of defensive behaviors. In Bouton, M. & Fanselow, M. S. (eds.) *Learning, Motivation and Cognition. The Functional Behaviorism of Robert C. Bolles*. Washington DC: American Psychological Association.

Blanchard, R. J. & Blanchard, D. C. (1989). Antipredator defensive behaviors in a visible burrow system. *Journal of Comparative Psychology*, **103**, 70–82.

Blanchard, D. C. & Blanchard, R. J. (2008). Defensive behaviors, fear and anxiety. In Blanchard, R. J., Blanchard, D. C., Griebel, G. & Nutt, D. J. (eds.) *Handbook of Anxiety and Fear*. Amsterdam: Elsevier Academic Press.

Blanchard, R. J., Taukulis, H. K., Rodgers, R. J., Magee, L. K. & Blanchard, D. C. (1993). Yohimbine potentiates active defensive responses to threatening stimuli in Swiss-Webster mice. *Pharmacology Biochemistry and Behavior*, **44**, 673–681.

Blanchard, R. J., Kaawaloa, J. N., Hebert, M. A. & Blanchard, D. C. (1999). Cocaine produces panic-like flight responses in mice in the mouse defense test battery. *Pharmacology Biochemistry and Behavior*, **64**, 523–528.

Blanchard, D. C., Griebel, G. & Blanchard, R. J. (2001). Mouse defensive behaviors: Pharmacological and behavioral assays for anxiety and panic. *Neuroscience and Biobehavioral Reviews*, **25**, 205–218.

Blanchard, D. C., Griebel, G. & Blanchard, R. J. (2003a). The Mouse Defense Test Battery: Pharmacological and behavioral assays for anxiety and panic. *European Journal of Pharmacology*, **463**, 97–116.

Blanchard, D. C., Markham, C., Yang, M. *et al.* (2003b). Failure to produce conditioning with low-dose trimethylthiazoline or cat feces as unconditioned stimuli. *Behavioral Neuroscience*, **117**, 360–368.

Blanchard, D. C., Litvin, Y., Pentkowski, N. S. & Blanchard, R. J. (2009). Defense and aggression. In Berntson, G. G. & Cacioppo, J. T. (eds.) *Handbook of Neuroscience for the Behavioral Sciences*. Hoboken, NJ: John Wiley & Sons.

Blanchard, D. C., Griebel, G., Pobbe, R. & Blanchard, R. J. (2011). Risk assessment as an evolved threat detection and analysis process. *Neuroscience Biobehavioral Reviews*, **35**, 991–998.

Borelli, K. G., Ferreira-Netto, C., Coimbra, N. C. & Brandao, M. L. (2005). Fos-like immunoreactivity in the brain associated with freezing or escape induced by inhibition of either glutamic acid decarboxylase or GABAA receptors in the dorsal periaqueductal gray. *Brain Research*, **1051**, 100–111.

Bourin, M., Baker, G. B. & Bradwejn, J. (1998). Neurobiology of panic disorder. *Journal of Psychosomatic Research*, **44**, 163–180.

Bovier, P., Broekkamp, C. L. & Lloyd, K. G. (1982). Enhancing GABAergic transmission reverses the aversive state in rats induced by electrical stimulation of the periaqueductal grey region. *Brain Research*, **248**, 313–320.

Brandao, M. L., De Aguiar, J. C. & Graeff, F. G. (1982). GABA mediation of the anti-aversive action of minor tranquilizers. *Pharmacology Biochemistry and Behavior*, **16**, 397–402.

Cannon, W. B. (1915). *Bodily Changes in Pain, Hunger, Fear and Rage*. New York, NY: D. Appleton & Company.

Cannon, W. B. (1927). The James-Lange theory of emotion: A critical examination and an alternative theory. *American Journal of Psychology*, **39**, 106–124.

Canteras, N. S. (2002). The medial hypothalamic defensive system: hodological organization and functional implications. *Pharmacology Biochemistry and Behavior*, **71**, 481–491.

Canteras, N. S. & Graeff, F. G. (2014). Executive and modulatory neural circuits of defensive reactions: Implications for panic disorder. *Neuroscience Biobehavioral Reviews*, **46**, 352–364.

Canteras, N. S., Kroon, J. A., Do-Monte, F. H., Pavesi, E. & Carobrez, A. P. (2008). Sensing danger through the olfactory system: The role of the hypothalamic dorsal premammillary nucleus. *Neuroscience Biobehavioral Review*, **32**, 1228–1235.

Cardoso, S. H., Coimbra, N. C. & Brandao, M. L. (1994). Defensive reactions evoked by activation of NMDA receptors in distinct sites of the inferior colliculus. *Behavioral Brain Research*, **63**, 17–24.

Carrasco, G. A. & Van De Kar, L. D. (2003). Neuroendocrine pharmacology of stress. *European Journal of Pharmacology*, **463**, 235–272.

Cezario, A. F., Ribeiro-Barbosa, E. R., Baldo, M. V. & Canteras, N. S. (2008). Hypothalamic sites responding to predator threats: The role of the dorsal premammillary nucleus in unconditioned and conditioned antipredatory defensive behavior. *European Journal of Neuroscience*, **28**, 1003–1015.

Coimbra, N. C. & Brandao, M. L. (1993). GABAergic nigro-collicular pathways modulate the defensive behaviour elicited by midbrain tectum stimulation. *Behavioral Brain Research*, **59**, 131–139.

Cox, B. J., Norton, G. R., Swinson, R. P. & Endler, N. S. (1990). Substance abuse and panic-related anxiety: A critical review. *Behavioral Research and Therapy*, **28**, 385–393.

De Bortoli, V. C., Nogueira, R. L. & Zangrossi, H., Jr. (2006). Effects of fluoxetine and buspirone on the panicolytic-like response induced by the activation of 5-HT1A and 5-HT2A receptors in the rat dorsal periaqueductal gray. *Psychopharmacology*, **183**, 422–428.

De Paula Soares, V. & Zangrossi, H., Jr. (2004). Involvement of 5-HT1A and 5-HT2 receptors of the dorsal periaqueductal gray in the regulation of the defensive behaviors generated by the elevated T-maze. *Brain Research Bulletin*, **64**, 181–188.

Deakin, J. F. & Graeff, F. G. (1991). 5-HT and mechanisms of defence. *Journal of Psychopharmacology*, **5**, 305–315.

Diamond, D. M., Bennett, M. C., Fleshner, M. & Rose, G. M. (1992). Inverted-U relationship between the level of peripheral corticosterone and the magnitude of hippocampal primed burst potentiation. *Hippocampus*, **2**, 421–430.

Dielenberg, R. A., Hunt, G. E. & Mcgregor, I. S. (2001). "When a rat smells a cat": The distribution of Fos immunoreactivity in rat brain following exposure to a predatory odor. *Neuroscience*, **104**, 1085–1097.

Du Vigneaud, V., Ressler, C. & Trippett, S. (1953). The sequence of amino acids in oxytocin, with a proposal for the structure of oxytocin. *Journal of Biological Chemistry*, **205**, 949–957.

Ferreira-Netto, C., Borelli, K. G. & Brandao, M. L. (2005). Neural segregation of Fos-protein distribution in the brain following freezing and escape behaviors induced by injections of either glutamate or NMDA into the dorsal periaqueductal gray of rats. *Brain Research*, **1031**, 151–163.

Fokkema, D. S. & Koolhaas, J. M. (1985). Acute and conditioned blood pressure changes in relation to social and psychosocial stimuli in rats. *Physiology and Behavior*, **34**, 33–38.

Graeff, F. G. (1990). Brain defence systems and anxiety. In Roth, M., Burrow, G. D. & Noyes, R. (eds.) *Handbook of Anxiety*, Vol. 3, 307–357. Amsterdam: Elsevier.

Graeff, F. G. (1997). Serotonergic systems. *Psychiatric Clinics of North America*, **20**, 723–739.

Graeff, F. G., Viana, M. B. & Tomaz, C. (1993). The elevated T maze: A new experimental model of anxiety and memory: effect of diazepam. *Brazilian Journal of Medical and Biological Research*, **26**, 67–70.

Griebel, G., Blanchard, D. C., Agnes, R. S. & Blanchard, R. J. (1995a). Differential modulation of antipredator defensive behavior in Swiss–Webster mice following acute or chronic administration of imipramine and fluoxetine. *Psychopharmacology*, **120**, 57–66.

Griebel, G., Blanchard, D. C., Jung, A. *et al.* (1995b). Further evidence that the mouse defense test battery is useful for screening anxiolytic and panicolytic drugs: Effects of acute and chronic treatment with alprazolam. *Neuropharmacology*, **34**, 1625–1633.

Griebel, G., Blanchard, D. C. & Blanchard, R. J. (1996). Predator-elicited flight responses in Swiss–Webster mice: An experimental model of panic attacks. *Progress in Neuro-Psychopharmacology & Biological Psychiatry*, **20**, 185–205.

Gross, C. T. & Canteras, N. S. (2012). The many paths to fear. *Nature Reviews Neuroscience*, **13**, 651–658.

Hahn, J. D. & Swanson, L. W. (2012). Connections of the lateral hypothalamic area juxtadorsomedial region in the male rat. *Journal of Comparative Neurology*, **520**, 1831–1890.

Herman, J. P., Ostrander, M. M., Mueller, N. K. & Figueiredo, H. (2005). Limbic system mechanisms of stress regulation: Hypothalamo-pituitary-adrenocortical axis. *Progress in Neuro-Psychopharmacology and Biological Psychiatry*, **29**, 1201–1213.

Hogg, S., Michan, L. & Jessa, M. (2006). Prediction of anti-panic properties of escitalopram in the dorsal periaqueductal grey model of panic anxiety. *Neuropharmacology*, **51**, 141–145.

Huhman, K. L., Bunnell, B. N., Mougey, E. H. & Meyerhoff, J. L. (1990). Effects of social conflict on POMC-derived peptides and glucocorticoids in male golden hamsters. *Physiology and Behavior*, **47**, 949–956.

Joels, M. & De Kloet, E. R. (1992). Control of neuronal excitability by corticosteroid hormones. *Trends in Neurosciences*, **15**, 25–30.

Johnson, M. R., Lydiard, R. B. & Ballenger, J. C. (1995). Panic disorder. Pathophysiology and drug treatment. *Drugs*, **49**, 328–344.

Johnson, P. L., Molosh, A., Fitz, S. D., Truitt, W. A. & Shekhar, A. (2012). Orexin, stress, and anxiety/panic states. *Progress in Brain Research*, **198**, 133–161.

Karatsoreos, I. N. & McEwen, B. S. (2013). Resilience and vulnerability: A neurobiological perspective. *F1000 Prime Reports*, **5**, 13.

Klein, D. F. (1993). False suffocation alarms, spontaneous panics, and related conditions. An integrative hypothesis. *Archives of General Psychiatry*, **50**, 306–317.

Litvin, Y. & Pfaff, D. W. (2013). The involvement of oxytocin and vasopressin in fear and anxiety. In Choleris, E., Pfaff, D. W. & Kavaliers, M. (eds.) *Oxytocin, Vasopressin and Related Peptides in the Regulation of Behavior.* Cambridge: Cambridge University Press.

Litvin, Y., Pentkowski, N. S., Pobbe, R. L., Blanchard, D. C. & Blanchard, R. J. (2008). Unconditioned models of fear and anxiety. In Blanchard, R. J., Blanchard, D. C., Griebel, G. & Nutt, D. J. (eds.) *Handbook of Anxiety and Fear.* Amsterdam: Elsevier Academic Press.

Lowry, C. A., Johnson, P. L., Hay-Schmidt, A., Mikkelsen, J. & Shekhar, A. (2005). Modulation of anxiety circuits by serotonergic systems. *Stress*, **8**, 233–246.

Lupien, S. J. & McEwen, B. S. (1997). The acute effects of corticosteroids on cognition: Integration of animal and human model studies. *Brain Research Reviews*, **24**, 1–27.

McEwen, B. S. (2007). Physiology and neurobiology of stress and adaptation: Central role of the brain. *Physiological Reviews*, **87**, 873–904.

McGaugh, J. L. & Roozendaal, B. (2002). Role of adrenal stress hormones in forming lasting memories in the brain. *Current Opinion in Neurobiology*, **12**, 205–210.

Melo, L. L., Cardoso, S. H. & Brandao, M. L. (1992). Antiaversive action of benzodiazepines on escape behavior induced by electrical stimulation of the inferior colliculus. *Physiology and Behavior*, **51**, 557–562.

Micheau, J., Destrade, C. & Soumireu-Mourat, B. (1984). Time-dependent effects of posttraining intrahippocampal injections of corticosterone on retention of appetitive learning tasks in mice. *European Journal of Pharmacology*, **106**, 39–46.

Mochcovitch, M. D. & Nardi, A. E. (2010). Selective serotonin-reuptake inhibitors in the treatment of panic disorder: A systematic review of placebo-controlled studies. *Expert Review of Neurotherapeutics*, **10**, 1285–1293.

Motta, S. C., Goto, M., Gouveia, F. V. *et al.* (2009). Dissecting the brain's fear system reveals the hypothalamus is critical for responding in subordinate conspecific intruders. *Proceedings of the National Academy of Sciences*, **106**, 4870–4875.

O'Keefe, J. & Nadel, L. (1978). *The Hippocampus as a Cognitive Map.* Oxford: Oxford University Press.

Pentkowski, N. S., Blanchard, D. C., Lever, C., Litvin, Y. & Blanchard, R. J. (2006). Effects of lesions to the dorsal and ventral hippocampus on defensive behaviors in rats. *European Journal of Neuroscience*, **23**, 2185–2196.

Petrovich, G. D., Canteras, N. S. & Swanson, L. W. (2001). Combinatorial amygdalar inputs to hippocampal domains and hypothalamic behavior systems. *Brain Research Reviews*, **38**, 247–289.

Pobbe, R. L. & Zangrossi, H., Jr. (2005). 5-HT(1A) and 5-HT(2A) receptors in the rat dorsal periaqueductal gray mediate the antipanic-like effect induced by the stimulation of serotonergic neurons in the dorsal raphe nucleus. *Psychopharmacology*, **183**, 314–321.

Pobbe, R. L., Zangrossi, H., Jr., Blanchard, D. C. & Blanchard, R. J. (2011). Involvement of dorsal raphe nucleus and dorsal periaqueductal gray 5-HT receptors in the modulation of mouse defensive behaviors. *European Neuropsychopharmacology*, **21**, 306–315.

Quintino-Dos-Santos, J. W., Muller, C. J., Bernabe, C. S. *et al.* (2014). Evidence that the periaqueductal gray matter mediates the facilitation of panic-like reactions in neonatally-isolated adult rats. *PLoS One*, **9**, e90726.

Risold, P. Y. & Swanson, L. W. (1995). Evidence for a hypothalamothalamocortical circuit mediating pheromonal influences on eye and head movements. *Proceedings of the National Academy of Sciences U S A*, **92**, 3898–3902.

Romero, L. M. (2004). Physiological stress in ecology: Lessons from biomedical research. *Trends in Ecology and Evolution*, **19**, 249–255.

Roncon, C. M., Biesdorf, C., Coimbra, N. C. *et al.* (2013). Cooperative regulation of anxiety and panic-related defensive behaviors in the rat periaqueductal grey matter by 5-HT1A and mu-receptors. *Journal of Psychopharmacology*, **27**, 1141–1148.

Roozendaal, B., Van Der Zee, E. A., Hensbroek, R. A. *et al.* (1997). Muscarinic acetylcholine receptor immunoreactivity in the amygdala–II. Fear-induced plasticity. *Neuroscience*, **76**, 75–83.

Roozendaal, B., Hahn, E. L., Nathan, S. V., De Quervain, D. J. & Mcgaugh, J. L. (2004). Glucocorticoid effects on memory retrieval require concurrent noradrenergic activity in the hippocampus and basolateral amygdala. *Journal of Neuroscience*, **24**, 8161–8169.

Rosen, J. B. (2004). The neurobiology of conditioned and unconditioned fear: A neurobehavioral system analysis of the amygdala. *Behavioral and Cognitive Neuroscience Reviews*, **3**, 23–41.

Spiess, J., Rivier, J., Rivier, C. & Vale, W. (1981). Primary structure of corticotropin-releasing factor from ovine hypothalamus. *Proceedings of the National Academy of Sciences*, **78**, 6517–6521.

Staples, L. G., McGregor, I. S., Apfelbach, R. & Hunt, G. E. (2008). Cat odor, but not trimethylthiazoline (fox odor), activates accessory olfactory and defense-related brain regions in rats. *Neuroscience*, **151**, 937–947.

Thaker, M., Vanak, A. T., Lima, S. L. & Hews, D. K. (2010). Stress and aversive learning in a wild vertebrate: The role of corticosterone in mediating escape from a novel stressor. *American Naturalist*, **175**, 50–60.

Tuppy, H. (1953). The amino-acid sequence in oxytocin. *Biochimica et Biophysica Acta*, **11**, 449–450.

Turner, R. A., Pierce, J. G. & Du, V. V. (1951). The purification and the amino acid content of vasopressin preparations. *Journal of Biological Chemistry*, **191**, 21–28.

Vale, W., Spiess, J., Rivier, C. & Rivier, J. (1981). Characterization of a 41-residue ovine hypothalamic peptide that stimulates secretion of corticotropin and beta-endorphin. *Science*, **213**, 1394–1397.

Viana, M. B., Tomaz, C. & Graeff, F. G. (1994). The elevated T-maze: a new animal model of anxiety and memory. *Pharmacology Biochemistry & Behavior*, **49**, 549–554.

Viken, R. J., Knutson, J. F. & Johnson, A. K. (1989). Effects of behavior and social condition on cardiovascular response to footshock stress. *Physiology and Behavior*, **46**, 961–966.

Yang, M., Farrokhi, C., Vasconcellos, A., Blanchard, R. J. & Blanchard, D. C. (2006). Central infusion of Ovine CRF (oCRF) potentiates defensive behaviors in CD-1 mice in the Mouse Defense Test Battery (MDTB). *Behavioral Brain Research*, **171**, 1–8.

Zangrossi, H., Jr. & Graeff, F. G.(2014). Serotonin in anxiety and panic: Contributions of the elevated T-maze. *Neuroscience Biobehavioral Reviews*, **46**, 397–406.

Zanoveli, J. M., Nogueira, R. L. & Zangrossi, H., Jr. (2003). Serotonin in the dorsal periaqueductal gray modulates inhibitory avoidance and one-way escape behaviors in the elevated T-maze. *European Journal of Pharmacology*, **473**, 153–161.

14 Maternal and genetic effects on escape: a prospective review

Lesley T. Lancaster

14.1 Introduction

Despite our understanding that escape behaviors are often optimized under strong and chronic selection, few studies have examined how these behaviors are transmitted, and this lack of information impedes knowledge of how escape behaviors can evolve. In this chapter, I review studies that have identified potential mechanisms of escape behavior transmission, from estimates of heritability of escape behavior and other quantitative genetic parameters, to family-, population-, and species-level effects on escape that are suggestive of heritability and local adaptation, to specific maternal effect mechanisms that organize escape behavior. This review provides an overview of the current state of the field, with discusion of how escape behavior may become adaptively integrated phenotypically with other components of an animal's biology, including morphology, life-history, and reproductive strategies. This chapter is intended as a foundation for further research directions and to identify the largest gaps in what is currently known. As predator–prey regimes are altered by human influences on the environment, it is becoming increasingly critical to determine whether and how prey animals will continue to optimize escape decisions. Understanding the evolvability of escape behavior is a critical component of this endeavor.

Predation imposes strong natural selection on individuals and populations of most animal species, resulting in evolution of antipredator traits that facilitate survival. Escape behavior is a particularly interesting component of any animal's antipredator syndrome (i.e., the animal's suite of traits that together facilitate survival against predation) because escape often represents the last line of defense. For example, most animals' antipredator syndromes comprise multiple predator-avoidance traits, such as altered activity patterns, cryptic or warning coloration and behavior, vigilance, defensive nest construction, or chemical defenses. However, for many individuals, these predator avoidance mechanisms at some point ultimately fail to prevent the prey animal from being targeted by a predator for attack (Pinheiro 1996). At this point, escape behavior becomes a critical determinant of an animal's survival, and the set of behaviors

Escaping From Predators: An Integrative View of Escape Decisions, ed. W. E. Cooper and D. T. Blumstein. Published by Cambridge University Press. © Cambridge University Press 2015.

comprising "escape" might therefore be predicted to be refined by selection into a highly context specific and reliably produced sequence of actions.

There are a number of ways by which adaptive and effective escape behaviors may be organized at the individual level, including cultural transmission, learning by experience, innate expression of an entirely genetically determined behavior, and more complex, higher-order modes of transmission in which predator cues experienced by the parental generation are translated into developmental cues that influence offspring behavior (i.e., adaptive maternal effects). It is commonly assumed that some combination of these modes of transmission is responsible for the expression of most adaptive escape behaviors: the requirement that effective escape behaviors must be context specific suggests that phenotypic plasticity and incorporation of environmental cues may be important influences on the expression of such behaviors. On the other hand, escape behaviors have an immediate life or death outcome, affording limited opportunity for these behaviors to be shaped by learning or experience, particularly in solitary animals that cannot learn from witnessing attacks on conspecifics. For this reason, it is predicted or assumed that most escape behaviors are also based on a system of early-developmental or intergenerational transmission such as cultural (i.e., non-genetic, horizontal transmission), maternal (i.e., the components of vertical transmission between mothers and offspring besides direct genetic transmission of traits), or direct genetic mechanisms.

Despite the expectation that escape behaviors are modified under natural selection and controlled by adaptive genetic × environmental interactions (G×E), little is known about how these behaviors are transmitted. This is on one hand because escape behaviors are higher order traits that rely on underlying physiological (Chapter 13) and morphological (Chapter 11) characteristics, which themselves each have complex environmental and genetic bases. On the other hand, lack of a comprehensive understanding of how escape behavior is transmitted, organized, and refined by selection is likely due to the scarcity of studies that have tackled this topic. Studies focusing on the evolution of reaction norms for escape behavior are particularly rare. In this chapter, I review studies that have investigated either quantitative genetic or mechanistic bases of escape behavior transmission to synthesize what is currently known and point to fruitful future directions for research. To facilitate evaluation and future synthesis, many of the reviewed studies are summarized in Table 14.1.

14.2   Empirical estimates of heritability

Because escape behavior has such a strong and direct link to survivorship with few opportunities for "practice," effective escape strategies should have evolved high heritabilities. In practice, remarkably few studies have directly estimated the heritability of escape behaviors. Often, heritabilities of escape strategies are assessed as a component of personality (Chapter 15; Sinn *et al.* 2006). Conversely, other studies report significant heritabilities for traits that commonly underlie escape behavior, such as aspects of locomotor performance (Chapter 11), including sprint speeds and

Table 14.1 Summary of reviewed studies that examine the inheritance of escape behavior.

Taxon	Behavior	Effect	Reference
Estimated heritability			
Scallops *Argopecten purpuratus*	Latency to flee	$h^2 = 0.45 \pm 0.18$	Brokordt (2012)
	Total number of claps (adductor muscle contractions)	$h^2 = 0.51 \pm 0.18$	
	Clapping time	$h^2 = 0.36 \pm 0.17$	
	Clapping rate	$h^2 = 0.57 \pm 0.18$	
Garter snakes *Thamnophis ordinoides*	Distance fled	$h^2 = 0.387 \pm 0.169 - 0.798 \pm 0.164$	Brodie (1989, 1993)
	Number of reversals	$h^2 = 0.225 \pm 0.110 - 0.783 \pm 0.184$	
	Escape speed	$h^2 = 0.419 \pm 0.196 - 1.173 \pm 0.163$	
Mamushi snakes *Gloydius blomhoffii*	Distance fled	$h^2 = 0.82 \pm 0.47$ (hunted site), 0.89 ± 0.50 (non-hunted site)	Sasaki *et al.* (2009)
Common fruit fly *Drosophila melanogaster*	Distance fled	$h^2 = 0.076 \pm 0.011$ (low line), 0.143 ± 0.021 (high line)	Grant & Mettler (1969)
Indirect evidence for heritability			
Alpine swifts *Apus melba*	Behavioral gradient from flee to attack	*Family-level effects (genetic or maternal)*	Bize *et al.* (2012)
Garter snakes *Thamnophis sirtalis*	Alert distance/flight initiation distance		King (2002)
Pea aphids *Acyrthosiphon pisum*	Dropping behavior		Andrade & Roitberg (1995)
Guppies *Poecilia reticulata*	Maneuverability/capture time	*Sire effects, non-maternal and likely genetic*	Evans *et al.* (2004)
Field crickets *Gryllus integer*	Hiding time	*Population-level effects in naïve progens, genetic or maternal*	Hedrick & Kortet (2006)
Desert grass spiders *Agelenopsis aperta*	Hiding time	*Population-level effects, likely genetic*	Riechert & Hedrick (1990)
Trinidadian guppies *Poecilia reticulata*	Capture time		O'Steen *et al.* (2002)
Streamside salamanders *Ambystoma barbouri*	Stimulus to initiate flight	*Population-level and gene flow effects, likely genetic*	Storfer & Sih (1998)
Checkered whiptail lizards *Aspidoscelis tesselata*	Flight initiation distance, distance fled	*Population-level differences; maternal, genetic or learned*	Punzo (2007)

Table 14.1 (cont.)

Taxon	Behavior	Effect	Reference
Garter snakes *Thamnophis sirtalis*	Proportion that flee	*Population-level effects, maternal-offspring correlation*	Placyk (2012)
Common frog *Rana temporaria*	Survival in predator presence	*Latitudinal cline*	Laurila *et al.* (2008)
159 bird species	Flight initiation distance		Diaz *et al.* (2013)
Sexual and unisexual whiptail lizards	Flight initiation distance	*Species-level differences, correlation with sexual system*	Hotchkin & Riveroll (2005), see text for additional references
Freshwater fish	Flight initiation distance	*Species-level differences,*	McLean & Godin (1989)
Lizards (family: Cordylidae)	Distance fled, proportion that enter refuge, escape speed, use of vertical surfaces in escape -	*correlation with body armor*	Losos *et al.* (2002)
	Maternal effects		
Side-blotched lizards *Uta stansburiana*	Vertical escape behaviors, evasive behaviors	*Egg size* ($V_M/V_P = 0.36$)	Lancaster *et al.* (2010)
Red drum *Sciaenops ocellatus*	Escape latency, flight initiation distance/alert distance, duration of escape	*Fatty acid content of eggs*	Fuiman & Ojanguren (2011)
Painted dragons *Ctenophorus pictus*	Latency to flee, assessment time	*Experimentally elevated yolk testosterone*	Tobler *et al.* (2012)
Pied flycatchers *Ficedula hypoleuca*	Proportion that flee		Ruuskanen & Laaksonen (2010)
Garter snakes *Thamnophis elegans*	Reversal behaviors	*Maternal ecotype × experimentally elevated maternal corticosterone*	Robert *et al.* (2009)
Common lizard *Zootoca vivipara*	Latency to flee	*Experimentally elevated maternal corticosterone*	Meylan & Clobert (2004)
Common lizard *Zootoca vivipara*	Hiding time	*Experimentally elevated yolk corticosterone*	Uller & Olsson (2006)
Grey partridge *Perdix perdix*	Proportion that flee, crouching behavior	*Yolk carotenoids – no effect*	Cucco *et al.* (2006)
Water pythons *Liasis fuscus*	Stimulation to sustain flight, vertical behaviors	*Incubation temperature regime*	Shine *et al.* (1997)
Keelback snakes *Tropidonophis mairii*	Pauses during flight, proportion of individuals that enter refuge		Webb *et al.* (2001)

Table 14.1 (cont.)

Taxon	Behavior	Effect	Reference
Oviparous scincid lizards (*Bassiana duperreyi* and *Nannoscincus maccoyi*)	Reversals	Incubation temperature regime	Shine (1995)
Three spine sticklebacks *Gasterosteus aculeatus*	Proportion that orient to predator, survival	*Maternal experience*	McGhee *et al.* (2012)
Fall crickets *Gryllus pennsylvanicus*	Hiding time		Storm & Lima (2010)
Skinks *Pseudemoia pagenstecheri*	Reversals	*Maternal condition*	Shine & Downes (1999)

stamina (Garland 1988, Shaffer & Formanowicz 2000, Watkins & McPeek 2006, Blumstein *et al.* 2010). However, it is often unclear how selection acting on either higher (i.e., personality) or lower order (i.e., locomotor performance) traits will affect the evolutionary response of escape behavior itself. Studies that directly estimate escape behavior heritability are often performed in the laboratory, which minimizes stochastic environmental effects on behavior, but which may present an artificial picture of how animals actually behave in the wild. Two examples in which thorough quantitative genetic analyses have been carried out are included below as case studies. These are followed by a review of other studies providing less complete evidence of heritable escape behaviors in section 14.3.

14.2.1   Case study 1: Flight in scallops

Juvenile scallops (*Argopecten purpuratus*) exhibit significant heritabilities for escape behaviors in response to controlled episodes of contact with a sea star, a natural predator (Brokordt *et al.* 2012; Figure 14.1). Brokordt *et al.* estimated heritabilities using offspring of wild-caught (but laboratory-reared) parents that were produced in a full/half-sib breeding design. Escape behaviors measured included latency to flee following predator contact, number of claps performed by the scallop during escape (claps = contractions of the phasic adductor muscle, producing valve closings and openings), and the rate and duration of clapping, which determine the speed and distance of the scallop's escape effort. Estimated heritabilities were high and significant for all behaviors (Table 14.1). In all cases, dam effects were near zero and non-significant, suggesting that escape is not strongly influenced by maternal effects in this system. Interestingly, when scallops were subjected to a repeat trial, heritabilities of escape behavior dropped considerably. Although behaviors were repeatable (R = 0.36–0.42), most were no longer significantly heritable when estimated from repeat performances. This suggests that naïve scallops exhibit innate and genetically based escape abilities

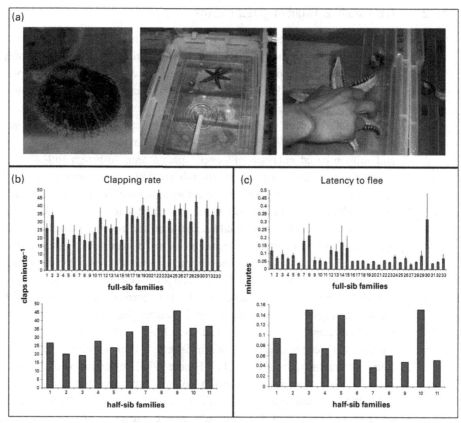

Figure 14.1   Heritable variation in scallop escape behavior (from Brokordt *et al.* 2012). (A) (left to right): Study organism, *A. purpuratus*. Escape trial arena. Escape trial in action (photo credits: Gabriela Núñez and Manuel Carmona). (B,C) Among-family variation in two of the measured escape behaviors, clapping rate (rate of contraction of phasic adductor muscle, providing an estimate of escape effort) and latency to flee following forced contact with a natural predator, a sea star. (Figures reproduced with premission from K. Brokordt unpublished)

that are subsequently influenced by experience or limiting energetic considerations (only five minutes rest time was allowed between trials).

Escape behaviors in scallops were not only highly heritable, but also exhibited significant genetic correlations with each other: reaction time exhibited significant genetic correlations with clapping time ($r_G = 0.79 \pm 0.21$) and with number of claps ($r_G = -0.74 \pm 0.26$), suggesting a genetic trade-off between fast reaction times and the ability to sustain the escape. Such a trade-off between speed and endurance has been commonly proposed (Garland 1988), but has not always been reported (Brodie 1993; Sorci *et al.* 1995). However, genetic correlations between different components of escape may be common, with some genetic correlations reflecting trade-offs and constraints, and others reflecting co-evolved suites of traits that work well together in an integrated escape strategy (see also section 14.2.2).

14.2.2   Case study 2: Flight in garter snakes

Garter snakes have become a model system for investigating the genetics of escape-related behavior (Arnold & Bennett 1984; Garland 1988) because they display a diversity of escape and defensive tactics combined with alternative antipredator markings (Jackson *et al.* 1976; Brodie 1989), and these traits each appear to be strongly genetically influenced. Brodie (1989, 1993) calculated heritabilities and genetic correlations among escape and other antipredator traits for individual garter snakes (*Thamnophis ordinoides*) based on laboratory behavioral trials of naïve, juvenile snakes and full-sib-based analyses of genetic parameters. Although full-sib analyses often conflate genetic and maternal effects, this conflation was partially removed by regressing behavior scores on potential indicators of maternal condition. Maternal effects that do not reflect maternal condition were not accounted for, however. As in Brokordt *et al.* (2012), significant and substantial heritabilities and genetic correlations were found for all escape and escape-related traits, including distance fled, number of reversals in direction of escape, and escape speed, with estimated heritabilities for escape behaviors ranging from 0.23 to 1.17. The highest and lowest estimates for each escape behavior's heritability are reported in Table 14.1. Genetic correlations were reported between the number of reversals that a snake performed during flight and its dorsal patterning in two out of four populations ($r_G = -0.328 \pm 0.116 - r_G = -0.499$ [s.e. not reported]). A significant genetic correlation between distance fled and speed was reported in one of the four populations ($r_G = 0.418 \pm 0.111$; Brodie 1993). In contrast with the scallop example above, faster garter snakes also exhibited more prolonged escapes.

Heritable variation in escape behavior of garter snakes is likely maintained under correlational selection favoring alternative escape syndromes: blotched snakes achieve high fitness by performing reversals to aid in crypsis whereas striped snakes survive best when escaping in a straight line to create an optical illusion of stasis (Brodie 1992; Figure 14.2A; see also section 14.5.1). Homogeneity of escape behavior × dorsal pattern G–matrices across diverged populations also suggests that these traits may be related by pleiotropy or linkage in addition to shared selection pressures (Brodie 1993) although much more work is needed to understand the genomic architecture of escape syndromes.

14.3   Other evidence for genetic basis of escape behaviors

Although formal quantitative genetic studies of escape behavior are rare, many studies present at least partially convincing evidence for genetic bases of escape behavior. These cover a broad array of taxa, and can be grouped by the methodologies used to infer heritability, from parent-offspring or among-sib comparisons to artificial selection experiments to population- or species-level comparisons. Parent-offspring and full-sib comparisons establish family-level effects on escape behavior, although how this genetic component of phenotypic variation is distributed among maternal, additive, dominance, epistatic, and G × E effects remains to be determined. Artificial selection

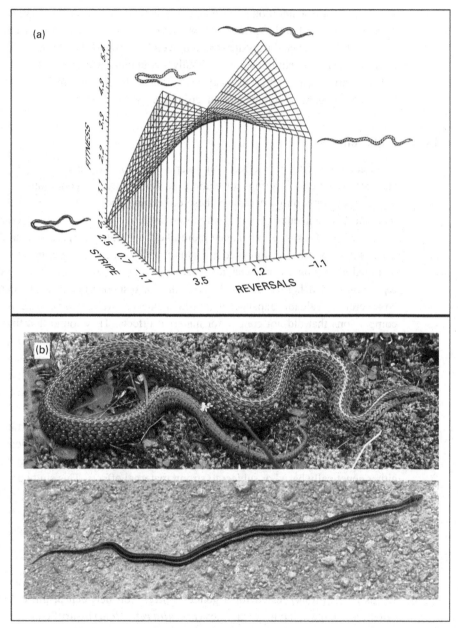

Figure 14.2   Genetic architecture of garter snake escape behavior (from Brodie 1989, 1993). (A) Correlational selection favors genetic correlations between dorsal patterning and escape behavior. Blotched snakes are selected to perform reversals, facilitating crypsis. Striped snakes are selected to escape in a straight line, facilitating an optical illusion of reduced speed. Figure reproduced with permission from Brodie (1992). (B) Escape behavior variation in *T. ordinoides*. Top panel: a blotched individual performing a reversal (photo by Gary Nafis). Bottom panel: a striped individual escapes in a straight line (photo by Jim Conrad).

studies provide the additional advantage of supplying evidence for additive effects on escape behaviors, but these often cannot rule out maternal and grand-maternal effects, and are often conducted in systems so removed from the wild that it is difficult to apply their conclusions to natural systems. Finally, population- and species-level comparisons indicate larger scale trends in local adaptation and trade-offs that can inform future studies of the genetic architecture underpinning escape.

14.3.1   Family effects

Most commonly, familial effects on escape behavior have been detected via full-sib analysis or parent-offspring correlations under controlled conditions (either cross-fostering or common garden), and these effects may be attributed to either genetic or maternal/environmental effects of parents on progeny. For instance, adult, cross-fostered alpine swifts (*Apus melba*) behaved more like their biological parents than their foster parents in response to a simulated predator attack, suggesting either genetic or prenatal maternal effects on escape behavior (Bize *et al.* 2012). Sasaki *et al.* (2009) studied the repeatability and heritability of distance fled in response to human predators in the commercially valuable Japanese mamushi snakes (*Gloydius blomhoffii*), using full-sib comparisons that did not control for maternal effects. They found that flight distance exhibited significant family effects in both hunted and non-hunted populations (Table 14.1).

Alert distance/flight initiation distance (assessed as the distance at which the snake reacted to a simulated predator by either orienting or fleeing) showed a significant family effect in garter snakes (*Thamnophis sirtalis*), in full-sib comparisons in lab-reared progeny of wild-caught dams (King 2002). King also found significant family × time and family × time × testosterone interactions, suggesting that the ontogeny of escape behavior and the response of escape behavior to circulating steroid hormones are also either genetically based or subject to strong maternal effects. This study provides base-line evidence for a heritable set of environmentally modified reaction norms for escape behavior, a mechanism of inheritance that allows escape responses to be both reliably produced over multiple generations (i.e., stereotyped) and also suited to current conditions (i.e., individual or maternal experiences of predator regime, habitat, or individual variation in trade-offs between escape and other activities).

In one of the more convincing examples of genetic effects on escape behavior, Evans *et al.* (2004) tested for a genetic correlation between bright coloration and effective escape behavior in guppies (*Poecilia reticulata*) by artificially inseminating females with sperm from brightly or dully colored males with which the females had not had prior contact. Artificial insemination prevented females from using male coloration as a signal to trigger maternal effects, while testing the hypothesis that coloration is a reliable indicator of male genetic quality (Hill 1991). More brightly colored males sired offspring with better maneuvering ability during escape, and thus longer times to capture (by a human using a net), suggesting a genetic sire effect on escape behavior, and a genetic correlation between escape behavior and sexually selected coloration (Evans *et al.* 2004).

14.3.2   Evidence of heritability from artificially selected lines

A response to artificial selection over multiple generations in a controlled environment is likely sufficient to dispel all but the most persistent of confounding maternal effects, and this methodology has provided some solid evidence of genetic effects on escape behavior. For instance, parthenogenic pea aphids (*Acyrthosiphon pisum*) exhibit variation in their tendency to drop from a perch in response to alarm pheromone emitted by clone-mates. Andrade and Roitberg (1995) created three to four generation, divergently selected lines for this escape behavior in three clones of pea aphids, resulting in significant divergence in phenotype in the majority of cases.

In a related study, divergently selected lines of *Drosophila melanogaster* exhibited phenotypic divergence in distance fled upward through an I-maze away from vibrations imparted to the bottom of the maze (Grant & Mettler 1969). Escape behavior that continued to diverge over 18 generations without plateau, and also resulted in a correlated evolutionary response in assortative mating behavior: individuals selected for non-fleeing behavior engaged more readily in courtship behavior and were thus more likely to pair with each other in mating trials. This result suggests that divergent selection on escape behavior imposed by predation may be sufficient to establish partial reproductive isolation. Significant realized heritabilities were calculated from these lines (Table 14.1). However, due to the highly artificial conditions of the behavioral trials, it is unclear how these results reflect true antipredator escape behaviors in a wild context.

14.3.3   Evidence for heritability and local adaptation from population comparisons

To infer local adaptation in escape behaviors, a number of investigators have examined the behaviors of lab-reared offspring of wild-caught mothers from populations subject to differing predation levels or regimes. Although these studies often cannot distinguish between genetic and maternal effects on offspring escape behaviors, it is possible in controlled rearing conditions to control for the effect of the offspring environment. Such controlled studies provide good evidence that at least some components of escape behaviors that vary among populations are organized before birth. Population comparisons represent the most abundant current evidence for heritability and local adaptation in escape behaviors.

Naïve, captive-reared offspring of wild-caught female field crickets (*Gryllus integer*) exhibited longer hiding times when their mothers had been captured from a population characterized by a greater diversity of predators than offspring from a population with fewer predator species (Hedrick & Kortet 2006). Subjects were obtained from two populations that differed in the number of predator species present and which were sufficiently geographically isolated to prevent high levels of gene flow, and escape behaviors were assessed in a controlled laboratory setting. A similar result for population level variation in hiding times was reported for lab-reared, F2 desert grass spiders *Agelenopsis aperta* from habitats characterized by differing avian predation intensities (Reichert & Hedrick 1990). Breeding to a second generation limits the influence of single-generation maternal effects, and provides strong evidence of genetic transmission and local adaptation in escape behavior. O'Steen *et al.* (2002), Punzo (2007), Placyk (2012), and Sasaki *et al.* (2009) have provided similar examples of population-level variation in escape behaviors in guppies, whiptail lizards, and snakes (Table 14.1).

Population-level comparisons are more convincing when couched in a formal population-genetics framework. Laboratory reared larval salamanders (*Ambystoma barbouri*) from populations with fish predators present required lower stimulus intensity (number of taps) to initiate flight than naïve larvae from populations in fishless habitats (Storfer & Sih 1998). Furthermore, the number of taps required to initiate escape depended on the degree of genetic isolation of the individual's source population from a population not exposed to fish, indicating that gene flow constrains local adaptation in escape behaviors. Survival rates in the presence of a cichlid predator were also higher among individuals from populations more genetically isolated from populations not exposed to predation by fish. This example clearly indicates a genetic effect on escape and suggests a trade-off between escape and some other aspect of performance that is favored in the absence of predators.

Clinal gradients in escape behavior can also indirectly implicate local adaptation over large-scale gradients in selective regimes. Latitudinal gradients in escape behavior, corresponding to decreases in predator densities at high latitudes, offer suggestive evidence of adaptive genetic effects on escape behavior in frogs (Laurila *et al.* 2008) and birds (Díaz *et al.* 2013).

14.3.4   Species-level comparisons

Species-level comparisons offer evidence complementary to that obtained from population-level comparisons, providing insight into the evolution of escape behavior at macroevolutionary scales. Studies reviewed above suggest that the maintenance of adaptive differences in escape behavior among populations may depend on low gene flow (Storfer & Sih 1998), and, in turn, population-level differences in escape behavior may contribute to reproductive isolation among populations (Grant & Mettler 1969; Nakayama & Miyatake 2010). When an ecologically relevant trait such as escape behavior varies among populations and contributes to reproductive isolation between populations, this trait may facilitate or drive ecological speciation and adaptive radiations. The evidence for effects of divergently selected escape behavior on reproductive isolation among conspecific populations indicates that escape behavior may drive speciation dynamics in some systems. In other cases, escape behavior may exhibit phylogenetic and niche conservatism. Phylogenetic conservatism could indicate that escape behavior is developmentally or ecologically constrained, and strongly suggests a genetic basis for escape behavior and its correlations and trade-offs with other traits.

In a comparison of three congeneric species of whiptail lizards (*Aspidoscelis* spp.), two parthenogenic and one gonochoristic, species-level differences in flight initiation distance and other defensive behaviors were reported (Hotchkin & Riveroll 2005), consistent with some previous observations (Milstead 1957; Schall & Pianka 1980; Price 1992). This suggests that escape behavior might be affected by genetic changes that occur in the transition to parthenogenesis or subsequent loss of genetic variability (Schall & Pianka 1980; Paulissen 1998) although more evidence is needed to confirm the cause of variation in escape behavior across these species.

Flight initiation distance in four populations from three species of freshwater fish was inversely correlated with degree of body armor (McLean & Godin 1989). The authors argued that this correlation reflects an evolved trade-off between behavioral and morphological defense (see also Abrahams 1995). These studies rely on relatively few species comparisons and do not consider effects of phylogeny or divergence times.

In a phylogenetically informed comparison of morphological defense and escape behavior in 15 cordylid lizard species, more heavily armored species ran shorter distances (distance fled), entered refuges more frequently (proportion of individuals that enter refuge), ran more slowly, and were less likely to utilize vertical surfaces during flight (Losos *et al.* 2002). Armor was concluded to be part of an evolved, genetically based antipredator syndrome that involves altered escape behavior and habitat use. Alternatively, differences in escape behavior could be non-genetic and result from behavioral plasticity producing similar behaviors in the habitats used by armored species. In general, Losos *et al.* found that phylogenetic comparisons provided similar results to non-phylogenetic tests of escape behavior and correlations with morphology, indicating a high degree of evolutionary lability. More phylogenetic tests of escape behavior are required to complement population-genetic analyses and within-population heritability estimates, in order to better understand the genetic architecture and evolutionary potential of escape behavior.

14.4 Conclusions based on case studies and other evidence of escape heritability

The genetics of escape behavior is currently a neglected field. Very few formal quantitative analyses of escape behavior have been conducted. Even among those, maternal effects are not always effectively excluded (e.g., Brodie, 1993), and dominance and epistasis have not yet been addressed. The recent advancements in computationally intensive methods for quantitative genetic and genomic analysis within the last decade mean that such studies are now much more feasible. However, most studies to date provide only partial or equivocal evidence for heritability of escape behavior. Collectively, these studies strongly indicate that escape behavior has a genetic basis in a wide variety of prey taxa, often exhibits local adaptation, and may be associated with predictable antipredator syndromes (such as degree of morphological defense) or sexual/genetic systems (e.g., parthenogenesis, sexually selected coloration). As predicted, many of these studies indicate that escape behavior is likely to exhibit evolved plasticity and ontogenetic modification, and high evolutionary potential.

14.5   Maternal effects

Adaptive maternal effects are predicted to arise when a female reliably experiences one of several different environments, and the environment that she experiences also reliably predicts conditions her offspring are likely to face (Mousseau & Fox 1998). Because predator regimes often persist at intermediate ecological scales of space and time and/or exhibit cyclical dynamics (May 1972), escape behaviors are ideal candidates for adaptive maternal modification. Theoretically, maternal effects can reliably produce a range of adaptive behaviors in offspring according to local cues, in contrast to locally adapted behaviors with a strictly genetic basis, which suffer from slower evolutionary responses to changing predator regimes, and from gene flow from areas having different predation regimes (Storfer & Sih 1998). Furthermore, adaptive maternal effects are predicted to appropriately adjust offspring behaviors according to phase of a predator–prey density cycle.

Many of the studies on familial effects may be most plausibly interpreted as partially or substantially due to maternal effects, but convincing evidence is lacking. In contrast, studies that specifically address maternal effects on escape behavior do not commonly include a formal quantitative genetic analysis of the maternal contribution to phenotypic variation (V_M). Instead, investigators of maternal effects on escape behavior have, to date, more often focused on behavioral and physiological mechanisms, including provisioning, incubation regimes, or other phenotypic interactions between mothers and their progeny that may or may not be adaptive. In these studies a combination of experimental manipulations and correlative approaches have been employed to identify specific effects of maternal traits on offspring escape behavior. Below I review a mechanism of maternal effects on escape behavior, with emphasis on a case study in which the role of maternal effects was assessed both mechanistically and in a quantitative genetics framework, and the maternal effect on escape behavior was placed in a broader context of an evolved character syndrome involving adaptive mating and antipredator strategies.

14.5.1   Case study: Egg size and alternative patterns of adaptive escape behavior in side-blotched lizards

Escape behaviors often exhibit adaptive variation within populations, where variation in escape behaviors prevents predators from matching their attack strategy to a single escape tactic (Schall & Pianka 1980). Furthermore, variable escape strategies are often most effective when paired with other traits that affect the success of each escape behavior in an integrated, multitrait antipredator strategy (e.g., adaptive correlations between particular escape behavior strategies and dorsal patterning or body size; Brodie 1989; DeWitt et al. 1999). Side-blotched lizards (*Uta stansburiana*) exhibit alternative throat colors that indicate alternative mating and reproductive tactics in each sex (Sinervo & Lively 1996). Throat color is correlated with egg size variation, with yellow-throated females laying larger eggs than orange-throated

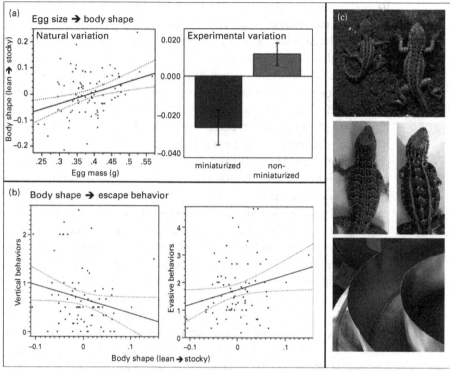

Figure 14.3   Effects of egg size on escape behavior (from Lancaster *et al.* 2010). (A) Egg size affects body shape in *U. stansburiana*. Left panel: regression of egg mass on body shape. Body shape, but not body size, effects persist throughout life (Figure 3C in original article, reproduced with permission). Right panel: experimental egg size manipulations also affect body shape. (B) Egg size effects on body shape direct alternative escape behaviors: leaner progeny are more likely to exhibit vertical behaviors (left panel), and stockier progeny are more likely to exhibit evasive behaviors (right panel). Experimental egg size manipulations produced similar effects on escape behavior (Figure 2C in original article, reproduced with permission). Data points in regressions represent full-sib means. (C) Top: effects of egg size manipulation on offspring body size and shape. Middle: examples of dorsal pattern variation; left = bars, right = stripes. Bottom: circular track for performing escape behavior trials (Photo 14.3C top: by Barry Sinervo; middle and bottom: by Lesley Lancaster)

females (Sinervo *et al.* 2000). This species also exhibits continuous variation in dorsal patterning, with patterns ranging from longitudinal stripes to horizontal bars (Lancaster *et al.* 2007; Figure 14.3C). Lancaster *et al.* (2010) found that survival selection favored two alternative trait combinations. Yellow-throated lizards, which exhibit a non-territorial, sneaker strategy in males, survived best with a barred dorsal pattern combined with evasive escape behaviors such as reversals and zigzags during flight. This result confirms earlier results that blotched and barred patterns are often co-selected with cryptic and evasive escape behaviors in reptiles (Jackson *et al.* 1976; Brodie 1992; Figure 14.2A) because this combination of traits facilitates crypsis, particularly when escaping into camouflaging vegetation. Territorial orange-throated lizards, in contrast, survived best when exhibiting a striped dorsal pattern and vertical (e.g., jumping, climbing) behaviors. These findings corroborate previous reports that stripes facilitate quick escape by creating an optical illusion of reduced speed (Brodie, 1992; see also section 14.2.2).

Adaptive combinations of such disparate traits as mating strategy, dorsal patterning, and escape behavior are rarely co-organized by a shared genetic pathway, and maternal effect plasticity may adaptively organize alternative character suites where linkage or pleiotropy are lacking (Lancaster *et al.* 2007, 2010). In side-blotched lizards, dorsal patterning and mating strategy are each heritable, but not genetically correlated with each other (Lancaster *et al.* 2007), and dorsal patterning is also under maternal control via yolk estradiol (Lancaster *et al.* 2007). In the context of a half-sib crossing design, escape behaviors were measured ten times in succession in all parents and progeny. Measured escape behaviors included vertical behaviors (number of jumping + climbing attempts within each trial), evasive behaviors (zigzags + reversals + pauses), hiding behaviors (crouches + burying attempts), and total distance fled. Behaviors were repeatable, but heritability was low and non-significant for all behaviors. However, escape behaviors were significantly phenotypically correlated with both natural and experimental variation in body shape, with "lean" body types more likely to engage in vertical behavior, and "stocky" body types more likely to engage in evasive behavior (Lancaster *et al.* 2010; Figure 14.3B). Body shape is controlled by egg size in this and other lizard species (Figure 14.3A; Sinervo & Huey 1990), a maternal effect. Egg size itself has both a genetic and environmental basis (Sinervo *et al.* 2000; Lancaster *et al.* 2008). Body shape was experimentally adjusted via egg size manipulations (Sinervo & Huey 1990; Lancaster *et al.* 2010) to confirm that egg size itself, and not a correlated direct-genetic or maternal effect, was causally responsible for inducing the alternative escape behaviors (Figure 14.3A). Furthermore, escape behavior was confirmed to be under maternal influence in a quantitative genetic analysis, which indicated that the maternal component of phenotypic variation (V_M, encompassing variance due to maternal effects and dominance) in progeny escape behavior was responsible for over a third of the total phenotypic variance (Table 14.1).

This study provides evidence that escape behavior may adaptively link alternative male and female reproductive strategies. In this study system, orange-throated males are territorial, inhabiting rock outcrops with good-quality nest sites. Orange-throated females tend to lay small eggs (resulting in lean hatchlings who perform vertical escape behaviors; these behaviors are beneficial in a three-dimensional, rocky habitat). Yellow-throated males are non-territorial sneakers that spend much of their time in the grass, and yellow-throated females tend to lay large eggs (resulting in stocky offspring that perform evasive behaviors that are beneficial in the between-territory vegetation). In the absence of an egg size effect on escape behaviors that are alternatively favored in habitats occupied by different mating strategy types, the genetic correlation between female egg size strategies and male mating strategies remains unexplained (egg size does not affect adult body size, but it does affect adult body shape; Lancaster *et al.* 2010). Similar correlations between mating and egg size strategies have been reported in other lizard species (Stapley & Keogh 2005), suggesting that escape behavior may commonly be responsible for observed correlations between alternative male mating strategies and female reproductive strategies.

14.5.2   Endocrine mechanisms of maternal effects on escape behavior

One of the most commonly studied ways that females can putatively affect the behavior of their progeny is by manipulating the prenatal endocrine environment, particularly by varying fetal exposure to steroid hormones. Prenatal glucocorticoid exposure (cortisol or corticosterone, depending on species) is a prime candidate for maternal organization of offspring escape behavior in vertebrates. This is because glucocorticoid levels, which function in vertebrate energy balance, are known to increase under stress and to affect behaviors requiring locomotion, such as activity level and dispersal (Dauphin-Villemant & Xavier 1987; De Fraipont *et al.* 2000). Glucocorticoids and other steroid hormones are easily transferred between mothers and developing offspring via the placenta or yolk of amniotic eggs (Hayward & Wingfield 2004). Therefore glucocorticoids provide a plausible, efficient mechanism by which mothers can communicate information about environmental stressors to offspring by using the same hormone that provides the cue to direct future offspring behavior (Uller & Olsson 2006), e.g., via known effects of glucocorticoids on energy distribution or muscle development (Chin *et al.* 2009).

Following this logic, several researchers have examined the effects of experimentally elevated maternal glucocorticoid levels on offspring escape behavior, mainly using reptilian study systems. Juvenile *Lacerta* (*Zootoca*) *vivipara* lizards from corticosterone-treated mothers exhibited increased latency to flee (required more stimulation to run) in comparison with offspring of control females (Meylan & Clobert 2004). Also in *Z. vivipara*, hatchlings from eggs that were directly injected with corticosterone exhibited significantly longer hiding times than control individuals (Uller & Olsson 2006). In the garter snake *Thamnophis elegans*, the effects of maternal corticosterone on escape behavior depended on maternal ecotype (Robert *et al.* 2009); specifically, experimentally elevated maternal corticosterone resulted in a reduced frequency of reversals in the "lakeshore" ecotype, which is characterized by a blotched dorsal pattern and frequent reversals. However, maternal corticosterone treatment had no effect on this behavior in the "mountain meadow" ecotype, which is characterized by stripes and few reversals. Ecotypes of *T. elegans* are correlated with alternative life-history strategies, and divergent naturally occurring corticosterone blood titers, suggesting that maternal effects on escape behavior may be closely tied to alternative life-history strategies (in addition to alternative mating and reproductive strategies; see sections 14.3 and 14.5.1). In each of these studies on maternal effects of glucocorticoids in reptiles, prenatal exposure to corticosterone was correlated with escape strategies involving lower energetic expenditure than in untreated controls.

Other steroid hormones have been investigated for potential maternal effects on escape behavior. Experimental prenatal exposure to androgens (testosterone injected into egg yolks) resulted in shorter assessment time and latency to flee in the painted dragon (*Ctenophorus pictus*), potentially indirectly via an effect on digit ratio (i.e., the relative lengths of individual digits on a single limb, which can affect locomotor performance; Tobler *et al.* 2011, 2012). Contrary to predicted effects of androgens on masculinized morphology and higher risk taking, experimentally elevated yolk testosterone in these studies resulted in a more feminized pattern of higher 3D:4D digit length ratios (ratio of the third to fourth digit length on a single limb), and a higher 3D:4D ratio was correlated with reduced risk-taking in escape behavior. In contrast, experimentally elevated yolk androgens (testosterone and androstenedione) resulted in the predicted pattern of increasingly risky escape behaviors in male pied flycatchers (*Ficedula hypoleuca*), which exhibited a decreased tendency to flee (~proportion that flee) (Ruuskanen & Laaksonen 2010).

The mechanism by which females increase offspring prenatal exposure to androgens in response to environmental cues is unknown, and likely involves a more complex physiological basis than glucocorticoid-based maternal effects, which can be transmitted as a passive response to maternal stress. Once androgens have been transferred to offspring, their effects on escape behavior are predicted to arise as downstream organizational effects on brain development, leading to increased overall levels of risk taking and aggressiveness (Partecke & Schwabl 2008). However, as Tobler *et al.* (2012) demonstrate, the effects of androgens on escape are often unpredictable and may have a more complex basis, including the aromatization of testosterone to estradiol by developing progeny (Crews *et al.* 1995). The potential effects of other (steroidal and non-steroidal) maternally derived hormones on escape behavior are currently unknown, with the exception of some preliminary evidence for no effect of maternal estradiol (Lancaster *et al.* 2010).

14.5.3   Other maternal provisioning effects on escape behavior

In addition to hormones, females provision offspring with varying quantities and qualities of many other nutrients and chemical cues that may have adaptive or incidental effects on offspring escape behavior. For instance, egg size influences escape behavior in side-blotched lizards via allometric body shape effects (section 14.5.1). Egg size is likely to commonly affect escape behavior in other species via its effect on offspring size because escape decisions are often size dependent (Wahle 1992, Shine *et al.* 1997, DeWitt *et al.* 1999). In addition to quantity of maternal provisioning, quality of provisioning may affect escape behaviors. The long-chain fatty acid content of eggs was correlated with offspring escape behaviors in red drum fish (*Sciaenops ocellatus*) although egg size itself had no effect (Fuiman & Ojanguren 2011). Long-chain fatty acids are usually associated with a high-quality diet and are important for nervous system function in vertebrates (Tocher 2003). Of 33 fatty acids tested, ten had significant effects on escape behavior. Effects were complex: some behaviors were influenced by multiple fatty acids, others by a single fatty acid type. In some cases, different fatty acids had opposing effects on the same escape variable. Understanding the generality and mechanisms of these effects will require further investigation.

Maternal investment in carotenoids represents an additional route by which females might increase offspring performance by increasing egg quality. Carotenoids are important in preventing damage due to oxidative stress and, like long-chain fatty acids, are obtained from high-quality diets (Sies 1997). Carotenoids are commonly invested in eggs (and are responsible for yellow yolk pigmentation), resulting in increased egg quality (Blount *et al.* 2002). However, carotenoid supplementation of laying females did not affect offspring escape behavior in the grey partridge, *Perdix perdix* (Cucco *et al.* 2006).

The putative link between compositional quality of eggs and escape behavior probably reflects an effect of provisioning on the overall condition and quality of offspring, with well-provisioned offspring better able to perform energetically costly or neurologically complex escape behaviors. Whether the quality of prenatal provisioning is in general an important contributor to effective escape performance is unknown. Furthermore, most studies of maternal provisioning effects have been conducted in egg-laying species, where provisioning is more easily quantified and characterized. In placental animals, the time interval available for prenatal provisioning is often more prolonged than in oviparous species. Therefore variation in the quantity and quality of resources provided by placental dams may reflect a broader range of conditions experienced by the mother. Although prenatal provisioning is more difficult to assess in placental species, such a study would provide a valuable comparison to existing information on egg-laying species.

14.5.4   Incubation regimes and maternal care

Incubation conditions, with or without maternal care, can affect escape behavior in reptiles. Nest site choice and incubation behaviors can introduce wide variation in the temperatures experienced by developing offspring, and incubation temperature has major effects on hatching time, offspring size, shape, sex, and behavior (Shine & Harlow 1996). Maternal choice of incubation temperature may be adaptively influenced by environmental cues, including predator density or predator type. Under natural selection, incubation temperature may be incorporated as a cue for offspring to develop appropriate escape strategies in response to the environment experienced by their mothers. Alternatively, variation in incubation temperature may have neutral or maladaptive effects on escape behavior if developmental conditions are suboptimal for neurological and musculoskeletal development.

Shine *et al.* (1997) investigated the effects of incubation regime on the amount of stimulation required by neonatal water pythons (*Liasis fuscus*) to sustain flight from a human predator through the water. Females exhibited alternative incubation strategies, choosing either to lay in varanid lizard burrows with hot, stable temperatures not requiring further attendance or to lay eggs in tree root boles having lower, more variable temperatures that require maternal attendance and shivering thermogenesis to maintain adequate incubation temperatures. Lab-reared hatchlings from eggs incubated in thermal regimes simulating (hot, stable) varanid burrow nests required more stimulation to sustain flight than hatchlings reared in conditions simulating (cooler, variable) tree bole nests, with or without maternal attendance. In contrast, hatchlings reared under root bole nest conditions, but without maternal attendance, exhibited increased vertical behaviors.

Incubation regimes reflecting natural variation in burrow depth affected escape behavior in a tropical natricine snake, the keelback, *Tropidonophis mairii* (Webb *et al.* 2001). Constant temperatures found in deep nests resulted in more pauses during flight, but a decreased tendency to hide, in comparison to the behavior of hatchlings incubated at the variable temperatures of shallow nests. The fitness consequences of offspring escape behaviors resulting from variation in incubation regimes, and whether these putative effects on offspring fitness have influenced the evolution of maternal incubation decisions, are unknown.

Shine (1995) investigated effects of incubation temperatures that mimic external nests vs. maternal body temperature in two oviparous scincid lizard species that are members of lineages in which viviparity has evolved. He found that cooler, nest-equivalent incubation temperatures resulted in hatchlings displaying more frequent reversals and defensive behaviors during flight. However, it is unknown whether the prenatal effects of maternal body temperature on offspring escape behavior are beneficial, or if they are involved in selection for viviparity.

14.5.5   Maternal environment and condition effects with unknown mechanisms

Several effects of maternal environment or condition on offspring escape behavior have been identified, but operate by unknown mechanisms. In a clear-cut example of a maladaptive maternal effect based on maternal experience, female three-spine stickle-backs that were exposed to predators produced offspring that were less likely to orient to the same predator type, and were therefore more likely to be eaten (McGhee *et al.* 2012). Conversely, female fall crickets (*Gryllus pennsylvanicus)* that were exposed to predators while gravid produced offspring with longer hiding times, which led to higher survival rates in the presence of predators (Storm & Lima 2010).

Maternal condition can also affect offspring escape behavior. For example, in the viviparous scincid lizard *Pseudemoia pagenstecheri*, offspring from females maintained with restricted food intake were more likely to perform reversals during escape, a behavior that was never seen in offspring from well-fed mothers (Shine & Downes 1999). The adaptive significance of this maternal effect is unknown.

14.5.6   Conclusions about maternal effects

Maternal effects on escape behavior have been reported in diverse taxa, albeit primarily in oviparous vertebrates. They operate by a wide variety of mechanisms, from effects of maternal behavior, experience, and condition to specific physiological effects of temperature and maternal provisioning. More studies are needed addressing the fitness effects of maternal effects on escape behavior in order to better discern adaptive maternal effects from maladaptive or neutral consequences of suboptimal prenatal and rearing conditions. More work is needed on viviparous vertebrates and invertebrates to complement existing studies, and to understand the generality of and interactions among different potential maternal effect mechanisms.

14.6   General conclusions

Evidence for a genetic basis or other prenatal organization of escape behavior has accumulated for diverse prey (Figure 14.4; Table 14.1) although data on invertebrates and mammals are sparse or lacking. One of the more interesting generalizations from findings to date is that escape behavior is often correlated with other aspects of an organism's biology, including mating and reproductive strategies, life history, sexually selected coloration, genetic systems, and morphology. These correlations suggest that escape behavior is often highly integrated with other aspects of an organism's biology, and that its heritability and mechanisms of transmission are strongly influenced and constrained by other, often non-predation related, traits. That escape behavior is often highly integrated with other traits also indicates its potential for use as an easily assessed indicator of the organism's overall behavioral syndrome.

The literature reviewed here also testifies to the breadth of genetic, maternal, and environmental mechanisms that can affect various components of escape behavior.

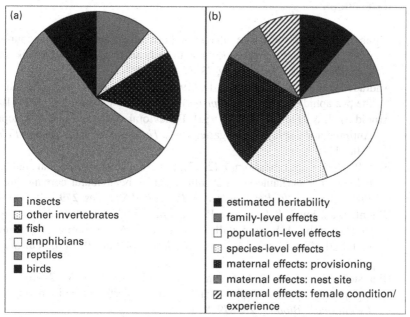

Figure 14.4   Summary of the current representation in the literature of studies examining the transmission of escape behavior, where each wedge represents the proportion of total papers reviewed: (A) by taxon; and (B) by mechanism. Studies were identified by searching Web of Science for combinations of the keywords and phrases: "maternal effect/s," "escape behavior/our," "antipredator behavior/our," "heritable/ility," "selection," and "genetic/s," and searching within cited articles and articles that cite keyword search results.

Overall, it confirms that escape behavior is subject to a wide range of influences affecting development, reflecting the dependence of variation in neurological and musculoskeletal development on the concerted action of a wide variety of underpinning genetic and physiological mechanisms. Because escape behavior is complex, many influences can potentially affect its effectiveness and/or adaptively direct its development. Further comparative studies are needed to determine how these trait associations evolve, and how escape is developmentally or ecologically constrained.

More research is needed to determine the generality of each of these mechanisms, to understand the genetic architecture of escape behavior evolution and to identify the evolutionary potential of escape behavior given correlations and trade-offs with other traits. Investigating the role of escape behavior in shaping macroevolutionary processes of speciation, facilitating niche evolution, and interacting with evolving sexual and genetic systems may prove fruitful. Further research is also needed to test for G × E interactions and specific genetic mechanisms that facilitate adaptive plasticity of escape behavior. Modern molecular ecological methods for identification of quantitative-trait loci (QTL), patterns of genome-wide association (GWA), and loci for adaptive traits in a landscape genetic framework are likely to be useful in determining maternal and genetic effects on escape behavior.

References

Abrahams, M. V. (1995). The interaction between antipredator behaviour and antipredator morphology: Experiments with fathead minnows and brook sticklebacks. *Canadian Journal of Zoology*, **73**, 2209–2215.

Andrade, M. C. B. & Roitberg, B. D. (1995). Rapid response to intraclonal selection in the pea aphid (*Acyrthosiphon pisum*). *Evolutionary Ecology*, **9**, 397–410.

Arnold, S. J. & Bennett, A. F. (1984). Behavioral variation in natural populations. 3. Antipredator displays in the garter snake *Thamnophis radix*. *Animal Behaviour*, **32**, 1108–1118.

Bize, P., Diaz, C. & Lindstrom, J. (2012). Experimental evidence that adult antipredator behaviour is heritable and not influenced by behavioural copying in a wild bird. *Proceedings of the Royal Society B-Biological Sciences*, **279**, 1380–1388.

Blount, J. D., Surai, P. F., Nager, R. G., *et al.* (2002). Carotenoids and egg quality in the lesser black-backed gull *Larus fuscus*: A supplemental feeding study of maternal effects. *Proceedings of the Royal Society B-Biological Sciences*, **269**, 29–36.

Blumstein, D. T., Lea, A. J., Olson, L. E. & Martin , J. G. A. (2010). Heritability of anti-predatory traits: Vigilance and locomotor performance in marmots. *Journal of Evolutionary Biology*, **23**, 879–887.

Brodie, E. D. (1989). Genetic correlations between morphology and antipredator behavior in natural populations of the garter snake *Thamnophis ordinoides*. *Nature*, **342**, 542–543.

Brodie, E. D. (1992). Correlational selection for color pattern and antipredator behavior in the garter snake *Thamnophis ordinoides*. *Evolution*, **46**, 1284–1298.

Brodie, E. D. (1993). Homogeneity of the genetic variance-covariance matrix for antipredator traits in 2 natural populations of the garter snake *Thamnophis ordinoides*. *Evolution*, **47**, 844–854.

Brokordt, K., Farias, W., Lhorente, J. P. & Winkler, F. (2012). Heritability and genetic correlations of escape behaviours in juvenile scallop *Argopecten purpuratus*. *Animal Behaviour*, **84**, 479–484.

Chin, E. H., Love, O. P., Verspoor, J. J., *et al.* (2009). Juveniles exposed to embryonic corticosterone have enhanced flight performance. *Proceedings of the Royal Society B-Biological Sciences*, **276**, 499–505.

Crews, D., Cantu, A. R., Bergeron, J. M. & Rhen, T. (1995). The relative effectiveness of androstenedione, testosterone, and estrone, precursors to estradiol, in sex reversal in the red-eared slider *(Trachemys scripta)*, a turtle with temperature-dependent sex determination. *General and Comparative Endocrinology*, **100**, 119–127.

Cucco, M., Guasco, B., Malacarne, G. & Ottonelli, R. (2006). Effects of beta-carotene supplementation on chick growth, immune status and behaviour in the grey partridge, *Perdix perdix*. *Behavioural Processes*, **73**, 325–332.

Dauphin-Villemant, C. & Xavier, F. (1987). Nychthemeral variations of plasma corticosteroids in captive *Lacerta vivipara* Jacquin: Influence of stress and reproductive state. *General and Comparative Endocrinology*, **67**, 292–302.

De Fraipont, M., Clobert, J., John-Alder, H. & Meylan, S. (2000). Increased pre-natal maternal corticosterone promotes philopatry of offspring in common lizards *Lacerta vivipara*. *Journal of Animal Ecology*, **69**, 404–413.

DeWitt, T. J., Sih, A. & Hucko, J. A. (1999). Trait compensation and cospecialization in a freshwater snail: Size, shape and antipredator behaviour. *Animal Behaviour*, **58**, 397–407.

Díaz, M., Møller, A. P., Flensted-Jensen, E., *et al.* (2013). The geography of fear: A latitudinal gradient in anti-predator escape distances of birds across Europe. *Plos One*, **8**, 7.

Evans, J. P., Kelley, J. L., Bisazza, A., Finazzo, E. & Pilastro, A. (2004). Sire attractiveness influences offspring performance in guppies. *Proceedings of the Royal Society B-Biological Sciences*, **271**, 2035–2042.

Fuiman, L. A. & Ojanguren, A. F. (2011). Fatty acid content of eggs determines antipredator performance of fish larvae. *Journal of Experimental Marine Biology and Ecology*, **407**, 155–165.

Garland, T. (1988). Genetic basis of activity metabolism – 1. Inheritance of speed, stamina, and antipredator displays in the garter snake *Thamnophis sirtalis*. *Evolution*, **42**, 335–350.

Grant, B. & Mettler, L. E. (1969). Disruptive and stabilizing selection on the escape behavior of *Drosophila melanogaster*. *Genetics*, **62**, 625–637.

Hayward, L. S. & Wingfield, J. C. (2004). Maternal corticosterone is transferred to avian yolk and may alter offspring growth and adult phenotype. *General and Comparative Endocrinology*, **135**, 365–371.

Hedrick, A. V. & Kortet, R. (2006). Hiding behaviour in two cricket populations that differ in predation pressure. *Animal Behaviour*, **72**, 1111–1118.

Hill, G. E. (1991). Plumage coloration is a sexually selected indicator of male quality. *Nature*, **350**, 337–339.

Hotchkin, P. & Riveroll, H. (2005). Comparative escape behavior of chihuahuan desert parthenogenetic and gonochoristic whiptail lizards. *Southwestern Naturalist*, **50**, 172–177.

Jackson, J. F., Ingram, W. & Campbell, H. W. (1976). Dorsal pigmentation pattern of snakes as an antipredator strategy: A multivariate approach. *American Naturalist*, **110**, 1029–1053.

King, R. B. (2002). Family, sex and testosterone effects on garter snake behavior. *Animal Behaviour*, **64**, 345–359.

Lancaster, L. T., McAdam, A. G., Wingfield, J. C. & Sinervo, B. R. (2007). Adaptive social and maternal induction of antipredator dorsal patterns in a lizard with alternative social strategies. *Ecology Letters*, **10**, 798–808.

Lancaster, L. T., Hazard, L. C., Clobert, J. & Sinervo, B. R. (2008). Corticosterone manipulation reveals differences in hierarchical organization of multidimensional reproductive trade-offs in r-strategist and K-strategist females. *Journal of Evolutionary Biology*, **21**, 556–565.

Lancaster, L. T., McAdam, A. G. & Sinervo, B. (2010). Maternal adjustment of egg size organizes alternative escape behaviors, promoting adaptive phenotypic integration. *Evolution*, **64**, 1607–1621.

Laurila, A., Lindgren, B. & Laugen, A. T. (2008). Antipredator defenses along a latitudinal gradient in *Rana temporaria*. *Ecology*, **89**, 1399–1413.

Losos, J. B., Mouton, P. L. N., Bickel, R., Cornelius, I. & Ruddock, L. (2002). The effect of body armature on escape behaviour in cordylid lizards. *Animal Behaviour*, **64**, 313–321.

May, R. M. (1972). Limit cycles in predator–prey communities. *Science*, **177**, 900–902.

McGhee, K. E., Pintor, L. M., Suhr, E. L. & Bell, A. M. (2012). Maternal exposure to predation risk decreases offspring antipredator behaviour and survival in threespined stickleback. *Functional Ecology*, **26**, 932–940.

McLean, E. B. & Godin, J. G. J. (1989). Distance to cover and fleeing from predators in fish with different amounts of defensive armor. *Oikos*, **55**, 281–290.

Meylan, S. & Clobert, J. (2004). Maternal effects on offspring locomotion: Influence of density and corticosterone elevation in the lizard *Lacerta vivipara*. *Physiological and Biochemical Zoology*, **77**, 450–458.

Milstead, W. W. (1957). Observations on the natural history of four species of whiptail lizard, *Cnemidophorus* (Sauria, Teiidae) in Trans-Pecos Texas. *Southwestern Naturalist*, **2**, 105–121.

Mousseau, T. A. & Fox, C. W. (1998). *Maternal Effects as Adaptations*. Oxford: Oxford University Press.

Nakayama, S. & Miyatake, T. (2010). Genetic trade-off between abilities to avoid attack and to mate: a cost of tonic immobility. *Biology Letters*, **6**, 18–20.

O'Steen, S., Cullum, A. J. & Bennett, A. F. (2002). Rapid evolution of escape ability in Trinidadian guppies (*Poecilia reticulata*). *Evolution*, **56**, 776–784.

Partecke, J. & Schwabl, H. (2008). Organizational effects of maternal testosterone on reproductive behavior of adult house sparrows. *Developmental Neurobiology*, **68**, 1538–1548.

Paulissen, M. A. (1998). Laboratory study of escape tactics of parthenogenetic and gonochoristic *Cnemidophorus* from southern Texas. *Copeia*, 240–243.

Pinheiro, C. E. G. (1996). Palatability and escaping ability in neotropical butterflies: Tests with wild kingbirds (*Tyrannus melancholicus*, Tyrannidae). *Biological Journal of the Linnean Society*, **59**, 351–365.

Placyk, J. S. (2012). The role of innate and environmental influences in shaping anti-predator behavior of mainland and insular gartersnakes (*Thamnophis sirtalis*). *Journal of Ethology*, **30**, 101–108.

Price, A. H. (1992). Comparative behavior in lizards of the genus *Cnemidophorus* (Teiidae), with comments on the evolution of parthenogenesis in reptiles. *Copeia*, 323–331.

Punzo, F. (2007). Sprint speed and degree of wariness in two populations of whiptail lizards (*Aspidoscelis tesselata*) (Squamata Teiidae). *Ethology Ecology & Evolution*, **19**, 159–169.

Riechert, S. E. & Hedrick, A. V. (1990). Levels of predation and genetically based antipredator behavior in the spider, *Agelenopsis aperta*. *Animal Behaviour*, **40**, 679–687.

Robert, K. A., Vleck, C. & Bronikowski, A. M. (2009). The effects of maternal corticosterone levels on offspring behavior in fast- and slow-growth garter snakes (*Thamnophis elegans*). *Hormones & Behavior*, **55**, 24–32.

Ruuskanen, S. & Laaksonen, T. (2010). Yolk hormones have sex-specific long-term effects on behavior in the pied flycatcher (*Ficedula hypoleuca*). *Hormones and Behavior*, **57**, 119–127.

Sasaki, K., Fox, S. F. & Duvall, D. (2009). Rapid evolution in the wild: Changes in body size, life-history traits, and behavior in hunted populations of the Japanese mamushi snake. *Conservation Biology*, **23**, 93–102.

Schall, J. J. & Pianka, E. R. (1980). Evolution of escape behavior diversity. *American Naturalist*, **115**, 551–566.

Shaffer, L. R. & Formanowicz, D. R. (2000). Sprint speeds of juvenile scorpions: Among family differences and parent offspring correlations. *Journal of Insect Behavior*, **13**, 45–54.

Shine, R. (1995). A new hypothesis for the evolution of viviparity in reptiles. *American Naturalist*, **145**, 809–823.

Shine, R. & Downes, S. J. (1999). Can pregnant lizards adjust their offspring phenotypes to environmental conditions? *Oecologia*, **119**, 1–8.

Shine, R. & Harlow, P. S. (1996). Maternal manipulation of offspring phenotypes via nest-site selection in an oviparous lizard. *Ecology*, **77**, 1808–1817.

Shine, R., Madsen, T. R. L., Elphick, M. J. & Harlow, P. S. (1997). The influence of nest temperatures and maternal brooding on hatchling phenotypes in water pythons. *Ecology*, **78**, 1713–1721.

Sies, H. (1997). Oxidative stress: Oxidants and antioxidants. *Experimental Physiology*, **82**, 291–295.

Sinervo, B. & Huey, R. B. (1990). Allometric engineering: An experimental test of the causes of interpopulational differences in performance. *Science*, **248**, 1106–1109.

Sinervo, B. & Lively, C. M. (1996). The rock–paper–scissors game and the evolution of alternative male strategies. *Nature*, **380**, 240–243.

Sinervo, B., Svensson, E. & Comendant, T. (2000). Density cycles and an offspring quantity and quality game driven by natural selection. *Nature*, **406**, 985–988.

Sinn, D. L., Apiolaza, L. A. & Moltschaniwskyj, N. A.(2006). Heritability and fitness-related consequences of squid personality traits. *Journal of Evolutionary Biology*, **19**, 1437–1447.

Sorci, G., Swallow, J. G., Garland, T. & Clobert, J. (1995). Quantitative genetics of locomotor speed and endurnace in the lizard *Lacerta vivipara*. *Physiological Zoology*, **68**, 698–720.

Stapley, J. & Keogh, J. S. (2005). Behavioral syndromes influence mating systems: Floater pairs of a lizard have heavier offspring. *Behavioral Ecology*, **16**, 514–520.

Storfer, A. & Sih, A. (1998). Gene flow and ineffective antipredator behavior in a stream-breeding salamander. *Evolution*, **52**, 558–565.

Storm, J. J. & Lima, S. L. (2010). Mothers forewarn offspring about predators: A Transgenerational maternal effect on behavior. *American Naturalist*, **175**, 382–390.

Tobler, M., Healey, M. & Olsson, M. (2011). Digit ratio, color polymorphism and egg testosterone in the Australian painted dragon. *Plos One*, **6**, 7.

Tobler, M., Healey, M. & Olsson, M. (2012). Digit ratio, polychromatism and associations with endurance and antipredator behaviour in male painted dragon lizards. *Animal Behaviour*, **84**, 1261–1269.

Tocher, D. R. (2003). Metabolism and functions of lipids and fatty acids in teleost fish. *Reviews in Fisheries Science*, **11**, 107–184.

Uller, T. & Olsson, M. (2006). Direct exposure to corticosterone during embryonic development influences behaviour in an ovoviviparous lizard. *Ethology*, **112**, 390–397.

Wahle, R. A. (1992). Body size dependent antipredator mechanisms of the American lobster. *Oikos*, **65**, 52–60.

Watkins, T. B. & McPeek, M. A. (2006). Growth and predation risk in green frog tadpoles (*Rana clamitans*): A quantitative genetic analysis. *Copeia*, **2006**, 478–488.

Webb, J. K., Brown, G. P. & Shine, R. (2001). Body size, locomotor speed and antipredator behaviour in a tropical snake (*Tropidonophis mairii*, Colubridae): The influence of incubation environments and genetic factors. *Functional Ecology*, **15**, 561–568.

15 The personality of escape

Pilar López and José Martín

15.1 Introduction

Experiments quantifying escape responses have revealed considerable inter-individual variation (Krause & Godin 1996; Jones *et al.* 2009), which might result from inter-individual differences in the ability to detect predators ("perceptual limit hypothesis"; Quinn & Cresswell 2005a), or in the time devoted to antipredator vigilance (Cresswell *et al.* 2003). Such inter-individual variation may be adaptive and represent different behavioral strategies (reviewed in Dall *et al.* 2004; Bell 2007; Réale *et al.* 2007; Smith & Blumstein 2008; Dingemanse & Wolf 2010). In behavioral and evolutionary ecology, the suites of behavioral traits with consistent individual differences across situations and contexts, or functional behavioral categories (e.g., foraging, social interactions, avoiding predators, etc.), are known as "behavioral syndromes" (Sih *et al.* 2004a,b; Sih & Bell 2008) or "animal personalities" (Dall *et al.* 2004; Groothuis & Carere 2005; Carere & Maestipieri 2013). In the past they were also referred to as temperament, coping styles, or coping strategies (Boissy 1995; Wechsler 1995; Koolhaas *et al.* 1999). Animal personalities have underlying genetic and physiological mechanisms (Koolhaas *et al.* 1999; Van Oers *et al.* 2004a), may be heritable (Van Oers *et al.* 2004b; Bell 2009) and have fitness consequences (Smith & Blumstein 2008).

We review individual differences in escape and hiding responses, and ask how the evolution of different personalities (i.e., the coexistence of different behavioral types in a population) is compatible with the theoretical prediction of a single optimal escape or hiding behavior response. Most work on personality in animals has focused on laboratory and field studies, considering variation in behaviors such as exploration, neophobia, and risk taking (reviewed in Sih *et al.* 2004a,b; Bell 2007; Réale *et al.* 2007). Particularly, escape responses and hiding behavior have often been used to characterize the personality of several animals (e.g., Sih *et al.* 2003; López *et al.* 2005; Hedrick & Kortet 2006, 2012; Cooper 2009; Carter *et al.* 2012a,b). Individuals that escape earlier from predators or spend longer times hidden in refuges can be considered as "shy" individuals. By contrast, "bold" individuals delay escape for longer or have shorter hiding times. However, the concept of personality or a

Escaping From Predators: An Integrative View of Escape Decisions, ed. W. E. Cooper and D. T. Blumstein. Published by Cambridge University Press. © Cambridge University Press 2015.

behavioral syndrome does not imply a simple dichotomy of behavioral types (e.g., proactive vs. reactive or shy vs. bold), but very often there is a continuous distributionof behavioral types and we should view personalities as existing along a continuum.

15.2   Is escape behavior a personality trait?

Behavioral syndromes or personalities were described as suites of correlated behaviors, with individual consistent differences being expressed in different behaviors in different situations and contexts (Sih *et al.* 2004a,b). A formal statistical definition, which has recently been proposed, suggests that mixed-effect statistical models can be applied to estimate a suite of between- and within-individual variance components of behavior (Dingemanse & Dochtermann 2013; see also Garamszegi & Herczeg 2012). Thus personalities could be identified if there is consistent repeatability in the interindividual differences between individuals. In other words, if the degree to which a behavioral trait differs between individuals (i.e., between individual variance) is greater than the degree to which a single observation differs from an individual's mean (i.e., within-individual variance). Repeatability represents the phenotypic variation attributable to differences between individuals, which is of key importance because it provides a standardized estimate of individuality that can be compared across studies. However, individuals can be consistent in their responses but also be plastic and change their responses between situations following behavioral reaction norms (Nusey *et al.* 2007; Biro & Stamps 2008; Dingemanse *et al.* 2010; see Figure 15.1). In that case, mixed-effect models allow the statistical definition of personality and plasticity as behavioral reaction norm intercepts and slopes respectively. When intercepts of these reaction norms differ between individuals in different situations, but slopes did not differ between individuals, we still could talk of personalities maintained across different situations. In addition, we can statistically define behavioral syndromes as non-zero between-individual correlations across behavioral attributes (Dingemanse & Dochtermann 2013).

Consider flight initiation distance (FID). We can imagine four different scenarios (Figure 15.1). On the one hand, individuals may react in a similar way to different risk levels and the average FID of the population may not change between risk levels (i.e., no plasticity; Figure 15.1b,d), but we will have different personalities if the variance of the FID responses of the same individual is consistently lower than the variance in FID between individuals (i.e., individuals differ in intercepts but not in slopes of the reaction norm; Figure 15.1d). We will not find different personalities if there are not consistent inter-individual differences in FID (Figure 15.1b). On the other hand, individuals may be sensitive and plastic and change their escape responses according to risk levels (Figure 15.1a,c), but they will still show different personalities in FID if the rank order differences between individuals is maintained consistently in both risk levels (i.e., individuals differ in intercepts but not in slopes; Figure 15.1c). Finally, individuals may be plastic and change their FID between risk levels, but with a lack of consistent

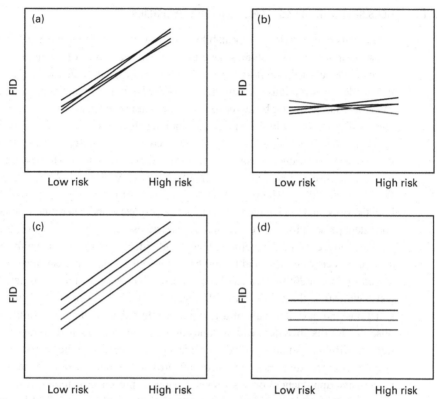

Figure 15.1   Consistency and plasticity in the escape response. Four hypothetical reaction norms of flight initiation distance (FID) responses of several individuals under two risk level situations. (a) The average FID increases when risk is high (plasticity) but there are not consistent personality differences between individuals. (b) The average FID response does not change between risk levels (no plasticity), and there is no consistency in the responses of the same individuals between risk levels. (c) The FID increases similarly in all individuals (plasticity), and the rank order differences between individuals (personality) is maintained consistently in both risk levels. (d) There are no changes in FID between risk levels (no plasticity) but there are consistent inter-individual differences in personality across risk levels. (Adapted from Nussey *et al.* 2007)

personality differences between individuals (i.e., individuals differ in slopes; Figure 15.1a).

Therefore if escape and hiding behavior were personality traits, we should expect that individuals differed consistently in their responses. However, individuals may show plasticity in different situations (e.g., different risk levels) while maintaining their personality rank in their responses. Moreover, when escaping from predators, bolder individuals might be also expected to show a behavioral syndrome and be bolder in other contexts, such as in conspecific agonistic interactions, foraging, etc. Although these predictions, and the existence of shy–bold escape syndromes, have been rarely tested specifically, we will review the evidence from several personality studies that have used escape and hiding behavior, or related antipredatory behaviors.

15.2.1   Consistency in the escape and hiding responses

To demonstrate individual repeatability, one must study the same subject repeatedly. However, relatively few studies have tested for repeatability of escape behavior in the same individuals in different situations. This is because most studies of escape behavior use independent observations (i.e., different individuals) in different treatments. Also, in most cases, measuring escape behavior requires simulating predatory attacks toward the tested animal. Thus most studies used different individuals to avoid the problem of habituation (see below) or sensitization, where animals decrease or increase, respectively, the magnitude of their subsequent responses to repeated risk situations. However, it would be possible to use a reaction norm approach (Biro & Stamps 2008; Dingemanse & Dochtermann 2013), whereby, by testing individuals repeatedly, it is possible to study both the slope and the intercept of their escape responses and determine whether there are consistent personality differences in responses across situations (see above, Figure 15.1).

One study examined whether reliable individual differences in boldness occur in several aspects of escape and hiding behavior in the striped plateau lizard, *Sceloporus virgatus* (Cooper 2009). Repeated measures of FID were positively correlated in several tests, indicating that individual differences in boldness were consistent in different situations and over intervals of a few minutes to a day or longer. A similar result was observed for distance fled. Hiding times of the same individuals (two repeated observations in different situations) were correlated in some tests where risk level changed (approach speed, directness, and predator proximity), but not in other tests where risk (successive approaches) or costs levels changed (presence of food outside the refuge; Cooper 2009, 2011). In this case, the latter result could be explained by uncontrolled differences between trials or small effect sizes.

Namibian rock agamas, *Agama planiceps*, have FIDs that are highly consistent within individuals (between 9 and 15 repeated measures) over a period of almost 50 days, and across situations (seasons). Also, there is more variation in FID between than within individuals, independently of other covariates such as body mass, temperature, and time of day (Carter *et al.* 2010, 2012a,b; Figure 15.2).

Similarly, within-individual repeatability in FID is very high in burrowing owls, *Athene cunicularia*, after controlling for several confounding effects (sex, territory). Furthermore, most individuals do not change their escape responses, and there are as many birds decreasing as increasing their FIDs across successive trials (Carrete & Tella 2010; Figure 15.3). In contrast, in yellow-bellied marmots, *Marmota flaviventris*, individual identity is not a significant predictor of FID (Runyan & Blumstein 2004). This negative result is probably explained by the very different situational contexts in which individuals were observed in different occasions.

In the field cricket, *Gryllus integer*, individual differences in latency to become active after defensive freezing and in hiding time inside a refuge are consistent (Hedrick & Kortet 2012; Niemelä *et al.* 2012a). However, individual differences in boldness are consistent only in a novel environment (control) but not after being exposed to a predator, which suggests the existence of a context-specific behavioral syndrome (Niemelä *et al.* 2012b). Moreover, hiding time is repeatable across metamorphosis stages in females, but not in

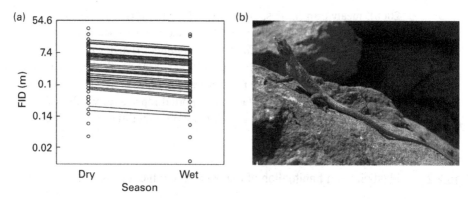

Figure 15.2   Consistency between seasons in the flight initiation distance (FID) of Namibian rock agamas, *Agama planiceps*. Each point represents an observation of an individual that was observed on multiple occasions in each season. Each line represents each individual's best linear unbiased predictor for the intercept. (Figure redrawn from Carter *et al.* 2012b; photograph by J. Martín)

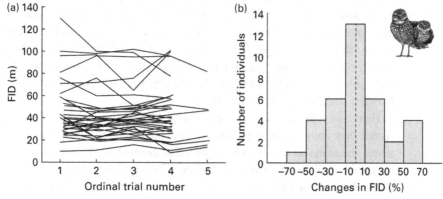

Figure 15.3   Consistency in the flight initiation distance (FID) of burrowing owls, *Athene cunicularia*. (a) Individual changes of FID across successive trials, for several individuals tested four or more times. (b) Percentage change in FID between the last and the first trial. (Figure redrawn from Carrete & Tella 2010)

males, which become shyer with maturation, probably because of the risk associated with calling for mates. Also, individuals have longer freezing times when they are nymphs than when they are adults (Hedrick & Kortet 2012).

In hermit crabs, *Coenobita clypeatus*, latency to hide and emerge from their shells are highly consistent in several contexts (i.e., when crabs were inverted, or in an open field, or when subjected to a predator visual stimulus, or to an electric shock). Moreover, there are correlations between the hiding time after suffering an electric shock and both the latency to hide and hiding time after presenting a visual predator stimulus (Watanabe *et al.* 2012). Similar individual consistency in hiding or tonic immobility responses is also found, for example, in other hermit crab species, *Pagurus bernhardus* (Briffa *et al.*

2008), mealworm beetles, *Tenebrio molitor* (Krams *et al.* 2014), larval salamanders, *Ambystoma barbouri* (Sih *et al.* 2003), and even in sea anemones (*Actinia equina*; Briffa & Greenaway 2011; *Condylactis gigantea*; Hensley *et al.* 2012).

Taken together, these studies suggest that escape and hiding behavior may be consistent repeatable personality traits in many animals, at least in some contexts or during some ontogenetic states. In fact, the reported repeatability values for FID and hiding times are in many cases among the highest repeatabilities observed for behaviors (Réale *et al.* 2007; Bell *et al.* 2009).

15.2.2   Plasticity and habituation of the escape and hiding response

Despite demonstrable individual consistent differences, animals may also modify their behavior to varying environmental conditions (Dingemanse *et al.* 2010). This behavioral plasticity could be either similar among individuals, hence maintaining personality differences across an environmental gradient, or vary among individuals and situations (Nussey *et al.* 2007; Dingemanse *et al.* 2010; Figure 15.1). Several studies have revealed that both behavioral plasticity and consistency between situations often coexist. For example, larval salamanders, *Ambystoma barbouri*, spend more time out of their refuges in the absence of a fish predator than when it is present, but individual responses are correlated between the two situations (Sih *et al.* 2003). Similarly, hermit crabs, *Pagurus bernhardus*, show variation in average startle hiding behavior responses between several predator-cue treatments, indicating that there is behavioral plasticity between situations, but crabs also show a high individual consistency in the ranks of individual hiding times between situations (Briffa *et al.* 2008).

Habituation to predators is a special case of behavioral plasticity by which animals reduce their antipredator responses to a potential predatory stimulus through a process in which the stimulus ceases to be regarded as dangerous after repeated non-threatening exposures to it (e.g., Hemmi & Merkle 2009; Rodríguez-Prieto *et al.* 2010, 2011). Habituation to low-risk predators is important because it may have fitness consequences. For example, individual Iberian wall lizards, *Podarcis hispanica*, that habituate (i.e., decrease their FID) more readily to a frequent low-risk predatory stimulus (a human, that does not attack, but passes by close to the lizard) are able to increase their body condition more than lizards that habituate less (Rodríguez-Prieto *et al.* 2010; Figure 15.4).

Several studies have used the progressive reduction in magnitude of FID in response to repeated predatory attacks as a measurable indicator of habituation (Lord *et al.* 2001; Runyan & Blumstein 2004; Magle *et al.* 2005; Hemmi & Merkle 2009; Rodríguez-Prieto *et al.* 2010, 2011; Carter *et al.* 2012b). For example, one study investigated the direct and indirect effects of boldness (estimated from refuge use, time being exposed, etc.), exploratory behavior in a novel environment and sociability (time spent hidden in a refuge with conspecific olfactory cues) on the inter-individual variability in habituation ability (i.e., reduction in FID) of Iberian wall lizards (Rodríguez-Prieto *et al.* 2011; Figure 15.4). Individual boldness was consistent across contexts, but it did not affect differences in habituation. However, exploration had a strong direct effect on habituation, with more exploratory individuals being able to habituate faster than less

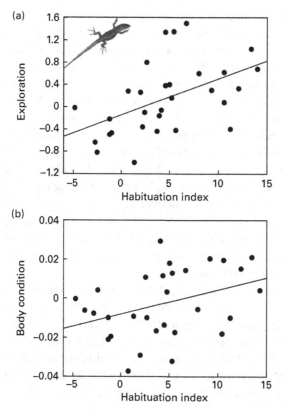

Figure 15.4 Inter-individual variation in habituation in Iberian wall lizards, *Podarcis hispanica*. Relationship between habituation index (higher values indicate a higher and quicker reduction of FID over the course of a six-day experiment with repeated approaches) and (a) exploration behavior (higher values indicate fast explorers) or (b) body condition change. (Redrawn from Rodríguez-Prieto *et al.* 2010, 2011)

exploratory ones, probably because they could gather more information from novel stimuli and were able to assess risk better. Individual variation in habituation was also indirectly affected by sociability, probably because less social individuals that avoided refuges with conspecific cues, increased exposure to the predator and eventually habituated.

In contrast, repeated observation of escape behavior of different individual male rock agamas revealed a small, but significant, decline in FID with time, which suggests habituation to the observer's approaches over the course of the study. However, individuals do not differ in the rate of habituation, which suggests that there are not inter-individual differences in behavioral plasticity (Carter *et al.* 2012a,b).

15.2.3   Correlations of escape and hiding behavior with other behavioral traits

Inter-individual variability in escape responses and hiding behavior from predators may be correlated with other personality traits such as activity level and exploration, thus providing strong evidence for a behavioral syndrome. For example, juvenile convict cichlids, *Amatitlania nigrofasciata*, that are more exploratory in a novel environment are slower to react to an attack by a simulated fish predator (Jones & Godin 2010). Similarly, great tits, *Parus major*, which are more willing to explore more of a novel environment, are also more likely to return to forage quicker after being startled (Van Oers *et al.* 2004b). And individual chaffinches, *Fringilla coelebs*, which are less active, are more likely to freeze than flee in response to a hawk attack and take longer to resume activity after the attack (Quinn & Cresswell 2005b). These syndromes could be explained by models of optimal escape behavior (Ydenberg & Dill 1986; Cooper & Frederick 2007b; see Chapter 2), with bolder, more exploratory individuals delaying their escape response and shortening hiding times to reduce the costs of missed foraging opportunities. Alternatively, consistent with the "perceptual limits hypothesis" (Quinn & Cresswell 2005a), individual prey differing in personality might have a different capacity to detect and react to predator attacks. Nevertheless, the latter may be tested in species that show alert responses before fleeing by looking at variation and consistency in alert distances.

Other studies have found a relationship between boldness toward predators and aggressive behavior toward conspecifics, although only in some populations of the same species but not in others (Huntingford 1976; Riechert & Hedrick 1993; Bell 2005). For example, individual breeding three-spined sticklebacks, *Gasterosteus aculeatus*, with higher levels of territorial aggression to intruders, are bolder toward a predator outside the breeding season (Huntingford 1976). In the spider *Agelenopsis aperta*, following a web disturbance that makes them hide, individuals that return more quickly to a foraging position at the funnel entrance of their webs are later more likely to win conspecific agonistic contests than spiders with longer return latencies (Riechert & Hedrick 1993). Male turtles, *Mauremsy leprosa*, that are bold in an antipredatory situation (i.e., with shorter hiding times inside the shell) avoid water with chemicals of unfamiliar competitor males, but not with chemicals of familiar males, whereas shy turtles avoid chemicals of both familiar and unfamiliar males (Ibañez *et al.* 2013). Bold individuals with respect to social interactions might also be bold under threatening situations because of high testosterone levels (Huntingford 1976; Tulley & Huntingford 1988). This may reflect a trade-off caused by the existence of behavioral correlations across functional contexts (Sih *et al.* 2003) because different traits have the same underlying physiological and genetic bases as pleiotropic effects of the same genes, which may not be necessarily adaptive in the context of predator avoidance. However, population comparisons and experimental work have shown that boldness and aggressiveness tend to covary in "high-predation" populations, where exposure to predation would generate this behavioral syndrome (Bell 2005; Dingemanse *et al.* 2007). One experimental study with sticklebacks, suggests that this relationship may be explained because while bolder individuals more willing to forage under predation risk are less likely to survive predation, those individuals that are more aggressive toward conspecifics are more likely to survive exposure to predators (Bell & Sih 2007), suggesting that this correlation between boldness and aggression may be adaptive in some environments.

However, boldness to predators is not necessarily correlated with boldness in other contexts. For example, in juvenile pumpkinseed sunfish, *Lepomis gibbosus*, individual consistent differences in responses to a threatening object do not correlate with individual consistent differences in response to a novel food source (Coleman & Wilson 1998). Similarly, dumpling squids, *Euprymna tasmanica*, that are bold in threat tests were not necessarily bold in feeding tests, and this lack of across-context correlations is observed across their entire life span (Sinn *et al.* 2008). These results suggest that shyness and boldness are context specific and may not exist as only a one-dimensional behavioral continuum, even within a single context. It is also possible that the lack of correlation tells us that responses to novel, non-threatening stimuli (neophobia) are not equivalent to responses to threatening predators or conspecifics.

15.3 Evolution of personalities and the optimal escape behavior

The economic or optimality models of escape and refuge use (Ydenberg & Dill 1986; Cooper & Frederick 2007a,b; see Chapter 2) do not explicitly consider inter-individual differences in personality. Such individual differences in boldness and other traits are a potentially important, but mostly neglected, source of variability in these antipredatory behaviors. The problem that arises is that if these models predict only one optimal escape response for each situation of risks and costs, we should initially expect that all individuals in the population will evolve to uniformly follow this optimal response. This is because individuals that fail to escape adequately from predators will incur higher predation risk, but individuals that have an exaggerated escape response will incur high costs in the form of missed foraging opportunities. Therefore natural selection would quickly favor individuals that show an optimal response (i.e., the one predicted by the models for each situation), and we should not expect to find inter-individual differences but rather a uniform escape strategy in all individuals of each population.

One possibility is that the optimality models are predicting what might be the average optimal response in each population, with observed differences being considered as the non-biologically important consequence of inaccurate measurements or small random non-adaptive variation around the adaptive mean (Wilson 1998). However, this does not exclude the fact that selection should eliminate those individuals with suboptimal responses. This would lead to uniform behavior after some time because survivors would be only those showing the single optimal response.

Other explanations for the existence of consistent inter-individual variability in personalities may be the existence of individual differences in state or life-history strategies (Dall *et al.* 2004; Wolf *et al.* 2007; Biro & Stamps 2008; Sih & Bell 2008; Luttberg & Sih 2010). Thus predictions of the models would apply separately to each individual because there is also variability in risk assessment (e.g., based on its escape abilities or life-history strategy) and costs of escape or refuge use (e.g., individuals with a better condition will have lower costs). These subtle differences in state or life-history strategies between individuals, which are not easy to measure, would explain the observed inter-individual variability in escape responses in apparently similar situations. We will expand and examine the empirical evidence for these hypotheses below.

15.3.1   State-dependent escape and hiding responses

Mathematical models suggest that among several state-dependent mechanisms, asset protection (i.e., individuals with more "assets" tend be more cautious) and starvation avoidance can explain short-term consistency in personality (Wolf *et al.* 2007, 2008), although not long-term stable personalities (McElreath *et al.* 2007). However, state-dependent safety (i.e., individuals with higher energy reserves, condition, or health are better at avoiding predators) can explain long-term stable differences in personality (Luttberg & Sih 2010). Therefore each individual would be optimizing its escape responses according to their own state and circumstances. In fact, many studies have shown that morphological and physiological factors, such as running speed, body weight, growth rates, tail loss, or health state, affect the escape responses and refuge use in many animals (Lindström *et al.* 2003; López *et al.* 2005; Biro & Stamps 2008; Jones *et al.* 2009; Cooper & Wilson 2010). Moreover, many of these state factors are permanent or of long-term duration in an individual, which will explain behavioral consistency through time, and their effects will be expressed across different contexts and correlated with other different behaviors, which in turn will result in behavioral syndromes (Dall *et al.* 2004). Therefore differences in the personality of escape behavior between otherwise apparently similar individuals can also be considered as adaptive.

Some studies support that inter-individual differences in escape behavior may reflect differences in state-dependent personalities between individuals. For example, when approached by skuas, *Catharacta* spp., unguarded old chinstrap penguin, *Pygoscelis antarctica*, chicks flee short distances and usually aggregate into a dense pack, which decreases individual predation risk. There is an apparently clear variability in the escape responses of different individual chicks under similar conditions. Some shy individuals flee sooner than others and even some bold individuals do not flee at all but remain still and face the approaching skua, threatening it with open bill and loud vocalizations (Martín *et al.* 2006). This variability might be related to the perceived vulnerability to predation of each individual chick. Simulated predatory attacks showed that inter-individual variability in escape behavior is partly explained by the social environment (i.e., the presence of some adults around that are able to deter a skua attack) and age (younger chicks do not escape because their parents are usually around to defend them). But in addition, chicks in relatively poor health, as indicated by their T-cell immune response, have greater FIDs and flee farther (Figure 15.5). Because health state affects general antipredatory behavior performance (Lindström *et al.* 2003), the ability of "poor" condition penguin chicks to defend themselves may be lower, forcing them to be shyer. Moreover, skuas and other avian predators might assess that bolder individual penguin chicks that escape relatively later or face the predator will be more difficult to capture, diverting their attacks to shyer individuals. Therefore bolder individuals might be signaling to predators their ability to escape and defend from a potential attack (see Chapter 10).

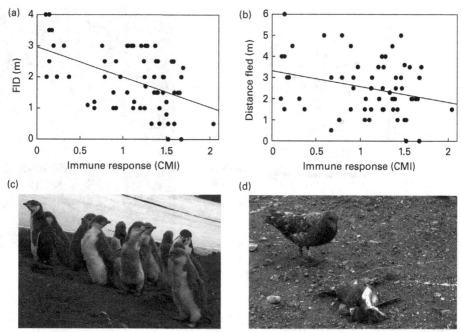

Figure 15.5 Inter-individual variability in state-dependent escape responses in unguarded chicks of chinstrap penguin, *Pygoscelis antarctica*. Relationships between the T-cell-mediated immune response (CMI) and (a) the flight initiation distance (FID) or (b) the distance fled of penguin chicks in response to a human predator attack simulating those naturally made by skuas, *Catharacta* spp. (c) Chinstrap penguins, *Pygoscelis antarctica*. (d) Skuas, *Catharacta antarctica* preying on a penguin chick. (Figure redrawn from Martín *et al.* 2006; photographs by J. Martín)

Similarly, the escape response of incubating female eiders, *Somateria mollissima*, is modulated by interactions between stress responsiveness and individual quality (Seltmann *et al.* 2012). Younger females with higher stress responses (those with higher handling-induced corticosterone blood concentrations) have greater FIDs, whereas the opposite is found in the oldest females, which are considered of higher quality because they have more breeding experience. Furthermore, the effect of stress on FIDs is less marked in females in good body condition.

The sources of individual variation in antipredator behavior of a homogeneous group of adult male rock lizards, *Iberolacerta cyreni*, were examined in another study (Figure 15.6). In a laboratory setting, experimenters simulated repeated predatory attacks of low or high risk and analyzed activity levels, escape decisions and refuge use of lizards in both risk situations (López *et al.* 2005). Results showed consistent inter-individual differences in the magnitude of the antipredator responses under similar conditions of risk and costs. These individual differences in propensity to take risk could be caused by the existence of two consistent and independent shy–bold continua. The first shy–bold continuum describes the time spent hidden in the refuge after predatory attacks, with shy lizards hiding for longer. The second shy–bold continuum describes the propensity to make false-alarm flights and hide before an actual predator

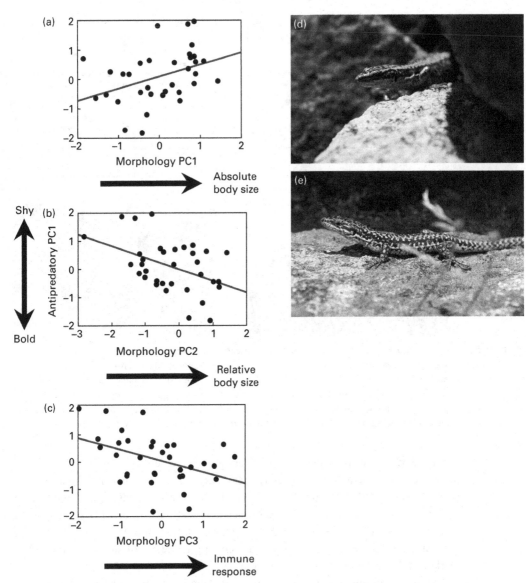

Figure 15.6   State-dependent hiding responses in adult male rock lizards, *Iberolacerta cyreni*. Relation between a shy–bold continuum (which describes a gradient from bold lizards that spent shorter times hidden in the refuge after predatory approaches to shy lizards with longer hiding times) and (a) absolute body size, (b) relative body size, and (c) immune response of lizards. (d, e) "Shy" and "bold" respectively, individual adult male rock lizards, *Iberolacerta cyreni*. (Figure redrawn from López *et al.* 2005; photographs by J. Martín)

attack occurs (López *et al.* 2005). These shy–bold gradients can be related to the morphology and health state of each individual lizard: shy individuals that spend more time hidden in refuges have greater absolute body sizes, but relatively smaller head sizes (an index of a lower social dominance) and a worse body condition and immune system.

(a) (b)

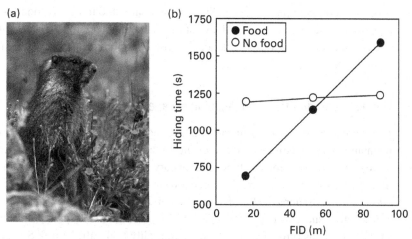

Figure 15.7 (a) A vigilant yellow-bellied marmot (*Marmot flaviventris*) monitoring an approaching predator. (b) The effect of FID (shy individuals have longer FIDs) on hiding time (mean ± SD) in their burrows by yellow-bellied marmots, *Marmota flaviventris*, as a function of whether supplementary food was presented or not. (Photograph by B. Hulsey; figure redrawn from Blumstein & Pelletier 2005)

However, shy individuals with a high propensity to hide when risk is low are those with smaller absolute body sizes, whereas their relative body size and the health state are not important (López *et al.* 2005). Interestingly, more dominant individuals were bolder. Similarly, territorial dominant males of the skink, *Eulamprus heatwolei*, were less likely than floater males to enter refuge when approached and returned to basking sites sooner after being attacked (Stapley & Keogh 2004). This may reflect the existence of a behavioral syndrome between boldness when using refuges and aggression toward conspecifics (see section 15.2.3 above).

In yellow-bellied marmots, the cost of lost foraging opportunities interacts with personalities to determine hiding times inside refuges (Blumstein & Pelletier 2005; Figure 15.7). Bolder individuals that had shorter FIDs before hiding had subsequently shorter hiding times when food had been experimentally placed outside of their burrows before the attack than when no food was added. In contrast, shy individuals with longer FIDs, had subsequent longer hiding times if there were food present. These results might be explained by state-dependent responses whereby bold individuals were hungrier, and thus delayed escaping and hid for shorter periods of time. Alternatively, if bold individuals were less alarmed by the attack, they could be more able to estimate more accurately the costs of escape. However, both shy and bold marmots had similar hiding times in the no-food treatment.

Results of these experiments suggest that the relative boldness of an individual when deciding escape or refuge use might be a function of state-dependent factors, such as its health and associated ability to evade predators. Moreover, all these characteristics can be considered as relatively fixed and phenotypically stable characteristics of an individual that might also be heritable. Persistence of personalities may emerge from positive feedback. For example, bolder individuals who are able to access food sooner, evade predators more easily, etc., and therefore maintain their higher states. In contrast, individuals in poor condition hide longer, lose opportunities to forage, and thus stay in a lower state.

15.3.2   Life history trade-offs when deciding escape responses

A meta-analysis (Smith & Blumstein 2008) suggests that the evolutionary mechanisms maintaining inter-individual variation in boldness may illustrate a trade-off between current and future reproduction (life history trade-offs hypothesis) with individual fitness varying depending on the context of the situation (Sih *et al.* 2004b; Wolf *et al.* 2007; Biro & Stamps 2008). Thus bolder individuals may have greater growth and reproductive success than shyer ones, but will suffer greater predation risk and have shorter life spans (productivity (growth)–mortality trade-off: Biro & Stamps 2008). In contrast, shy individuals may have reduced short-term reproductive success but will live longer by reducing predation risk, and therefore have the same overall life-time fitness as bold individuals (see models in Stamps 2007; Wolf *et al.* 2007). This trade-off may affect animal escape decisions.

Empirical evidence for the "life history trade-off hypothesis" (Wolf *et al.* 2007; Biro & Stamps 2008) with respect to escape responses is suggested from a field study of rock agamas (Carter *et al.* 2010). Bolder male agamas (those with consistently shorter FIDs) spend more time exposed in basking or moving and less time hidden than shyer males, suggesting the existence of a behavioral syndrome. These differences may have fitness consequences; bolder males benefit by having larger home ranges, which increase access to females and food, and higher feeding rates than shyer males. However, given that bolder males spent more time being conspicuous, they should suffer a higher predation risk, as inferred from a higher rate of tail loss (Carter *et al.* 2010). These observations suggest that bolder males may have higher reproductive success, but being bold may increase predation risk at a younger age, making their lifetime reproductive success equal to that of shyer males.

15.3.3   Negative frequency-dependent selection on escape responses

Although differences in state or life-history strategies may provide an explanation for personality differences (Dall *et al.* 2004; Biro & Stamps 2008; Sih & Bell 2008), there are many cases where individuals do not seem to differ in state, and it is not clear why a state-dependent response should be correlated with other behaviors in other contexts. Some alternative or complementary explanations to the evolution of personalities have been suggested, including negative frequency-dependent selection, spatio-temporal variations in the environment, or non-equilibrium dynamics, which could promote the coexistence of phenotypic variation in the population in stable frequencies (see review in Wolf *et al.* 2013). Nevertheless, these explanations account only for the existence of different personalities within a population but they do not explain why personality is consistent within an individual.

One study examined the role of negative frequency-dependent selection in inter-individual variations in antipredatory behavior of flocks of red knots, *Calidris canutus*, in response to a model sparrowhawk, *Accipiter nisus* (Mathot *et al.* 2011). Although flocks of knots differed in their escape behavior in relation to risk level, there was no between-individual variation in escape flight duration within flocks. In contrast, individuals differed in their degree of plasticity for the proportion of time spent vigilant across risk levels. These results support the prediction that traits with negative frequency-dependent payoffs (vigilance) may favor individual variation in plasticity (Wolf *et al.* 2008, 2013), while traits with positive frequency state-dependent payoffs (escape flights) may favor cohesiveness among group members.

15.4   Future directions

Although we have a relatively good understanding of the various trade-offs between avoiding predators and costs of the escape response and refuge use that an individual prey can face, we need to fully explain the causes of the inter-individual variation in escape strategies. However, most studies are based on single observations of each individual, while we need to track the same individuals in multiple occasions to test for consistency and repeatability of personalities in the different components of escape behavior and refuge use, and for the existence of plasticity and correlations between the different behaviors.

Also, to develop a comprehensive understanding of the evolutionary and ecological significance of personalities in escape responses, we need more integrative studies that follow a Tinbergian multidisciplinary approach (Sih *et al.* 2004b; Bell 2007). Thus we need to determine: (1) the proximate mechanisms (hormonal and neurological pathways, health state, etc.) underlying variation in escape responses; (2) the genetic basis of personalities, which may depend on both inherited and environmentally responsive genes, and may also suffer maternal effects (Bell 2009); (3) the factors that influence whether the escape responses and other behaviors (e.g., exploration, aggression) are decoupled or correlated as behavioral syndromes (Sih & Bell 2008); and (4) the fitness consequences of different escape strategies to test whether individuals with different personalities have similar success in evading predators, or whether, even if risk of predation is higher for some personality types, this is compensated for higher benefits in other contexts (foraging, reproduction, etc.) leading to similar lifetime fitness.

Finally, future theoretical models of optimal escape behavior and refuge use will have to incorporate relevant individuality into their structure/logic. Delaying escape or spending longer times hidden in a refuge than other individuals should not be considered as always maladaptive, but may simply represent alternative adaptive personalities, which may be understood when knowing the whole suite of behavioral responses and ecological demands of an animal.

References

Bell, A. M. (2005). Behavioral differences between individuals and populations of threespined stickleback. *Journal of Evolutionary Biology*, **18**, 464–473.

Bell, A. M. (2007). Future directions in behavioural syndromes research. *Proceedings of the Royal Society of London Series B, Biological Sciences*, **274**, 755–761.

Bell, A. M. (2009). Approaching the genomics of risk-taking behavior. *Advances in Genetics*, **68**, 83–104.

Bell, A. M. & Sih, A. (2007). Exposure to predation generates personality in threespined sticklebacks (*Gasterosteus aculeatus*). *Ecology Letters*, **10**, 828–834.

Bell, A. M., Hankison, S. J. & Laskowski, K. L. (2009). The repeatability of behaviour: a meta-analysis. *Animal Behaviour*, **77**, 771–783.

Biro, P. A. & Stamps, J. A. (2008). Are animal personality traits linked to life-history productivity? *Trends in Ecology and Evolution*, **23**, 361–368.

Blumstein, D. T. & Pelletier, D. (2005). Yellow-bellied marmot hiding time is sensitive to variation in costs. *Canadian Journal of Zoology*, **83**, 363–367.

Boissy, A. (1995). Fear and fearfulness in animals. *Quarterly Review of Biology*, **70**, 165–191.

Briffa, M. & Greenaway, J. (2011). High *in situ* repeatability of behaviour indicates animal personality in the beadlet anemone *Actinia equina* (Cnidaria). *PLoS ONE*, **6** (7), e21963.

Briffa, M., Rundle, S. D. & Fryer, A. (2008). Comparing the strength of behavioural plasticity and consistency across situations: Animal personalities in the hermit crab *Pagurus bernhardus*. *Proceedings of the Royal Society of London Series B, Biological Sciences*, **275**, 1305–1311.

Carere, C. & Maestipieri, D. (eds.) (2013). *Animal Personalities. Behavior, Physiology and Evolution*. Chicago, IL: University of Chicago Press.

Carrete, M. & Tella, J. L. (2010). Individual consistency in flight initiation distances in burrowing owls: A new hypothesis on disturbance induced habitat selection. *Biology Letters*, **6**, 167–170.

Carter, A. J., Goldizen, A. W. & Tromp, S. A. (2010). Agamas exhibit behavioral syndromes: bolder males bask and feed more but may suffer higher predation. *Behavioral Ecology*, **21**, 655–661.

Carter, A. J., Heinsohn, R., Goldizen, A. W. & Biro, P. A. (2012a). Boldness, trappability and sampling bias in wild lizards. *Animal Behaviour*, **83**, 1051–1058.

Carter, A., Goldizen, A. & Heinsohn, R. (2012b). Personality and plasticity: Temporal behavioural reaction norms in a lizard, the Namibian rock agama. *Animal Behaviour*, **84**, 471–477.

Coleman, K. & Wilson, D. S. (1998). Shyness and boldness in pumpkinseed sunfish: individual differences are context-specific. *Animal Behaviour*, **56**, 927–936.

Cooper, W. E., Jr. (2009). Variation in escape behavior among individuals of the striped plateau lizard *Sceloporus virgatus* may reflect differences in boldness. *Journal of Herpetology*, **43**, 495–502.

Cooper, W. E., Jr. (2011). Risk, escape from ambush, and hiding time in the lizard *Sceloporus virgatus*. *Herpetologica*, **68**, 505–513.

Cooper, W. E., Jr. & Frederick, W. G. (2007a). Optimal flight initiation distance. *Journal of Theoretical Biology*, **244**, 59–67

Cooper, W. E., Jr. & Frederick, W. G. (2007b). Optimal time to emerge from refuge. *Biological Journal of The Linnean Society*, **91**, 375–382.

Cooper, W. E., Jr. & Wilson, D. S. (2010). Longer hiding time in refuge implies greater assessed risk after capture and autotomy in striped plateau lizards (*Sceloporus virgatus*). *Herpetologica*, **66**, 425–431.

Cresswell, W., Quinn, J. L., Whittingham, M. J. & Butler, S. (2003). Good foragers can also be good at detecting predators. *Proceedings of the Royal Society of London Series B, Biological Sciences*, **270**, 1069–1076.

Dall, S. R. X., Houston, A. I. & McNamara, J. M. (2004). The behavioural ecology of personality: Consistent individual differences from an adaptive perspective. *Ecology Letters*, **7**, 734–739.

Dingemanse, N. J. & Dochtermann, N. A. (2013). Quantifying individual variation in behaviour: mixed effect modelling approaches. *Journal of Animal Ecology*, **82**, 39–54.

Dingemanse, N. J. & Wolf, M. (2010) A review of recent models for adaptive personality differences. *Philosophical Transactions of the Royal Society of London Series B*, **365**, 3947–3958.

Dingemanse, N. J., Thomas, D. K., Wright, J. *et al.* (2007). Behavioural syndromes differ predictably between twelve populations of three-spined stickleback. *Journal of Animal Ecology*, **76**, 1128–1138.

Dingemanse, N. J., Kazem, A. J. M., Réale, D. & Wright, J. (2010). Behavioural reaction norms: Animal personality meets individual plasticity. *Trends in Ecology and Evolution*, **25**, 81–89.

Garamszegi, L. Z. & Herczeg, G. (2012). Behavioural syndromes, syndrome deviation and the within- and between-individual components of phenotypic correlations: When reality does not meet statistics. *Behavioral Ecology and Sociobiology*, **66**, 1651–1658.

Groothuis, T. G. G. & Carere, C. (2005). Avian personalities: characterization and epigenesis. *Neuroscience & Biobehavioral Reviews*, **29**, 137–150.

Hedrick, A. V. & Kortet, R. (2006). Hiding behaviour in two cricket populations that differ in predation pressure. *Animal Behaviour*, **72**, 1111–1118.

Hedrick, A. V. & Kortet, R. (2012). Sex differences in the repeatability of boldness over metamorphosis. *Behavioral Ecology and Sociobiology*, **66**, 407–412.

Hemmi, J. & Merkle, T. (2009). High stimulus specificity characterizes anti-predator habituation under natural conditions. *Proceedings of the Royal Society of London Series B, Biological Sciences*, **276**, 4381–4388.

Hensley, N. M., Cook, T. C., Lang, M., Petelle, M. B. & Blumstein, D. T. (2012). Personality and habitat segregation in giant sea anemones (*Condylactis gigantea*). *Journal of Experimental Marine Biology and Ecology*, **426–427**, 1–4.

Huntingford, F. A. (1976). The relationship between anti-predator behaviour and aggression among conspecifics in the three-spined stickleback, *Gasterosteus aculeatus*. *Animal Behaviour*, **24**, 245–260.

Ibáñez, A., Marzal, A., López, P. & Martín, J. (2013). Boldness and body size of male Spanish terrapins affect their responses to chemical cues of familiar and unfamiliar males. *Behavioral Ecology and Sociobiology*, **67**, 541–548.

Jones, K. A. & Godin, J.-G. J. (2010). Are fast explorers slow reactors? Linking personality type and anti-predator behaviour. *Proceedings of the Royal Society of London. Series B: Biological Sciences*, **277**, 625–632.

Jones, K. A., Krebs, J. R. & Whittingham, M. J. (2009). Heavier birds react faster to predators: Individual differences in the detection of stalking and ambush predators. *Behavioral Ecology and Sociobiology*, **63**, 1319–1329.

Koolhaas, J. M., Korte, S. M., De Boer, S. F. *et al.* (1999). Coping styles in animals: Current status in behavior and stress-physiology. *Neuroscience and Biobehavioral Reviews*, **23**, 925–935.

Krams, I., Kivleniece, I., Kuusik, A. *et al.* (2014). High repeatability of anti-predator responses and resting metabolic rate in a beetle. *Journal of Insect Behavior*, **27**, 57–66.

Krause, J. & Godin, J.-G. J. (1996). Influence of prey foraging posture on flight behavior and predation risk: Predators take advantage of unwary prey. *Behavioral Ecology*, **7**, 264–271.

Lindström, K. M., Van de Veen, I. T., Lagault, B. A. & Lundström, J. O. (2003). Activity and predator escape performance of common greenfinches *Carduelis chloris* infected with sindbis virus. *Ardea*, **91**, 103–111.

López, P., Hawlena, D., Polo, V., Amo, L. & Martín, J. (2005). Sources of interindividual shy–bold variations in antipredatory behaviour of male Iberian rock-lizards. *Animal Behaviour*, **69**, 1–9.

Lord, A., Waas, J. R., Innes, J. & Whittingham, M. J. (2001). Effects of human approaches to nests of northern New Zealand dotterels. *Biological Conservation*, **98**, 233–240.

Luttbeg, B. & Sih, A. (2010). Risk, resources and state-dependent adaptive behavioural syndromes. *Philosophical Transactions of the Royal Society of London. Series B: Biological Sciences*, **365**, 3977–3990.

Magle, S., Zhu, J. & Crooks, K. R. (2005). Behavioral responses to repeated human intrusion by black-tailed prairie dogs (*Cynomys ludovicianus*). *Journal of Mammalogy*, **86**, 524–530.

Mathot, K. J., van den Hout, P. J., Piersma, T. *et al.* (2011). Disentangling the roles of frequency- vs. state-dependence in generating individual differences in behavioural plasticity. *Ecology Letters*, **14**, 1254–1262.

Martín, J., de Neve, L., Fargallo, J. A., Polo, V. & Soler, M. (2006). Health-dependent vulnerability to predation affects escape responses of unguarded chinstrap penguin chicks. *Behavioral Ecology and Sociobiology*, **60**, 778–784.

McElreath, R., Luttbeg, B., Fogarty, S. P., Brodin, T. & Sih, A. (2007). Communication arising: Evolution of animal personalities. *Nature*, **450**, e5–e6.

Niemelä, P. T., Vainikka, A., Hedrick, A. V. & Kortet, R. (2012a). Integrating behaviour with life history: Boldness of the field cricket, *Gryllus integer*, during ontogeny. *Functional Ecology*, **26**, 450–456.

Niemelä, P. T., DiRienzo, N. & Hedrick, A. V. (2012b). Predator-induced changes in the boldness of naïve field crickets, *Gryllus integer*, depends on behavioural type. *Animal Behaviour*, **84**, 129–135.

Nussey, D. H., Wilson, A. J. & Brommer, J. E. (2007). The evolutionary ecology of individual phenotypic plasticity in wild populations. *Journal of Evolutionary Biology*, **20**, 831–844.

Quinn, J. L. & Cresswell, W. (2005a). Escape response delays in wintering redshank, *Tringa totanus*, flocks: Perceptual limits and economic decisions. *Animal Behaviour*, **69**, 1285–1292.

Quinn, J. L. & Cresswell, W. (2005b) Personality, anti-predation behaviour and behavioural plasticity in the chaffinch *Fringilla coelebs*. *Behaviour*, **142**, 1377–1402.

Réale, D., Reader, S. M., Sol, D., McDougall, P. T. & Dingemanse, N. J. (2007). Integrating animal temperament within ecology and evolution. *Biological Reviews*, **82**, 291–318.

Riechert, S. E. & Hedrick, A. V. (1993). A test for correlations among fitness-linked behavioural traits in the spider *Agelenopsis aperta* (Araneae, Agelinidae). *Animal Behaviour*, **46**, 669–675.

Rodríguez-Prieto, I., Martín, J. & Fernández-Juricic, E. (2010). Habituation to low risk predators improves body condition in lizards. *Behavioral Ecology and Sociobiology*, **64**, 1937–1945.

Rodríguez-Prieto, I., Martín, J. & Fernández-Juricic, E. (2011). Individual variation in behavioural plasticity: Direct and indirect effects of boldness, exploration and sociability on habituation to predators in lizards. *Proceedings of the Royal Society of London. Series B: Biological Sciences*, **278**, 266–273.

Runyan, A. & Blumstein, D. T. (2004). Do individual differences influence flight initiation distance? *Journal of Wildlife Management*, **68**, 1124–1129.

Seltmann, M. W., Ost, M., Jaatinen, K. *et al.* (2012). Stress responsiveness, age and body condition interactively affect flight initiation distance in breeding female eiders. *Animal Behaviour*, **84**, 889–896.

Sih, A. & Bell, A. M. (2008). Insights from behavioral syndromes for behavioral ecology. *Advances in the Study of Behavior*, **38**, 277–281.

Sih, A., Kats, L. B. & Maurer, E. E. (2003). Behavioural correlations across situations and the evolution of antipredator behaviour in a sunfish–salamander system. *Animal Behaviour*, **65**, 29–44.

Sih, A., Bell, A. & Johnson, J. C. (2004a). Behavioral syndromes: an ecological and evolutionary overview. *Trends in Ecology and Evolution*, **19**, 372–378.

Sih, A., Bell, A. M., Johnson, J. C. & Ziemba, R. E. (2004b). Behavioral syndromes: An integrative overview. *Quarterly Review of Biology*, **79**, 241–277.

Sinn, D. L., Gosling, S. D. & Moltschaniwskyj, N. A. (2008). Development of shy/bold behaviour in squid: Context-specific phenotypes associated with developmental plasticity. *Animal Behaviour*, **75**, 433–442.

Smith, B. R. & Blumstein, D. T. (2008). Fitness consequences of personality: A meta-analysis. *Behavioral Ecology*, **19**, 448–455.

Stamps, J. A. (2007). Growth-mortality tradeoffs and "personality traits" in animals. *Ecology Letters*, **10**, 355–363.

Stapley, J. & Keogh, J. S. (2004). Exploratory and antipredator behaviours differ between territorial and nonterritorial male lizards. *Animal Behaviour*, **68**, 841–846.

Tulley, J. J. & Huntingford, F. A. (1988). Additional information on the relationship between intra-specific aggression and antipredator behaviour in the three-spined stickleback *Gasterosteus aculeatus*. *Ethology*, **78**, 219–222.

Van Oers, K., De Jong, G., Drent, P. J. & Van Noordwijk, A. J. (2004a). Genetic correlations of avian personality traits: Correlated response to artificial selection. *Behavior Genetics*, **34**, 611–619.

Van Oers, K., Drent, P. J., De Goede, P. & Van Noordwijk, A. J. (2004b). Realized heritability and repeatability of risk-taking behaviour in relation to avian personalities. *Proceedings of the Royal Society of London Series B, Biological Sciences*, **271**, 65–73.

Watanabe, N. M., Stahlman, W. D., Blaisdell, A. P. *et al.* (2012). Quantifying personality: Different measures, different inferences. *Behavioral Processes*, **91**, 133–140.

Wechsler, B. (1995). Coping and coping strategies: A behavioural view. *Applied Animal Behaviour Science*, **43**, 123–134.

Wilson, D. S. (1998). Adaptive individual differences within single populations. *Philosophical Transactions of the Royal Society of London Series B, Biological Sciences*, **353**, 199–205.

Wolf, M., van Doorn, G. S., Leimar, O. & Weissing, F. J. (2007). Life-history trade-offs favour the evolution of animal personalities. *Nature*, **447**, 581–584.

Wolf, M., van Doorn, G. S. & Weissing, F. J. (2008). Evolutionary emergence of responsive and unresponsive personalities. *Proceedings of the National Academy of Sciences of the United States of America*, **105**, 15825–15830

Wolf, M., van Doorn, G. S., Leimar, O. & Weissing, F. J. (2013). The evolution of animal personalities. In Carere, C. & Maestipieri, D. (eds.) *Animal Personalities. Behavior, Physiology and Evolution*. Chicago: University of Chicago Press, pp. 252–275.

Ydenberg, R. C. & Dill, L. M. (1986). The economics of fleeing from predators. *Advances in the Study of Behavior*, **16**, 229–249.

Part IV

The application and study of escape

16 Best practice for the study of escape behavior

Daniel T. Blumstein, Diogo S. M. Samia, Theodore Stankowich, and William E. Cooper, Jr.

Escape decisions have been studied in a remarkably Tinbergian way that has included examination of both proximate and ultimate questions, including questions about the evolution of escape behavior. Evolutionary studies have been made possible by developing large comparative data sets. Methodological differences, however, may impede our ability to combine studies to create comparative databases that can be, and have been, used to ask both evolutionary questions and questions of management relevance. Evolutionary comparative studies and meta-analyses both depend on animals being studied in relatively consistent ways, yet astute readers of the primary literature will have noticed that there is great variation in the ways in which studies of escape have been conducted. We wish to discuss some of the variation in how escape has been studied, and to recommend best practices for moving forward. We discuss several key details below, focusing primarily on flight initiation distance (FID).

In part because escape theory is now capable of predicting many aspects of escape behavior and in part because hypothesis-driven research is an efficient way to advance our understanding, the use of focused hypotheses and predictions is a fundamental feature of best practices for escape studies. Beyond this key feature, we make many recommendations that apply to a wide range of studies. Our recommendations, however, do not apply universally. In some cases, researchers should ignore our suggestions if, for instance, they wish to study the consequences of a recommendation. In other cases it may be essential to alter the approach protocol to ask other focused questions. Thus researchers should view our recommended practices as guidelines, not scripture.

16.1 Behavior of prey as a trial begins

Before measuring the escape of an individual, many key data must be collected. What animals are doing before they are experimentally approached influences both flight decisions (e.g., level of alertness, fighting with conspecifics, foraging in a profitable patch, sleeping or lying down: reviewed in Stankowich & Blumstein 2005) and hiding time decisions (Blumstein & Pelletier 2005). *We suggest that animals be relaxed yet not*

Escaping From Predators: An Integrative View of Escape Decisions, ed. W. E. Cooper and D. T. Blumstein. Published by Cambridge University Press. © Cambridge University Press 2015.

sleeping, as opposed to highly vigilant, when initiating an experimental approach. Relaxed behavior might include sitting and looking, or being perched, singing or producing other non-alarm vocalizations or signals, self-grooming, or foraging. Some protocols (including some of ours) require humans to identify a subject from a given distance and then wait quietly for five to ten seconds before initiating an experimental approach. In theory this is fine, but some species (e.g., browsing ungulates) move quickly through an area and the opportunity to approach might be lost if there is a lengthy delay before approach. In practice, animals may continue monitoring us, albeit in a relaxed way, and animals that were alert to the approacher prior to the initiation of the approach may make flight decisions differently than unaware subjects with different information about the approacher (Stankowich & Coss 2006). This requires a decision about whether or not to include immediate flushes when the experimental approach begins. Ultimately, this decision may rest on the exact question being asked. For example, immediate flushes may be of particular interest when testing the flush early and avoid the rush (FEAR) hypothesis (Blumstein 2010; Chapter 2).

These recommendations apply to many birds and mammals, but cannot be followed readily in some other taxa, including lizards, especially those that are ambush foragers in which it is often not possible to discern signs of vigilance (Cooper 2008a, b). For such prey, an experimenter approaches to some starting distance (SD) and position at which the prey is presumed to have detected the experimenter, stops for a brief interval, and then begins an experimental approach. Thus, SD equals alert distance (AD), and only questions related to zones I and II (Blumstein 2003) can be studied because the subject is already aware of the threat. It would be preferable to include approaches beginning at longer SDs when the examination of effects of spontaneous movements and the flushing early hypothesis are of interest. Inclusion of longer SDs would make lizard studies more comparable to those on birds and mammals, but the issue of degree of vigilance remains problematic. This might be addressed by monitoring focal animals for physiological correlates of vigilance (*sensu* Blumstein & Bouskila 1996). Another advantage of including long SDs is that in FID should begin to asymptote at the boundary of zone II, where prey monitor predators, and zone III, where they do not.

16.2   Number of humans

The vast majority of FID experiments have used a single experimenter to flush individuals. Unless the objective is to study the effects of multiple observers (Geist *et al.* 2005; Cooper *et al.* 2007*), we suggest that future studies use a single observer.* By doing so, we ensure that future data will be maximally comparable to previously collected data. Sometimes a second person is called in to watch the animals from afar and record behavior. This practice should be fine as long as there is only a single person experimentally approaching the subject. Ideally, the second person is at a distance far enough to not influence the escape behavior of the animal (since the number of predators can affect the subject's flight decision), but close enough to guarantee the accuracy of their records.

16.3   Group size

The prey's group size can influence antipredator behavior and escape responses. Models of predation risk assessment predict that FID decreases as group size increases for two possible reasons: (1) either risk to the individuals decreases as group size increases because the predator has more choices (risk dilution hypothesis; Roberts 1996) or (2) an individual's risk decreases because at least one group member will detect the predator before it can overtake any member of the group (many-eyes hypothesis; Roberts 1996), permitting escape. These hypotheses are not mutually exclusive. Indeed, a variety of studies demonstrate that group size influences FID (Fernández-Juricic et al. 2004; Stankowich & Coss 2006), but the strength of the effect is widely variable, even within taxa (Stankowich & Blumstein 2005; Stankowich 2008). As species get larger, the area around them that they monitor increases (Blumstein et al. 2004). *Thus it is essential to collect information on the number of conspecifics and, if interested, heterospecifics, within a biologically relevant distance and use these values as covariates in subsequent analyses.*

16.4   Starting distance and alert distance

Starting distance has one of the largest effects on FID for many species (Samia et al. 2013), and serves as a proxy for the real biologically relevant measure, alert distance (Blumstein 2003). The main difference between these variables is that SD is determined by the experimenter, whereas AD is determined by the focal animal. Despite this key difference, it is impossible to test the effect of AD without varying the SD because of a mathematical constraint that links these two variables (i.e., $SD \geq AD$; see detailed discussion in section 16.9 below). In some studies of lizards, SDs have been systematically varied to include observations over a wide range of values (Cooper 2005, 2008; Cooper et al. 2009). And while some large data sets exist on birds and mammals that have a variety of SDs, many of these have been collected in an *ad hoc* manner; systematic variation in their collection is needed. Indeed, it is desirable to include approaches beginning at longer SD when studying the effects of spontaneous movements or when testing the FEAR hypothesis. Inclusion of longer SDs would make lizard studies more comparable to those on birds and mammals, but the issue of degree of vigilance (AD) remains problematic as does the ability to observe a relatively tiny lizard in shrubby habitat. This might be addressed by monitoring focal animals for physiological correlates of vigilance.

We recognize that several issues arise when initiating experimental approaches at variable distances. There may be distances beyond which animals will not flee from an approaching person, possibly because it is simply not worth it or because the human is not detected (zone III: Blumstein 2003; Chapter 3). Thus initiating experimental flushes at relatively long distances may mean that the experimenter walks toward an animal until s/he is detected or enters a "zone of awareness" where the animal begins assessing risk (zone II). Given that animals are constrained in their ability to scan in all directions at all times, an approacher starting from outside the zone of awareness (D_{max}) and walking directly toward the animal may be able to approach nearer the subject before it becomes alert than an approacher milling around at D_{max}, where the subject might eventually become alert before approach begins. This effect could lead to shorter ADs in zone II and a general quadratic effect between SD and FID (Stankowich & Coss 2006; Chapter 3: Figure 3.1). In addition to this effect, a predator approaching in a prey's field of view may well be detected while farther from the prey than one that is out of the field of view. Similarly, prey may detect predators farther away if they approach from within a binocular vs. monocular field of view, in taxa that have both, such as birds. In lizards, detection is easier when the predator is in one of the lateral fields of view than when in front of or behind the lizards (Cooper 2008a, b).

Because animals may look up and move at the start of natural bouts of vigilance and intermittent locomotion (here named as "spontaneous behaviors"), mistakenly scoring spontaneous behaviors as AD or FID is theoretically more likely for experiments with large SD (Cooper 2008a, b; Cooper & Blumstein 2014). *As long as the experimenter is attuned to eventual natural threats or distractions (such as social behavior), long approaches will likely not produce spurious data.* Despite their potential to confound the study of escape, we do not believe these are often "real" issues because it is usually very obvious when an animal alerts or flees from an approaching human. *We recommend that if an observer is unsure of whether the animal is responding to their experimental approach, they should simply not record data for that approach.* Although some models have shown that spontaneous behaviors could potentially bias the conclusions that are drawn (Chamaillé-Jammes & Blumstein 2012), our experience with over 15,000 experimental approaches on lizards, birds, and mammals, suggests that it is very unlikely that we have been making systematic mistakes scoring escape decisions. Moreover, the influence of spontaneous behaviors on final results may be in itself of particular interest. With knowledge of natural patterns of vigilance and locomotion, it is possible to develop null models (Williams *et al.* 2014) that allow one to eliminate those experimental approaches that are possibly "tainted." Even without such knowledge, it is possible to develop null models that eliminate the suspicion of spurious relationship caused by tainted observations (Samia *et al.* 2013).

Some investigators have used a fixed or narrow range of SDs to study effects of factors that affect the cost of not fleeing and the cost of fleeing. These distances are intended to be long enough to avoid creating situations in which escape is immediate (Cooper 1998, 2012), yet short enough to ensure that the prey has detected the predator before the approach begins (e.g., Møller & Garamszegi 2012 and almost all lizard studies). *If SD is fixed or has a narrow range, there must be some justification for selecting a particular distance and the experimenters must clearly describe their rationale for selecting this distance. When working with an unfamiliar species or situation, we recommend that pilot data be collected to ensure that the SD is appropriate.* It is important to ensure the prey is monitoring the predator during the entire approach, which is necessary for the predator–prey encounter to match the scenario of the economic escape models of Ydenberg and Dill (1986) and Cooper and Frederick (2007).

16.5   Flight initiation distance

Many of our recommendations are designed to properly measure FID. When animals are on the ground, FID is readily measured as the straight line separating the experimenter and the animal when the escape begins. To identify the exact point at which FID (and other variables) occurs, many experimenters drop weighted flags or other objects along the path of approach. Typically markers are placed (1) at the starting point of the experimental approach; (2) at the approacher's position when the prey becomes alert and responds to the approacher; (3) at the point where the prey began to flee; and (4) at the point where prey was located at the start of the experiment. The distance between markers 1 and 4 is SD; that between markers 2 and 4 is AD, and that between markers 3 and 4 is FID. Additionally, beyond the preferred method of measuring FID using a measuring-tape or laser rangefinder, it is also a common practice for experimenters to convert the number of paces into meters to record the escape variables (e.g., SD, AD, FID; Blumstein 2006).

However, when studying many birds, lizards, or arboreal mammals, the focal animal may be perched above the ground. Two procedures have been developed to measure the FID for animals off the ground.

The first is to test all individuals, and then determine the boundary height, which is assumed to represent the maximum height at which the animals perceive themselves to be at risk (c. two to three meters for some lizards approached by human investigators; Cooper 1997; Cooper & Avalos 2010). Flight initiation distance is calculated as if all individuals are at ground level (i.e., no adjustment is made for differences in predator–prey distance among perch heights). The relationship between perch height and FID is studied in the range 0 m to boundary height. At typical SDs and FIDs, this has a relatively small effect on estimates of distance. However, as perch height increases, the proportion of the Euclidean distance between predator and prey that is attributable to perch height increases substantially. To our knowledge, only lizards have been tested using this boundary height approach to date.

A second, more generally correct, method has been used to study many birds and arboreal mammals that flee when perched at greater heights, where perch height may account for a large portion of the Euclidean distance. Birds are usually tested using the "direct" FID, which is calculated as the Euclidian distance between experimenter and focal animal (i.e., the square root of the sum of the squared horizontal distance and the squared height of perch; Blumstein 2006). Because height in tree may (or may not) affect risk perception (Blumstein *et al.* 2004), *our conservative suggestion is that height should be estimated and the direct FID (FID$_{direct}$) should be calculated using the Pythagorean theorem*. It should be noted, however, that because FID$_{direct}$ depends on the height an individual is in a tree, it is possible that when there are immediate or near immediate flushes, FID$_{direct}$ may be greater than SD. This would contradict the envelope constraint (where SD > AD > FID).

16.6   Approach speed and angle

We know that the speed at which an individual is approached may influence both the decision to flee and the decision to hide. Thus it is important for researchers to report clearly the approach speed. Many data have been collected by approaching animals between 0.5 and 1.0 m/s (Blumstein 2006; Gulbransen *et al.* 2006). As humans speed up (e.g., 0.5 to 1.0 m/s vs. 2 to 3 m/s in Stankowich & Coss 2006; Chapter 5), speed has detectable effects on escape. While it is essential to vary approach speed to determine whether animals are maintaining a spatial margin of safety or a temporal margin of safety (Cárdenas *et al.* 2005), and to study joint effects of approach speed and other factors that may affect FID, *we recommend a default approach speed of 0.5 to 1.0 m/s to ensure data are maximally comparable with other studies.* In comparative studies, if animals are approached at different speeds, approach speed could be used as a covariate (e.g., Cooper *et al.* 2014). And speed can be varied during approach to study effects of changes during approach on FID (Cooper 2006), but investigators should realize that these will not be generally comparable with other studies.

The angle and directness of approach also may affect escape decisions (Fernández-Juricic *et al.* 2005; Cooper *et al.* 2010; Chapter 5). Interestingly, while many species are more tolerant of tangential approaches compared to direct approaches, birds studied in a high-elevation grassland in Argentina were more sensitive to tangential approaches (Fernández-Juricic *et al.* 2005). *Unless it is of interest to study the effect of directness of approach or the approacher is restricted to established trails in sensitive wildlife areas, we recommend that researchers directly approach experimental subjects.* In some cases it may be prudent to add the bypass distance (for tangential approaches) as a covariate in models explaining variation in FID.

16.7   When to stop approaching

Once an animal flees, a relevant question is whether to stop approaching toward the location where animal was, continuing to walk up to its initial location, or continue approaching the prey past its initial location. Pragmatically, to properly measure SD, it is important to know precisely the location of the subject. Additionally, if it is desirable to measure the distance fled, or the distance to the nearest refuge, it is essential to go to the subject's initial location. *Our recommendation is that approaches should be terminated in one of two places, the predator's location when escape begins or the prey's location when escape begins. If the predator continues to the initial position where the subject was at the start of the experimental approach, the prey will likely flee a longer distance and/or be more likely to enter refuge than if the predator stops moving as soon as the prey flees.* The choice between these stopping points sometimes may be dictated by the escape tendencies of the prey, the need to continue observations on the animal (i.e., escape into refuge or out of the area is undesirable), or the need to maintain comparability with previously collected data.

If the approacher continues to the prey's initial location, distance fled will depend on the additional risk implied by the continued approach and will very likely vary with the directness of approach during flight (i.e., on the angle between the approach path and the flight path). With continued approach, distance fled, probability of refuge entry, and hiding time may increase. The correlation between distance to refuge and distance fled may also be greater than when the predator stops approaching when escape begins. We also note that sometimes it may be essential to follow an animal *until* it hides, if the goal is to study hiding time. Stopping as soon as the prey flees may be realistic in portraying reactions of predators that stop approaching when they assess that they will not be able to capture the prey. Experimentally pursuing prey might be the most realistic way to simulate attacks by pursuing predators, but pursuit introduces uncontrolled variation in risk and costs that may affect distance fled and hiding time. Continuing to approach, but only to the prey's initial location, may be a compromise between these extremes and has the advantage of being more likely to induce prey to enter refuge if hiding time is of interest.

16.8   Data to collect

At the very minimum, data sheets should permit the collection of location, date, time, species, sex, initial behavior, starting distance, alert distance, flight initiation distance, and the number of conspecifics (and potentially heterospecifics) within a biologically relevant distance. Of course, additional questions can be asked with additional data and some researchers (and for some questions) have collected data on how far animals were from refugia when an experimental approach began, details about the type of movement during escape, and the distance fled. Some researchers have examined subsequent escape decisions that have included the dynamics of the second flush (which sometimes happens), and the dynamics of hiding, the type of escape behavior performed, the distance fled, or the latency to resume initial behavior. Analyses that include such additional information can provide a richer understanding of escape, but we recommend that investigators also collect the initial data to ensure maximum comparability.

16.9   Statistical analysis of FID data

16.9.1   Use of SD or AD as covariate or study of interactions involving the SD x FID relationship

There are many statistical issues associated with analyzing FID data. A key feature of the analysis of FID data is that variance in both AD and FID increases as a function of SD. This happens because these variables are subject to a constraint envelope relationship where $SD \geq AD \geq FID$. Logically, a prey cannot flee from a predator (FID) at a greater distance than where it was detected (AD) and, similarly, prey cannot become alert to a predator before the predator initiates its approach (SD). We note that there are situations where AD > SD are possible, but, because true AD is not measurable when animals are alerted to the experimenter prior to the start of the approach, such observations do not typically exist in FID data sets or AD is set to equal SD. For example, SD = AD in experiments in which all approaches begin at relatively short SDs at which prey are already aware of the predator's presence. The constraint envelope is an unavoidable statistical issue in FID studies and has implications as to how data may be analyzed.

Our first statistical recommendation is: *if starting distances vary and alert distances are not available, starting distance must be added as covariate in subsequent statistical models. However, starting distance is unrelated to FID in some species, especially at slow approach speeds. For studies of single species for which it is known that SD and FID are unrelated, SD should not be used as a covariate.* Starting distance is a proxy for AD and it likely explains a considerable proportion of the variance in FID (Blumstein 2010; Samia *et al.* 2013; Samia & Blumstein 2014). This creates a statistical issue about whether the effect of other variables should be tested as main effects or as interactions between SD and the other variables. When interpreting a two-way interaction, the question becomes "does a variable of interest influence the expected relationship between SD and FID?" Researchers have tested these both ways and *we recommend thorough examination leading to an understanding of the nature of a data set before making a decision about whether to focus on interpreting main effects or interactions.*

16.9.2   Should the FID x SD regression be forced through the origin?

Another important decision one must make is whether or not to include an intercept in statistical models of data sets that include SD. Because FID cannot be greater than the distance where an experimental approach begins, FID is zero when SD is zero. Some investigators prefer to force though the origin and other do not when using regression models. It is important to note that the slopes and estimated intercepts of fitted regression models likely differ in zones I, II, and III (Blumstein 2003; Stankowich & Coss 2006; Chapter 3), and that it may be more appropriate to conduct separate regressions in the different zones. *If you know your data are exclusively in zone I, you should force the fitted model through the origin (i.e., exclude the intercept – unless you want to test the hypothesis that the intercept differs from 0). If you suspect that your data spans zones I and II, you should consider fitting a piecewise linear regression where you can look for a breakpoint. If you suspect your data spans only zones II and III, you should consider exploring both linear and non-linear models (e.g., logarithmic) with intercepts included, as the predicted relationship between SD and FID changes with increasing SD.* The remaining residual error can then be used to test for whatever factor effects were included in the study. Please note that while the idea of three zones is conceptually useful, focused empirical studies are needed to properly define these zones in a given species.

16.9.3 Spontaneous movements and the decision to keep observations of immediate flight

Another issue is whether or not to remove values where SD = FID. In zone I immediate flushing is predicted, but in zone II prey are predicted to monitor the predator's approach prior to fleeing. Situations where SD = FID may be the result of animals flushing immediately at the start of the experimental approach if the SD happens to be the FID for that individual, which occurs at the boundary of zones I and II or may occur if an animal is particularly wary. At longer SDs, flushing may also be attributable to spontaneous movements (Williams *et al.* 2014). *We generally suggest that investigators only remove data if they believe that the movement is not in response to a predator and to otherwise keep cases where SD = FID.*

In cases where SD varies considerably, *FID studies can profitably employ quantile regression*, particularly if one is concerned that long SD values may influence the relationship between SD or AD and FID (Chamaillé-Jammes & Blumstein 2012). Quantile regression estimates how subsets of the data vary. Thus if one is concerned that at large SDs, larger FIDs may reflect spontaneous movement (see below), one could focus on quantiles that did not include these data. Quantile regression cannot be used if SD is fixed. And quantile regression requires a substantial amount of data to profitably employ it.

16.9.4 Other statistical issues associated with studying FID

Because correlational statistics are sensitive both to expected heteroscedasticity (caused by the constraint envelope) and to outliers with high leverage, such effects can lead to potentially erroneous conclusions about whether observations support the FEAR hypothesis or not. Samia and Blumstein (2014) developed an index (phi, Φ) designed to test the 1:1 expectation in an SD–FID or an AD–FID relationship in a way that avoids the above statistical pitfalls. Moreover, in addition to allowing the proper evaluation of the FEAR hypothesis, the index permits one to determine if a species is flushing later or with no predetermined strategy.

Recently, there have been some concerns about the use of SD as proxy for AD (Dumont *et al.* 2012). If SD is not a good proxy for AD, conclusions drawn from studies using SD rather than AD might be suspect. It could be even more critical to studies of lizards for which AD is difficult to determine. However, a further comparative study with 75 avian species showed that the use of SD is a conservative alternative to using AD as a covariate in FID studies (Samia & Blumstein 2014). By conservative, we mean that while a low and/or non-significant SD–FID relationship is inconclusive, a large and/or significant SD–FID is robust support of the influence that AD has on FID.

Computational simulations and null models have been recently used to study FID. Specifically, computational simulations have been used to model the effect of spontaneous behaviors on FID (Chamaillé-Jammes & Blumstein 2012), to filter the data according with a baseline rate of spontaneous behaviors observed in natural conditions (Williams *et al.* 2014), to eliminate the suspicion of spurious data in the AD–FID relationship caused by the envelope constraint (Dumont *et al.* 2012; Samia *et al.*

2013), and to simulate null distributions of metrics developed to test the FEAR hypothesis (Samia & Blumstein 2014). The already available algorithms can be valuable when one tests the FEAR hypothesis, but we argue that further benefits can be obtained by using computational simulations. For example, the conceptual zones that Blumstein (2003) proposed influence escape behavior. Because it is difficult to identify such zones in natural conditions, mathematical and computational models can help us better understand their roles in dynamic decision-making of prey. *We expect that future advances in our understanding of escape will rely on developing specific null models and using computational simulations to evaluate empirical data.*

16.10   Comparative studies and meta-analyses: a complementary way to study escape

Many hypotheses about escape theory have been studied using a comparative or meta-analytical approach (Stankowich & Blumstein 2005; Blumstein 2006; Møller 2008; Samia *et al.* 2013). Because the evolutionary history of taxa renders species not statistically independent, most of these studies use phylogenetically informed models to account for the non-independence (Garland & Ives 2000; Felsenstein 2004; Lajeunesse 2009; Nakagawa & Santos 2012). Some recent studies, however, show remarkable plasticity in escape behavior that seems rather unconstrained by phylogeny (e.g., Cooper *et al.* 2014) and different populations of the same species often vary greatly in their flight responses based on their experience with natural predators or humans. *Thus we recommend that in comparative studies, authors provide a measure of the phylogenetic signal of the FID.* To date, we have little evidence to assess whether FID is a conserved or a species-specific trait. This is because, although most interspecific studies control the phylogenetic effect, few studies provide a measure of phylogenetic signal such as Pagel's lambda or Bloomberg's K (for exceptions, see Møller & Garamszegi 2012; Samia *et al.* 2013). In the absence of such measures, the superiority of phylogenetic models, as indicated by adjusted r^2 or Akaike's information criterion, indicates that a phylogenetic signal occurs, but does not quantify its strength (Cooper *et al.* 2014). It is also important to realize that phylogenetic models are not indicated when there is no phylogenetic signal present because there is increased uncertainty about parameter estimates (Revell 2010).

Our final suggestion is one that has brought us all together. We think that while there is a lot to learn from single-species studies of escape, *we encourage others to present their findings either in the context of meta-analysis or to present them in ways that facilitate future meta-analyses* ("meta-analytic thinking"; Cumming & Finch 2001; Nakagawa & Cuthill 2007; Borenstein *et al.* 2009). This requires a bit of a paradigm shift and we have two recommendations to facilitate this shift. *In primary studies, we suggest that inferences should be based on the magnitude of the effect; thus researchers should present the effect size along with its confidence interval. Second, we encourage researchers to present results in sufficient detail so that the calculation of the effect size can be made easily (e.g., provide the sample size and the exact P-values of statistics).*

16.11 Conclusions

We are thrilled and excited by both the number of studies and the diversity of studies of escape behavior. We hope that our suggestions for standardizing some of the ways that escape is studied will lead to even more comparative studies and meta-analyses. Indeed, we believe that it is through these sorts of studies that generalizations emerge. Creating such data sets is typically beyond the scope of a single researcher or a single study. As we also wrote, there are reasons to ignore some of our suggestions and researchers that do so will invariably discover new ways that animals manage predation risk through the dynamics of their escape behavior. We look forward to reading those studies in the future!

References

Blumstein, D. T. (2003). Flight initiation distance in birds is dependent on intruder starting distance. *Journal of Wildlife Management*, **67**, 852–857.

Blumstein, D. T. (2006). Developing an evolutionary ecology of fear: How life history and natural history traits affect disturbance tolerance in birds. *Animal Behaviour*, **71**, 389–399.

Blumstein, D. T. (2010). Flush early and avoid the rush: A general rule of antipredator behavior? *Behavioral Ecology*, **21**, 440–442.

Blumstein, D. T. & Bouskila, A. (1996). Assessment and decision making in animals: A mechanistic model underlying behavioral flexibility can prevent ambiguity. *Oikos*, **77**, 569–576.

Blumstein, D. T. & Pelletier, D. (2005). Yellow-bellied marmot hiding time is sensitive to variation in costs. *Canadian Journal of Zoology*, **83**, 363–367.

Blumstein, D. T., Runyan, A., Seymour, M. *et al.* (2004). Locomotor ability and wariness in yellow-bellied marmots. *Ethology*, **110**, 615–634.

Borenstein, M., Hedges, L. V., Higgins, J.P.T. & Rothstein, H.R. (2009). *Introduction to Meta-Analysis*. John Wiley & Sons, Ltd., Chichester, UK.

Cárdenas, Y. L., Shen, B., Zung, L. & Blumstein, D. T. (2005). Evaluating temporal and spatial margins of safety in galahs. *Animal Behaviour*, **70**, 1395–1399.

Chamaillé-Jammes, S. & Blumstein, D.T. (2012). A case for quantile regression in behavioral ecology: Getting more out of flight initiation distance data. *Behavior Ecology and Sociobiology*, **66**, 985–992.

Cooper, W. E., Jr. (1997). Escape by a refuging prey: The broad-headed skink (*Eumeces laticeps*). *Canadian Journal of Zoology*, **75**, 943–947.

Cooper, W. E., Jr. (1998). Direction of predator turning, a neglected cue to predation risk. *Behaviour*, **135**, 55–64.

Cooper, W. E., Jr. (2005). When and how do predator starting distances affect flight initiation distances? *Canadian Journal of Zoology*, **83**, 1045–1050.

Cooper, W. E., Jr. (2006). Dynamic risk assessment: Prey rapidly adjust flight initiation distance to changes in predator approach speed. *Ethology*, **112**, 858–864.

Cooper, W. E., Jr. (2008a). Visual monitoring of predators: Occurrence, cost and benefit for escape. *Animal Behaviour*, **76**, 1365–1372.

Cooper, W. E., Jr. (2008b). Strong artifactual effect of starting distance on flight initiation distance in the actively foraging lizard *Aspidoscelis exsanguis*. *Herpetologica*, **64**, 200–206.

Cooper, W. E., Jr. (2012). Risk, escape from ambush, and hiding time by the lizard *Sceloporus virgatus*. *Herpetologica*, **68**, 505–513.

Cooper, W. E., Jr. & Avalos, A. (2010). Escape decisions by the syntopic congeners *Sceloporus jarrovii* and *S. virgatus*: comparative effects of perch height and of predator approach speed, persistence, and direction of turning. *Journal of Herpetology*, **44**, 425–430.

Cooper, W. E., Jr. & Blumstein, D. T. (2014). Novel effects of monitoring predators on costs of fleeing and not fleeing explain flushing early in economic escape theory. *Behavioral Ecology*, **25**, 44–52.

Cooper, W. E., Jr. & Frederick, W. G. (2007). Optimal flight initiation distance. *Journal of Theoretical Biology*, **244**, 59–67.

Cooper, W. E., Jr., Pérez-Mellado, V. & Hawlena, D. (2007). Number, speeds, and approach paths of predators affect escape behavior by the Balearic lizard, Podarcis lilfordi. *Journal of Herpetology*, **41**, 197–204.

Cooper, W. E., Jr., Hawlena, D. & Pérez-Mellado, V. (2009). Interactive effect of starting distance and approach speed on escape behavior challenges theory. *Behavioral Ecology*, **20**, 542–546.

Cooper, W. E., Jr., Hawlena, D. & Pérez-Mellado, V. (2010). Influence of risk on hiding time by Balearic lizards (*Podarcis lilfordi*): Predator approach speed, directness, persistence, and proximity. *Herpetologica*, **66**, 131–141.

Cooper, W. E., Jr., Pyron, R. A. & Garland, J. T. (2014). Island tameness: living on islands reduces flight initiation distance. *Proceedings of the Royal Society of London, Series B, Biological Sciences*, **281**, 20133019.

Cumming, G. & Finch, S. (2001). A Primer on the understanding, use, and calculation of confidence intervals that are based on central and noncentral distributions. *Educational Psychology and Measurement*, **61**, 532–574.

Dumont, F., Pasquaretta, C., Réale, D., Bogliani, G. & Hardenberg, A. (2012). Flight initiation distance and starting distance: Biological effect or mathematical artefact? *Ethology*, **118**, 1–12.

Felsenstein, J. (2004). *Inferring Phylogenies*. Sunderland, MA: Sinauer Associates, Inc.

Fernández-Juricic, E., Vaca, R. & Schroeder, N. (2004). Spatial and temporal responses of forest birds to human approaches in a protected area and implications for two management strategies. *Biological Conservation*, **117**, 407–416.

Fernández-Juricic, E., Venier, M. P., Renison, D. & Blumstein, D. T. (2005). Sensitivity of wildlife to spatial patterns of recreationist behavior: A critical assessment of minimum approaching distances and buffer areas for grassland birds. *Biological Conservation*, **125**, 225–235.

Garland, T. & Ives, A. R. (2000). Using the past to predict the present: Confidence intervals for regression equations in phylogenetic comparative methods. *American Naturalist*, **155**, 346–364.

Geist, C., Liao, J., Libby, S. & Blumstein, D. T. (2005). Does intruder group size and orientation affect flight initiation distance in birds? *Animal Biodiversity and Conservation*, **28**, 69–73.

Gulbransen, D., Segrist, T., del Castillo, P. & Blumstein, D.T. (2006). The fixed slope rule: An inter-specific study. *Ethology*, **112**, 1056–1061.

Lajeunesse, M. J. (2009). Meta-analysis and the comparative phylogenetic method. *American Naturalist*, **174**, 369–381.

Møller, A. P. (2008). Flight distance and blood parasites in birds. *Behavioral Ecology*, **19**, 1305–1313.

Møller, A. P. & Garamszegi, L. Z.(2012). Between individual variation in risk-taking behavior and its life history consequences. *Behavioral Ecology*, **23**, 843–853.

Nakagawa, S. & Cuthill, I. C. (2007). Effect size, confidence interval and statistical significance: A practical guide for biologists. *Biological Reviews of the Cambridge Philosophical Society*, **82**, 591–605.

Nakagawa, S. & Santos, E. S. A. (2012). Methodological issues and advances in biological meta-analysis. *Evolutionary Ecology*, **26**, 1253–1274.

Revell, L. J. (2010). Phylogenetic signal and linear regression on species data. *Methods in Ecology and Evolution*, **1**, 319–329.

Roberts, G. (1996). Why individual vigilance declines as group size increases. *Animal Behaviour*, **51**, 1077–1086.

Samia, D. S. M. & Blumstein, D. T. (2014). Phi index: A new metric to test the flush early and avoid the rush hypothesis. *PLoS One*, **9**, e113134.

Samia, D. S. M., Nomura, F. & Blumstein, D. T. (2013). Do animals generally flush early and avoid the rush? A meta-analysis. *Biology Letters*, **9**, 20130016.

Stankowich, T. (2008). Ungulate flight responses to human disturbance: a review and meta-analysis. *Biological Conservation*, **141**, 2159–2173.

Stankowich, T. & Blumstein, D. T. (2005). Fear in animals: A meta-analysis and review of risk assessment. *Proceedings of the Royal Society B*, **272**, 2627–34.

Stankowich, T. & Coss, R. G. (2006). Effects of predator behavior and proximity on risk assessment by Columbian black-tailed deer. *Behavioral Ecology*, **17**, 246–254.

Williams, D. M., Samia, D. S. M., Cooper, W. E., Jr. & Blumstein, D. T. (2014). The flush early and avoid the rush hypothesis holds after accounting for spontaneous behavior. *Behavioral Ecology*, **25**, 1136–1147.

Ydenberg, R. C. & Dill, L. M. (1986). The economics of fleeing from predators. *Advances in the Study of Behavior*, **16**, 229–247.

17 Afterword

Daniel T. Blumstein and William E. Cooper, Jr.

17.1 Introduction

As the chapters in this volume have shown, the field of escape behavior is both active and diverse. What has particularly excited us while editing this book is how a simple economic framework, pioneered by Ydenberg and Dill (1986) that (as they wrote in the forward) had problems getting published, has stimulated so much work about so many different aspects of escape. Theoretical advances have been coupled with empirical study. Indeed, we suggest that the study of escape provides a textbook example of the reciprocally illuminating interplay between theoretical models, observational and experimental empirical studies, and comparative studies, including meta-analyses. Many, but not all, escape decisions can be studied without specialized equipment. This simplicity and elegance puts the emphasis on clear thinking and focused hypothesis testing. We have taught classes and short courses on quantifying escape behavior. Students learn the methods quickly and are able to produce high-quality data soon. Thus we believe that the study of escape will continue to be a highly productive field. This is good because while we have learned a lot, as our authors have noted, there's much room for future discovery! In this afterword, we will briefly highlight five themes or questions that have emerged from this book, and touch on a sixth theme that we did not have sufficient room to properly discuss.

17.2 The importance of studying individuals

The field of behavioral ecology has fully embraced the importance of understanding individual variation (Carere & Maestripieri 2013). Indeed, the publication of papers showing that individuals behave in consistently different ways – they have personalities – has exploded over the past decade. However, many of the studies of escape behavior, especially those of FID and hiding time conducted in the field, do not follow individually identified animals. There are some notable exceptions (Carrete & Tella 2010; Ibáñez et al. 2014; Williams et al. 2014).

Escaping From Predators: An Integrative View of Escape Decisions, ed. W. E. Cooper and D. T. Blumstein. Published by Cambridge University Press. © Cambridge University Press 2015.

The study of unmarked individuals has permitted remarkably large comparative data sets to be produced. This is a particularly notable characteristic of the escape literature. However, by not following individually identified animals, we are prevented from asking some sorts of questions. Individually marked animals are required to properly study the processes of habituation or sensitization to repeated exposure to predators (Runyan & Blumstein 2004). Individually marked animals are required to study the maintenance of personality variation (FID is a metric of boldness – Petelle *et al.* 2013). Without individually marked animals we cannot understand the importance of individual variation for escape decisions. Without studies of marked individuals we cannot study the quantitative genetics of escape behavior and understand selection and evolutionary dynamics.

We encourage others to continue to study unmarked animals when such data permit answers to salient questions, and when such studies also help expand large comparative data sets. However, we strongly encourage future researchers to study escape decisions of marked animals. By doing so, we will be able to address unanswered, but addressable, questions, that will reveal a level of complexity and nuance heretofore just hinted at.

17.3   The interplay between interspecific studies and intraspecific studies

This brings us to a second emergent question – the interplay between comparative results and results from single species. Meta-analyses and comparative analyses have shown that body size is an important determinant of escape decisions (Stankowich & Blumstein 2005; Blumstein 2006; Chapter 3). However, the range of body size across species is much greater than the range of body size within a species. Intraspecific studies often yield much smaller effect sizes than meta-analyses or do not find significant effects of body size on escape decisions (Petelle *et al.* 2013).

It is therefore relevant to ask: what can we learn from interspecific studies with respect to understanding decisions that individuals of a single species make? We encourage future researchers to test specific hypotheses about trade-offs and constraints identified from comparative studies using data from focused, single-species studies to conduct comparisons of multiple species. By doing so, we will better understand the limits of interspecific conclusions for understanding individual decisions. Furthermore, comparative studies permit detection of phylogenetic trends and important effects of ecology, life history, morphology, and physiology that may not be detectable using studies limited to single species.

17.4   Using physiology to define decision-making mechanisms

The third theme emerged from a careful reading of Chapter 13. In that chapter Litvin *et al.* highlighted the huge disconnect between field studies of escape and the detailed, and nuanced, insights that emerge from studies of escape behavior in laboratory rodents.

The studies they discussed have begun to identify specific neurophysiological pathways underlying specific escape behaviors. In some cases they have shown us that what a field-oriented biologist may assume is one type of escape behavior is actually controlled in a very proximate sense by different mechanisms and thus is a more complex behavior than initially realized. Clearly, detailed neurophysiological studies will shed light on different decision-making mechanisms and, by doing so, will enable us to better understand the drivers of escape decisions. Much work remains to be done in this exciting field and future field investigators who draw insights from laboratory studies have the potential to make fundamental advances in understanding decision-making in natural situations.

Much of this book is focused on FID, but effects of physiology on FID have only rarely been studied in the field. One study cited in Chapter 13 detected a relationship between corticosterone level and FID in a lizard (Thaker *et al.* 2009). We know of only two other studies of the physiology of FID, both of which confirm the importance of corticosterone in lizards (Berger *et al.* 2007; Rödl *et al.* 2007). Although these studies cover only a single aspect of the diverse neuroendocrine mechanisms that modulate escape behavior, the findings of the few field studies are as predicted from our knowledge of the physiological underpinnings of other aspects of escape behavior gained from laboratory studies. This suggests that other previously identified neuroendocrine mechanisms of escape behaviors may similarly affect FID and perhaps other aspects of escape in the field. An almost entirely unexplored avenue of research, that promises to be extremely fruitful, awaits future investigation.

17.5   The importance of sensory physiology

As Chapter 12 so clearly demonstrated, a fundamental understanding of sensory physiology is important to create realistic assumptions when modeling escape decisions. Tyrrell and Fernández-Juricic clearly showed us in Chapter 12 how it is essential to understand, at a fundamental level, what animals can see, hear, and smell, if we are to understand how they make escape decisions. For instance, it is essential to know about an animal's visual field to properly understand if individuals engaged in searching for food pay a cost in terms of reduced vigilance. This reminds us that models of decision-making may be flawed if assumptions do not properly capture sensory constraints on acquisition of information. These warnings should stimulate considerable work, and it will be exciting to see its outcomes.

17.6   Utility, range, and testability of theory

The escape theory described extensively in Chapter 2 provides the basis for predicting effects of many factors discussed in later chapters. The economic models of FID and hiding time, including optimality models and other models in which escape and hiding decisions are based on costs and benefits of fleeing, have been very successful in the sense that their predictions have been broadly supported for many factors affecting escape by diverse prey taxa. Despite their successes, current models are limited in scope, and critical tests to distinguish between predictions of alternative models have not been forthcoming.

Current escape models describe decisions about escape behavior for only limited aspects of the range of predator–prey interactions that are the most amenable to empirical study. They apply primarily to decisions to flee by an immobile prey monitoring a predator as it approaches and to emerge from refuge after some interval spent hiding. Recently, the latency to flee from an immobile predator by an immobile prey has been modeled successfully. In Chapter 2 these models are extended to another scenario in which the prey approaches the predator and the more complex scenario in which both predator and prey are moving is discussed, but models of these scenarios remain to be tested. Indeed, the latter scenario will be more difficult to study than the others, and will likely require video and computer equipment to measure movements of predator and prey simultaneously. Current economic models also do not predict escape strategies or changes in strategy discussed in the chapter on escape strategy (Chapter 8) and some of the taxonomically oriented chapters. These will be important topics for future theoretical exploration.

Two types of models, some with extensions, have been used to predict decisions involving distance and time. Ydenberg and Dill's (1986) original graphical escape model predicted that prey flee when the cost of not fleeing equals the cost of fleeing. This model was later adapted by Martín and López (1999) to predict hiding time in a refuge. Cooper and Frederick (2007a,b) developed optimality models for both FID and hiding time. In the optimality models, prey make decisions that afford them greater fitness at the end of the encounter than do the other models.

Although the quantitative predictions of the two types of models differ, we are currently unable to perform the critical tests needed to choose the better sort of model because we have not measured the effects of relevant variables on fitness, which is the currency of all of these models. In studies of escape behavior, behavioral ecologists are confronted by the same inability to measure fitness, and therefore the same inability to adequately test quantitative predictions, that has plagued fitness-based models in studies of foraging and other behaviors. A second general problem that applies to all current escape models is that animals may not be capable of making decisions that are exactly optimal or of determining the exact distance between predator and prey. It is to be expected that they reach approximations of such decisions by using rules of thumb to gauge predation risk (Bouskila & Blumstein 1992), cost of fleeing, and their own initial fitness.

Despite these handicaps, both types of models are useful. The mathematical functions implied by their graphs, or stated explicitly by their equations, were selected to meet some criteria for the escape and hiding scenarios. However, they are merely illustrative because the shapes of the fitness functions are unknown. Therefore empirical determinations of the distance and time functions cannot distinguish between the models. New methods are needed to measure fitness directly or to equate fitness units among variables such as cost of fleeing, cost of not fleeing, and initial fitness. One of the most difficult challenges for empiricists using escape theory will be to untangle the effects of factors such as body size, autotomy, and female reproductive status on multiple variables in the models.

Fortunately, the models are very useful despite these limitations. The qualitative predictions of both models are similar with slight alterations of the original graphical models to incorporate the effect of the prey's fitness at the start of a predator–prey encounter. Tests of the qualitative predictions support the models equally well. They continue to provide useful frameworks for future advances in understanding effects of numerous factors on escape behavior and seem well suited for extensions predicting simultaneous effects of multiple variables and modification to make predictions for other escape variables and changes in escape strategy.

17.7   Application to wildlife conservation and management

The application of escape behavior to improve wildlife conservation and management, the last major theme of this chapter, is an important field that has already begun to yield insights and can be expected to produce more useful aids to conservation and wildlife management. The chapters in this volume have shown, in exquisite detail, how the rules dictating when and how to escape are the outcome of natural selection and sexual selection that have traded off costs and benefits of escape. Such rules have evolved to be "optimal" in the environment in which they were selected. Sadly, humans have had a remarkably huge impact on the natural world. Animals may now find themselves in situations where old decision rules are no longer adaptive (Candolin & Wong 2012; Gill & Brumm 2014). Such evolutionary mismatches have consequences for fitness.

Thus, there is a need to properly understand the environmental drivers of decisions about escape. Doing so may permit us to understand and identify which key environmental drivers (such as habitat type, predator density or diversity, patch size, food type, etc.) have a disproportionate impact on escape behavior. Much of the field of conservation behavior is focused on managing decisions individuals make. Thus armed with this knowledge we may identify what to conserve or manage.

However, knowledge of escape behavior can be used more directly. As has been discussed elsewhere (Blumstein & Fernández-Juricic 2010), by quantifying AD and FID, we can develop set-back zones that aim to reduce the impact of humans on sensitive wildlife. Physiological effects of being approached and of escaping on prey may become important considerations in the establishment of set-back distances. By understanding the costs and benefits of hiding, we can begin to quantify disturbance in ways that may be particularly useful to managers tasked with reducing human impacts on sensitive wildlife.

17.8   Conclusions

The questions we ask about escape are not without controversy. As our chapter on best practice (Chapter 16) illustrates, there are unresolved methodological questions. And there are unresolved mechanistic hypotheses. For instance, what is the magnitude of attentional costs? Is the flush early and avoid the rush (FEAR) hypothesis supported? Which theoretical models best describe prey behavior? We hope that the rapid rate that new results are generated will, in another decade, allow us to look back and not only have answers to some of these and more questions, but also have developed new and unforeseen questions.

We have written much about escape behavior in the hope that it will be interesting to you, our readers, and to provide enough information to stimulate new research. We know that the book will have some heuristic value because writing and editing it has given us many new ideas, some of which we have already begun to explore. Our overarching goal has been to present the information, but we have neglected to convey a major motivation that drives our work. The sheer joy of developing new ideas, designing experiments and observational studies, analyzing data statistically to test predictions, writing to share our findings, are our rewards, as well as working with colleagues at all of these stages of the scientific process. New ideas flow when writing about the findings. For many of us, the most exciting times are spent in the field in beautiful natural habitats. Enough writing: it's clearly time to get back into the field, scare some animals, and reveal the wonderful complexity by which animals escape their predators!

References

Berger, S., Wikelski, M., Romero, L. M., Kalko, E. K. V. & Rödl, T. (2007). Behavioral and physiological adjustments to new predators in an endemic island species, the Galápagos marine iguana. *Hormones and Behavior*, **52**, 653–663.

Blumstein, D. T. (2006). Developing an evolutionary ecology of fear: How life history and natural history traits affect disturbance tolerance in birds. *Animal Behaviour*, **71**, 389–399.

Blumstein, D. T. & Fernández-Juricic, E. (2010). *A Primer of Conservation Behavior*. Sunderland, MA: Sinauer.

Bouskila, A. & Blumstein, D. T. (1992). Rules of thumb for predation hazard assessment: Predictions from a dynamic model. *American Naturalist*, **139**, 161–176.

Candolin, U. & Wong, B. (eds.) (2012). *Behavioural Responses to a Changing World*. Oxford: Oxford University Press.

Carere, C. & Maestripieri, D. (eds.) (2013). *Animal Personalities: Behavior, Physiology, and Evolution*. Chicago, IL: University of Chicago Press.

Carrete, M. & Tella, J. L.(2010). Individual consistency in flight initiation distances in burrowing owls: A new hypothesis on disturbance-induced habitat selection. *Biology Letters*, **6**, 167–170.

Cooper, W. E., Jr. & Frederick, W. G. (2007a). Optimal flight initiation distance. *Journal of Theoretical Biology*, **244**, 59–67.

Cooper, W. E., Jr. & Frederick, W. G. (2007b). Optimal time to emerge from refuge. *Biological Journal of the Linnaean Society*, **91**, 375–382.

Gil, D. & Brumm, H. (eds.) (2014). *Avian Urban Ecology*. Oxford: Oxford University Press.

Ibáñez, A., López, P. & Martín, J. (2014). Inter-individual variation in antipredator hiding behavior of Spanish terrapins depends on sex, size, and coloration. *Ethology*, **120**, 1–11.

Martín, J. & López, P. (1999). When to come out from a refuge: Risk-sensitive and state-dependent decisions in an alpine lizard. *Behavioral Ecology*, **10**, 487–492.

Petelle, M. B., McCoy, D. E., Alejandro, V., Martin, J. G. A. & Blumstein, D. T. (2013). Development of boldness and docility in yellow-bellied marmots. *Animal Behaviour*, **86**, 1147–1154.

Rödl, T., Berger, S., Romero, L. M. & Wikelski, M. (2007). Tameness and stress physiology in a predator-naïve island species confronted with novel predation threat. *Proceedings of the Royal Society of London, Series B*, **274**, 577–582.

Runyan, A. & Blumstein, D. T. (2004). Do individual differences influence flight initiation distance? *Journal of Wildlife Management*, **68**, 1124–1129.

Stankowich, T. & Blumstein, D. T. (2005). Fear in animals: A meta-analysis and review of risk assessment. *Proceedings of the Royal Society of London, Series B, Biological Sciences*, **272**, 2627–2634.

Thaker, M., Lima, S. L. & Hews, D. K. (2009). Alternative antipredatory tactics in tree lizard morphs: Hormonal and behavioural responses to a predator encounter. *Animal Behaviour*, **77**, 395–401.

Williams, D. M., Samia, D. S. M., Cooper, W. E. Jr. & Blumstein, D. T. (2014). The flush early and avoid the rush hypothesis holds after accounting for spontaneous behavior. *Behavioral Ecology*, **25**, 1136–1147.

Ydenberg, R. C. & Dill, L. M. (1986). The economics of fleeing from predators. *Advances in the Study of Behavior*, **16**, 229–249.

Index

Locators in **bold** refer to figures and tables.

Species appear under their *Latin* names with cross-references from common names when these are used in the text. Broader phylogenetic groupings are also gathered together under common names where these come from different or unspecified genera (e.g., frogs).

Printed in the United States
By Bookmasters